Frontiers in Anti-Cancer Drug Discovery

(Volume 10)

Edited by

Atta-ur-Rahman, *FRS*
Honorary Life Fellow,
Kings College, University of Cambridge, Cambridge, UK

&

M. Iqbal Choudhary
H.E.J. Research Institute of Chemistry, International Center for Chemical
and Biological Sciences, University of Karachi, Karachi, Pakistan

Frontiers in Anti-Cancer Drug Discovery

Volume # 10

Editors: Atta-ur-Rahman and M. Iqbal Choudhary

ISSN (Online): 1879-6656

ISSN (Print): 2451-8395

ISBN (Online): 978-981-14-0071-1

ISBN (Print): 978-981-14-0191-6

©2019, Bentham eBooks imprint.

Published by Bentham Science Publishers Pte. Ltd. Singapore. All Rights Reserved.

BENTHAM SCIENCE PUBLISHERS LTD.
End User License Agreement (for non-institutional, personal use)

This is an agreement between you and Bentham Science Publishers Ltd. Please read this License Agreement carefully before using the ebook/echapter/ejournal (**"Work"**). Your use of the Work constitutes your agreement to the terms and conditions set forth in this License Agreement. If you do not agree to these terms and conditions then you should not use the Work.

Bentham Science Publishers agrees to grant you a non-exclusive, non-transferable limited license to use the Work subject to and in accordance with the following terms and conditions. This License Agreement is for non-library, personal use only. For a library / institutional / multi user license in respect of the Work, please contact: permission@benthamscience.net.

Usage Rules:

1. All rights reserved: The Work is the subject of copyright and Bentham Science Publishers either owns the Work (and the copyright in it) or is licensed to distribute the Work. You shall not copy, reproduce, modify, remove, delete, augment, add to, publish, transmit, sell, resell, create derivative works from, or in any way exploit the Work or make the Work available for others to do any of the same, in any form or by any means, in whole or in part, in each case without the prior written permission of Bentham Science Publishers, unless stated otherwise in this License Agreement.
2. You may download a copy of the Work on one occasion to one personal computer (including tablet, laptop, desktop, or other such devices). You may make one back-up copy of the Work to avoid losing it.
3. The unauthorised use or distribution of copyrighted or other proprietary content is illegal and could subject you to liability for substantial money damages. You will be liable for any damage resulting from your misuse of the Work or any violation of this License Agreement, including any infringement by you of copyrights or proprietary rights.

Disclaimer:

Bentham Science Publishers does not guarantee that the information in the Work is error-free, or warrant that it will meet your requirements or that access to the Work will be uninterrupted or error-free. The Work is provided "as is" without warranty of any kind, either express or implied or statutory, including, without limitation, implied warranties of merchantability and fitness for a particular purpose. The entire risk as to the results and performance of the Work is assumed by you. No responsibility is assumed by Bentham Science Publishers, its staff, editors and/or authors for any injury and/or damage to persons or property as a matter of products liability, negligence or otherwise, or from any use or operation of any methods, products instruction, advertisements or ideas contained in the Work.

Limitation of Liability:

In no event will Bentham Science Publishers, its staff, editors and/or authors, be liable for any damages, including, without limitation, special, incidental and/or consequential damages and/or damages for lost data and/or profits arising out of (whether directly or indirectly) the use or inability to use the Work. The entire liability of Bentham Science Publishers shall be limited to the amount actually paid by you for the Work.

General:

1. Any dispute or claim arising out of or in connection with this License Agreement or the Work (including non-contractual disputes or claims) will be governed by and construed in accordance with the laws of Singapore. Each party agrees that the courts of the state of Singapore shall have exclusive jurisdiction to settle any dispute or claim arising out of or in connection with this License Agreement or the Work (including non-contractual disputes or claims).
2. Your rights under this License Agreement will automatically terminate without notice and without the

need for a court order if at any point you breach any terms of this License Agreement. In no event will any delay or failure by Bentham Science Publishers in enforcing your compliance with this License Agreement constitute a waiver of any of its rights.

3. You acknowledge that you have read this License Agreement, and agree to be bound by its terms and conditions. To the extent that any other terms and conditions presented on any website of Bentham Science Publishers conflict with, or are inconsistent with, the terms and conditions set out in this License Agreement, you acknowledge that the terms and conditions set out in this License Agreement shall prevail.

Bentham Science Publishers Pte. Ltd.
80 Robinson Road #02-00
Singapore 068898
Singapore
Email: subscriptions@benthamscience.net

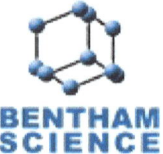

CONTENTS

PREFACE	i
LIST OF CONTRIBUTORS	ii

CHAPTER 1 CHALLENGES IN THE MANAGEMENT OF HEPATOBLASTOMA ... 1
Ioannis A. Ziogas and Georgios Tsoulfas

INTRODUCTION	1
GENETICS & PROGNOSIS	2
HISTOPATHOLOGY & PROGNOSIS	2
PRETREATMENT EXTENT OF DISEASE & RISK STRATIFICATION	3
SURGICAL RESECTION	4
CHEMOTHERAPY	6
TRANSARTERIAL CHEMOEMBOLIZATION (TACE) & HIGH-INTENSITY FOCUSED ULTRASOUND (HIFU)	10
LIVER TRANSPLANTATION (LT)	11
THE ROLE OF AFP	13
CONCLUSION	14
CONSENT FOR PUBLICATION	15
CONFLICT OF INTEREST	15
ACKNOWLEDGEMENT	15
REFERENCES	15

CHAPTER 2 THE EMERGING ROLE OF MONOCARBOXYLATE TRANSPORTER-1 IN CANCER: OVERVIEW AND THERAPEUTIC OPPORTUNITIES ... 23
Gouthami Thumma, Kiran Gangarapu, Anvesh Jallapally and Anil Kumar Mondru

INTRODUCTION	24
MCTs and their Isoforms	25
MCT1 Inhibitors	26
Other MCT's	27
SYNTHETIC MCT 1 INHIBITORS	28
Targeting MCTs in Cancer	30
NATURAL MCT1 INHIBITORS	33
Flavonoid Analogues [46]	33
Mechanism of MCT1 Inhibition	36
CONCLUSION AND FUTURE DIRECTIONS	38
AREA OF INTEREST	38
KEY FEATURES	38
READERSHIP	38
CONSENT FOR PUBLICATION	38
CONFLICT OF INTEREST	39
ACKNOWLEDGEMENTS	39
REFERENCES	39

CHAPTER 3 IN-VITRO ANTI-PROLIFERATIVE ASSAYS AND TECHNIQUES USED IN PRE-CLINICAL ANTI-CANCER DRUG DISCOVERY ... 43
Meran Keshawa Ediriweera, Kamani Hemamala Tennekoon and Sameera Ranganath Samarakoon

INTRODUCTION	43
Assays Based on Cellular Enzymes and Proteins	45
General Assay Procedures for Tetrazolium-Based Anti-proliferative Assays	48
General Assay Procedure for the sulforhodamine B (SRB)	49
Electric Cell-substrate Impedance Sensing (ECIS)	49
Assays Based on DNA Synthesis	49

    General Assay Procedure for the 3H-thymidine incorporation assay 50
    General Assay Procedure for the BrdU assay 50
    Dye Exclusion Assays 51
    General Assay Procedure for the Trypan Blue Cell Viability Assay 51
    Colony Formation Assay 52
    General Assay Procedure for the Colony Formation Assay 52
    Real-time Monitoring and Live Cell Imaging Techniques 52
CONCLUDING REMARKS 54
CONSENT FOR PUBLICATION 55
CONFLICT OF INTEREST 55
ACKNOWLEDGEMENT 55
REFERENCES 55

CHAPTER 4 POLYPHENOLS AND CANCER 62
Peramaiyan Rajendran, Abdullah M. Alzahrani, Thamaraiselvan Rengarajan, Ravi Kaushik, Palanisamy Arulselvan and Arthanari Umamaheswari
    INTRODUCTION 63
        Types of Polyphenol 63
            Flavonoids 65
            Stilbenes 65
            Lignans 65
            Phenolic Acids 65
            Other Polyphenols 65
            Bioavailability of Polyphenol 66
        Polyphenol and Inflammation 67
            Polyphenol on Cytokines 67
            Polyphenols Modulate Nitric Oxide Synthase Family 68
            Polyphenols Interact with The Mitogen-Activated Protein Kinase Pathway 71
            Polyphenols Modulate NFκB Pathway 73
        Polyphenols in Cancer 76
            Anticancer Properties and Mechanisms 77
            Anticancer Effect of Polyphenol Structure and Activity 79
            Preclinical Studies on Anti-Metastatic Activities 81
            Polyphenols on Epithelial–Mesenchymal Transition 81
            Polyphenols in Clinical Trials 84
        Risks and Safety of Polyphenol Utilization 85
        Epigenetics Mechanism of Polyphenols 87
            Epigenetic Modification in Mammals 88
            DNA Methylation 88
            Histone Modifications and Chromatin Remodeling 91
            Sulforaphane 93
            Genistein 94
            Curcumin 96
            Resveratrol 97
            EGCG 98
            Lycopene 100
        CONCLUSION AND FUTURE DIRECTIONS 101
    ABBREVIATIONS 101
    CONSENT FOR PUBLICATION 103
    CONFLICT OF INTEREST 103
    ACKNOWLEDGEMENTS 103

| REFERENCES | 103 |

CHAPTER 5 GLIOBLASTOMA MULTIFORME; DRUG RESISTANCE & COMBINATION THERAPY 111
Megha Gautam, Saumya Singh, Mehak Aggarwal, Manish K Sharma, Shweta Dang and Reema Gabrani

INTRODUCTION	112
CLASSIFICATION OF ASTROCYTIC TUMORS	113
Diffusive Astrocytomas and Anaplastic Astrocytomas	113
DRUG RESISTANCE	114
COMBINATION THERAPY AGAINST GLIOBLASTOMA	115
MGMT Inhibitors	117
Anti-angiogenic Compounds	118
Bcl-2 Family Inhibitors	118
Histone Deacetylase Inhibitors	119
Epidermal Growth Factor Receptor Inhibitor	119
Targeting Hedgehog Pathway	120
Other Target Mechanisms	120
Psychotropic Drugs	121
Beta-Blockers	121
Anti-Metabolites	122
CONCLUSION	122
CONSENT FOR PUBLICATION	123
CONFLICT OF INTEREST	123
ACKNOWLEDGEMENTS	124
REFERENCES	124

CHAPTER 6 RECENT ADVANCES IN THE DEVELOPMENT OF MESOPOROUS ANTI-CANCER DRUG NANOCARRIERS 131
Jessica Flood-Garibay, Lucila I. Castro-Pastrana and Miguel A. Méndez-Rojas

INTRODUCTION	132
Tackling the Global Cancer Burden	132
Present and Future of Cancer Medications	133
Reaching Cancerous Tissues More Efficiently	134
Nanomaterials: Types and Potential Uses in Drug Delivery	139
Mesoporous Nanomaterials: Characteristics, Advantages, and Promising Role as Nanocarriers	145
A) Mesoporous Silica Nanocarriers	149
B). Mesoporous Magnetic Nanocarriers	154
C). Other Mesoporous Inorganic and Organic Nanocarriers	157
CONCLUDING REMARKS	161
ABBREVIATIONS	162
CONSENT FOR PUBLICATION	164
CONFLICT OF INTEREST	164
ACKNOWLEDGEMENT	164
REFERENCES	165

CHAPTER 7 CUTTING EDGE TARGETING STRATEGIES UTILIZING NANOTECHNOLOGY IN BREAST CANCER THERAPY 180
Samipta Singh, Priyanka Maurya and Shubhini A. Saraf

| INTRODUCTION | 181 |

DIFFERENT NANO DELIVERY SYSTEMS USED FOR THE TREATMENT OF BREAST CANCER 182
    Spherical Nanoparticles 182
    Micelles 183
    Self-emulsifying Systems 183
    Dendrimers 184
    Nanotubes 184
    Vesicular Systems 184
        Liposomes 184
        Niosomes 185
        Exosomes 185
        Polymerosomes 185
        Miscellaneous 186
    Hybrid Nanosystems 186
    Layer by Layer Nanoparticles 186
    Drug Polymer/Lipid Conjugates 186
    External Field Based Delivery 187
    Nanostars 187
    Nanorods 187
MATERIALS USED IN PREPARATION OF NANO-FORMULATIONS FOR BREAST CANCER 188
    Viruses or Capsid 188
    Cells 188
    Metals 188
        Gold 188
        Silver 189
        Other Metals 189
    Metal Oxide 189
        Copper Oxide 189
        Iron Oxide 189
        Other Metal Oxide 190
    Polymers 190
    Ceramics 190
    Carbon 191
    Lipids 191
    Proteins 191
DIFFERENT SURFACE MODIFICATIONS OF THE DELIVERY SYSTEM FOR TARGETING OF DRUGS 192
    Antibody-antigen Active Targeting 193
        Anti HER2 194
        SM51 194
        Other MABs/Antibody Fragments 194
    Aptamer-Molecules 195
        AS1411 196
        EpCAM Aptamers 196
        Thioaptamer 196
        Other Aptamers 196
    Lectin-Carbohydrate 199
        Fucose 199
        Glucose 199
        Mannose 200

  Ligand-Receptor 200
   Vitamin-based Ligand Targeting 200
   Hyaluronic Acid 203
   Amino Acid 204
   Protein 204
  Peptide 206
   LHRH 206
   RGD Peptide 207
   TMT Peptide 207
   Other Peptides 207
   Miscellaneous 208
 NANOFORMULATIONS AT CLINICAL LEVEL 208
 RECENT CLINICAL TRIALS 208
 CHALLENGES 210
 RECENT PATENTS 210
 DISCUSSION 211
 CONCLUSION 212
 CONSENT FOR PUBLICATION 213
 CONFLICT OF INTEREST 213
 ACKNOWLEDGEMENTS 213
 REFERENCES 213

SUBJECT INDEX 229

PREFACE

Cancers are among the most fearful human diseases. This has attracted the attention of scientists, policy makers, media, and general publica alike. There are dozens of different types of cancers, with complex etiologies, heterogenicities and complex risk factors. This makes the treatment of cancer a major challenge. Recent advances in the field of anti-cancer drug discovery and development is largely based on a better understanding of cancer biology and molecular genetics. This book series entitled, *"Frontiers in Anti-Cancer Drug Discovery"* is regularly publishing excellent articles in this field and has gained reputation of being thorough, up-to-date and inclusive.

The present 10th volume contains seven excellent chapters focusing on various aspects of cancer biology, and advances in anti-cancer drug development. Ziogas and Tsoulfas have focused their article on general characteristics of hepatoblastoma, the third most common pediatrics tumor of the abdomen. They have reviewed various treatment options in different stages of the disease. The review by Gangarapu *et al.*, is focused on the importance of monocarboxylate transporters (MCT) as a novel anti-cancer drug target. They summarize the recent developments in the field of MCT inhibitors, a new class of drugs against various cancers.

Biological screenings play an important role in initial drug discovery process. For pre-clinical anticancer drug lead discovery, a large number of in vitro cell-based anti-proliferative assays have been developed which are critically reviewed in the next chapter by Ediriweera *et al*. The nexus between diet and the onset of malignancies is the central theme of the article by Rajendran *et al.*, They have reviewed the anticancer effects of major polyphenolic compounds found in common foods, in the context of their molecular mechanisms. Glioblastoma multiforme (GBM) is an aggressive lethal form of brain tumor, with poor prognosis. The chapter Review of Gabrani *et al.*, is focused on recent development of synergistic combinations various classes of drugs with temozolomide, which provide substantial survival advantages to GBM patients. The central theme of the last two reviews is recent developments of anti-cancer drug delivery systems by using nanocarriers. Mendez-Rojas *et al* have reviewed recent progress on the development of mesoporous nanocarriers as efficient systems for controlled transport and delivery of various anti-cancer drugs, whereas the last review by Saraf *et al.*, mainly deals with the active targeting of anti-breast cancer drugs by using various kinds of nanomaterials, and the challenges faced in these processes.

We are grateful to all contributors for their excellent scholarly contributions, and for the timely submissions of their reviews. We would like to express our gratitude to the excellent coordination of Ms. Fariya Zulfiqar (Manager Publications), Mr. Shehzad Naqvi (Editorial Manager Publications) and Mr. Mahmood Alam (Director Publications) of Bentham Science Publishers for the timely completion of the volume in hand. We sincerely hope that the efforts of the authors and the production team will help readers in a better understanding of the subject and motivate them to conduct further good quality research.

Prof. Dr. Atta-ur-Rahman, *FRS*
Honorary Life Fellow,
Kings College,
University of Cambridge,
Cambridge
UK

Prof. Dr. M. Iqbal Choudhary
H.E.J. Research Institute of Chemistry,
International Center for Chemical and Biological Sciences,
University of Karachi,
Pakistan

List of Contributors

Anvesh Jallapally	Department of Pharmaceutical Sciences, University of Antwerp, Antwerp, Belgium
Anil Kumar Mondru	Department of Molecular and Clinical Cancer Medicine, Institute of Translational Medicine, University of Liverpool, Liverpool, United Kingdom
Abdullah M Alzahrani	Department of Biological Sciences, College of Science, King Faisal University, Hufouf, Al Hassa, Saudi Arabia
Arthanari Umamaheswari	Department of Plant Biology and Plant Biotechnology, Presidency College, Chennai, Tamilnadu, India
Georgios Tsoulfas	1st Department of Surgery, Aristotle University of Thessaloniki, Thessaloniki, Greece
Gouthami Thumma	Department of Pharmaceutics, Mother Theresa College of Pharmacy, Hyderabad, 500 088, Telangana, India
Ioannis A. Ziogas	School of Medicine, Aristotle University of Thessaloniki, Thessaloniki, Greece
Jessica Flood-Garibay	Department of Chemical & Biological Sciences and Laboratory of Nanotechnology and Molecular Biomedicine Research, School of Sciences, Universidad de las Américas Puebla, San Andrés Cholula, Puebla, México
Kiran Gangarapu	School of Pharmacy, Anurag Group of Institutions, Hyderabad, 500 088, Telangana, India
Kamani Hemamala Tennekoon	Institute of Biochemistry, Molecular Biology and Biotechnology, University of Colombo, 90, Cumaratunga Munidasa Mawatha, Colombo 03, Sri Lanka
Lucila I. Castro-Pastrana	Department of Chemical & Biological Sciences and Laboratory of Nanotechnology and Molecular Biomedicine Research, School of Sciences, Universidad de las Américas Puebla, San Andrés Cholula, Puebla, México
Miguel A. Méndez-Rojas	Department of Chemical & Biological Sciences and Laboratory of Nanotechnology and Molecular Biomedicine Research, School of Sciences, Universidad de las Américas Puebla, San Andrés Cholula, Puebla, México
Meran Keshawa Ediriweera	Institute of Biochemistry, Molecular Biology and Biotechnology, University of Colombo, 90, Cumaratunga Munidasa Mawatha, Colombo 03, Sri Lanka
Megha Gautam	Jaypee Institute of Information Technology, A-10, Sector 62, Noida, Uttar Pardesh, India
Mehak Aggarwal	Jaypee Institute of Information Technology, A-10, Sector 62, Noida, Uttar Pardesh, India
Manish K Sharma	Pioneer Center of Biosciences, Mohan Nagar, Ghaziabad, Uttar Pardesh, India

Priyanka Maurya	Department of Pharmaceutical Sciences, Babasaheb Bhimrao Ambedkar University, Lucknow, India
Peramaiyan Rajendran	Department of Biological Sciences, College of Science, King Faisal University, Hufouf, Al Hassa, Saudi Arabia
Palanisamy Arulselvan	Scigen Research & Innovation, Periyar Technology Business Incubator, Periyar Nagar, Vallam, Thanjavur, Tamilnadu, India Muthayammal Centre for Advanced Research, Muthayammal College of Arts and Science, Rasipuram, Namakkal, Tamilnadu, India
Ravi Kaushik	ICMR-National Institute of Cancer Prevention and Research, Noida, Uttar Pradesh, India
Reema Gabrani	Jaypee Institute of Information Technology, A-10, Sector 62, Noida, Uttar Pardesh, India
Sameera Ranganath Samarakoon	Institute of Biochemistry, Molecular Biology and Biotechnology, University of Colombo, 90, Cumaratunga Munidasa Mawatha, Colombo 03, Sri Lanka
Samipta Singh	Department of Pharmaceutical Sciences, Babasaheb Bhimrao Ambedkar University, Lucknow, India
Saumya Singh	Jaypee Institute of Information Technology, A-10, Sector 62, Noida, Uttar Pardesh, India
Shweta Dang	Jaypee Institute of Information Technology, A-10, Sector 62, Noida, Uttar Pardesh, India
Shubhini A. Saraf	Department of Pharmaceutical Sciences, Babasaheb Bhimrao Ambedkar University, Lucknow, India
Thamaraiselvan Rengarajan	Scigen Research & Innovation, Periyar Technology Business Incubator, Periyar Nagar, Vallam, Thanjavur, Tamilnadu, India

CHAPTER 1

Challenges in the Management of Hepatoblastoma

Ioannis A. Ziogas[1] and Georgios Tsoulfas[2,*]

[1] School of Medicine, Aristotle University of Thessaloniki, Thessaloniki, Greece
[2] 1st Department of Surgery, Aristotle University of Thessaloniki, Thessaloniki, Greece

Abstract: Hepatoblastoma is the third most common pediatric tumor of the abdomen with an incidence of about 1.2-1.5 cases/million population/year. It has been associated with various genetic conditions, such as familial adenomatous polyposis, Beckwith-Wiedemann syndrome and Edwards syndrome, while genetic mutations of the Wnt signaling pathway are also frequently seen. The different staging systems and treatment approaches of the four hepatoblastoma study groups, International childhood liver tumors strategy group, Children's Oncology Group, German Society for Pediatric Oncology, and Japanese Study Group for Pediatric Liver Tumors, led to different outcomes among the various trials published over the years. Some groups tended to follow a protocol of an upfront surgical resection, while others suggested neoadjuvant chemotherapy to all patients. Now these groups try to come on the same page by initiating an international collaborative attempt to pool previously published data, as well as to classify future patients into risk-stratified groups that would determine treatment options and facilitate improved survival outcomes. The aim of this chapter is to review the general characteristics of hepatoblastoma, the various treatments implemented over the last years, as well as the challenges in management that its rarity and discrepancies among the study groups pose.

Keywords: Chemotherapy, Hepatoblastoma, Liver Malignancy, Liver Surgery, Liver Transplantation, Liver Tumor, Pediatric Oncology, Pediatric Surgery, Pediatric Tumor, Pediatric Solid Tumor.

INTRODUCTION

Hepatoblastoma (HB) is the third most frequently reported solid tumor of the abdominal cavity in very young children and the most common pediatric malignancy of the liver [1]. In fact, currently the incidence is 1.2-1.5 cases/million population/year [2], thus representing around 1% of the malignant tumors in childhood. HB usually presents in children between 6 months and 4 years old with a median age of 18 months [3]. It is an embryonal malignancy, thought to be

---

[*] Corresponding author Georgios Tsoulfas: 1st Department of Surgery, Aristotle University of Thessaloniki, 66 Tsimiski Street, Thessaloniki 54622, Greece; Tel: +306971895190; Email: tsoulfasg@gmail.com

Atta-ur-Rahman and M. Iqbal Choudhary (Eds.)
All rights reserved-© 2019 Bentham Science Publishers

derived from the hepatoblast (precursor of hepatocyte) during embryogenesis of the liver [4]. Many factors have been accused of increasing the risk of HB development, such as low birth weight, prematurity, oxygen therapy, total parenteral nutrition, medication (furosemide) and radiation, but the exact pathogenetic mechanisms are yet to be unveiled [2]. Additionally, parental exposure to tobacco or metals, increased maternal weight before pregnancy, preeclampsia, previous treatment for infertility and either poly- or oligohydramnios can be such risk factors [5].

GENETICS & PROGNOSIS

Although HB mostly presents in a sporadic manner, it has been associated with familial adenomatous polyposis, Beckwith-Wiedemann syndrome and Edwards syndrome [6]. These associations indicate that genes in chromosomes 5, 11 and 18 may pose important assets in the development of HB. At the same time, the Wnt signaling pathway, and the beta-catenin gene in particular, is the cascade exhibiting the highest rate of genetic mutations (70-80%) [7]. Those aberrations result in the accumulation of beta-catenin inside the nucleus, which has been linked to poorly differentiated cellular components [7]. The same finding has been demonstrated in other liver malignancies (*i.e.* cholangiocarcinoma) and appears to have an association with the status of differentiation [8]. Alterations in the beta-catenin gene can also lead to the overexpression of some target genes, such as cyclin D and fibronectin [7]. Telomerase, a reverse transcriptase enzyme, prevents the shortening of telomeres hence rendering normal stem cells, as well as cancer cells, immortal. This process is closely regulated by the expression of TERT (human telomerase reverse transcriptase) [9]. Notably, MYC, a target gene of the Wnt pathway, upregulates the expression of TERT, while the latter one simultaneously participates in the activation process of the Wnt signaling cascade. Together, active TERT and MYC signaling tends to be found in more aggressive HB phenotypes [10, 11]. Hippo, a tumor-suppressor signaling pathway, and one of its downstream effectors called Yes-associated protein (Yap) also play a vital role in cell growth and differentiation. Even though the implications about its oncogenic properties have only recently been described, it has already been found that it intersects with the Wnt cascade, thus leading to tumorigenesis in general [12], but also in HB specifically [13]. Further evaluation of the genetic features of HB, may lead to more solid conclusions regarding the genetic associations of HB, while by intervening in those pathways we may be able to improve overall prognosis.

HISTOPATHOLOGY & PROGNOSIS

Another important factor associated with prognosis is histopathology. To elaborate this, there are two HB subtypes, the epithelial one and the epithelial mixed with mesenchymal tissues, such as skeletal muscle, bone or cartilage [14]. The epithelial group can be further subclassified into well-differentiated fetal (WDF), crowded or mitotically active fetal, embryonal, macrotrabecular (fetal or embryonal), small cell undifferentiated (SCU) and cholangioblastic. 30-60% of the HB cases are mixed fetal and embryonal with the rest of the epithelial group comprising less than 10% of the total cases [15]. On the other hand, the epithelial mixed with mesenchymal elements group accounts for 20-56% of the specimens [16, 17]. In terms of prognosis, it has been reported by the Children's Oncology Group (COG) that when complete resection was facilitated prior to chemotherapy, children with WDF histology and low mitotic activity could be solely treated with surgical resection without the need for chemotherapy [18]. Although those patients represented only 7% of the cases, their event-free survival (EFS) was 100%. Additionally, the SCU histopathology, which usually presents with low alpha-fetoprotein (AFP) levels and is nonresponsive to chemotherapy, has been linked to worse prognosis [2, 19]. Limited data from immunohistochemical staining showed that INI1 nuclear negative SCU HBs are linked to more unfavorable prognosis [20], but on the same time classical HB SCU cells retain the INI1 stain [21]. A study reported that the SCU HBs that retained INI1 may be not be linked to poor prognosis [22]. Unfortunately, due to the rarity of HB and the scarcity of prechemotherapy resections, histopathology data were not commonly implemented in the management plan of HB, hence compromising the importance of biologic studies. Recently, consensus has been reached on the importance of HB sampling before the initiation of chemotherapy, thus facilitating diagnosis based on histopathological analysis, as well as HB classification [21]. Nevertheless, clinical data, such as patient age, AFP levels at diagnosis, underlying liver disease and liver reserve and results of imaging studies, should be provided to those reviewing the specimen [21].

PRETREATMENT EXTENT OF DISEASE & RISK STRATIFICATION

As in most pathologic entities, management varies according to risk stratification. Consequently, the therapeutic approach is determined not only by imaging and histopathology results, as well as by the presence or not of distant metastasis. Another crucial factor, apart from the tumor itself, is the extent of the liver remaining unaffected, as the vast majority of HBs require surgical resection. The four major study groups, International childhood liver tumors strategy group (SIOPEL), COG, German Society for Pediatric Oncology (GPOH), and Japanese Study Group for Pediatric Liver Tumors (JPLT), used to follow different risk stratification stages, hence rendering it impossible to pool cumulative data on the outcomes. Auspiciously, most US and European centers follow the presurgical extent of disease (PRETEXT) grading system to predict tumor resectability established by SIOPEL, which is based on imaging data. According to that, stage I is defined as one involved section and three free adjoining sections, while stage II is defined as one or two involved sections, but two free adjoining sections. Furthermore, stage III is described as two or three involved sections, while no two adjoining sections are free and in stage IV all sections are involved [23]. As adjuvant chemotherapy may usually afflict the anatomy of the area, the PRETEXT classification system is also used about 10 days after every two cycles of chemotherapy to reevaluate the anatomy (post-treatment extent/POST-TEXT). Even though the above-mentioned groups have launched many trials based on PRETEXT grading system, they still had many differences in terms of the annotation factors, which define involvement of the vena cava (V) or the portal vein (P), contiguous extrahepatic intra-abdominal tumor extension (E), multifocal liver tumor (F), rupture of the tumor at diagnosis (R), and metastasis (M). It was the Children's Hepatic tumors International Collaboration (CHIC) that tried to pool the data from all those trials, follow a standardization process and conclude to the most useful individual prognostic factors regarding EFS [3]. They also utilized multivariate analyses in order to hierarchically prioritize prognostic factors, and as a result come up with a more accurate risk stratification system [24]. CHIC takes into consideration the PRETEXT radiologic groups and annotation factors, in combination with age and AFP levels, so as to define treatment groups for the ongoing "Paediatric Hepatic International Tumour Trial (PHITT) (NCT03017326)" [25]. It is therefore profound that dealing with HB is a real challenge and although its management has been through different approaches, the future seems promising based on collaborative initiatives.

SURGICAL RESECTION

As previously stated HB is a malignant tumor, and as such resection is the cornerstone of treatment. In fact, complete surgical resection determines the prognosis of the HB patients. Unfortunately, only one-third of the tumors are resectable at the time of diagnosis [26]. However, the great challenge of effectively treating HB laid for many years on the discrepancies between the different study groups. The most historically significant was the one between COG and SIOPEL in terms of the endeavor to completely resect HB at the time of diagnosis. The SIOPEL group followed a protocol of four neoadjuvant chemotherapy sessions before attempting surgical resection [27]. On the contrary, the COG collaboration group used to pursue complete surgical resection if possible upfront based on the Evan's system and limit the administration of chemotherapy, if this goal was achieved [28, 29]. According to this staging system, surgeons would perform an exploratory laparotomy and, if the tumor could be resected, it was classified as stage I and IIwith microscopically negative and positive margins, respectively. If the tumor was considered unresectable, it was classified at stage III and IV without and with metastasis, respectively. At the same time, GPOH and JPLT used their own hybrid refined staging systems to determine tumor resectability [30]. Subsequently, COG also abandoned the exploratory surgery protocol at the time of diagnosis and implemented their own PRETEXT-based hybrid system (current COG protocol, AHEP0731) [27]. They suggested performing surgery upfront at diagnosis only in PRETEXT I or II HBs with more than 1 cm free margin, which were not concerning for macrovascular involvement. Apparently, JPLT multicenter studies followed the same rule for early stage HB (PRETEXT I and II) complete resection at diagnosis, but according to their protocols the majority of HBs should be treated not only with resection but also with liver transplantation (LT) and neoadjuvant chemotherapy [31 - 33]. In the same manner, COG also suggested that PRETEXT III (or POST-TEXT, V and P: negative) patients should be treated with neoadjuvant chemotherapy before resection, while PRETEXT IV (and POST-TEXT III with V and P: positive) may require either radical resection or liver transplant [27]. The need for referral to an LT center for PRETEXT IV was also highlighted by SIOPEL [1]. On the other hand, the upfront complete resection adopted by the COG group led to the identification of the WDF HBs, for which resection is enough [18]. Fortunately, it was reported that complete resection contributes significantly in non-WDF HBs as well, by decreasing the necessity for adjuvant chemotherapy [18, 29].

The resectability of the HB is not only stage-dependent, but also technique-dependent. Top-notch expertise is required in order to yield optimal outcomes. The only acceptable surgical resection techniques are the non-extended lobectomy and segmentectomy, so that complete tumor resection is achieved. On the same wavelength, according to the two trials launched by GPOH (HB89 and HB94), near 40% of the patients receiving an atypical resection can have residual tumor postoperatively [16]. Obviously, residual disease is associated with worse outcomes and this may be due to the fact that atypical resection leads to dissemination of tumor cells in the liver [34]. It is clearly articulated, therefore, that atypical, wedge and non-anatomic resections should be abandoned when it comes to surgical resection of HB. They could be considered appropriate only in multifocal HB, and particularly when metastases and lack of donor graft render LT unfeasible. The utilization of intraoperative ultrasonography is useful in identifying those multiple foci, as well as in achieving 1 cm resection margins. Biopsy and marginal resection should be attempted if residual macroscopic lesions are present [27]. The surgeons should be accustomed to liver anatomy and vessel variations, as well as follow the basic principles of surgical oncology. The technological advances in surgical equipment, such as Ligasure, harmonic scalpel, argonbeam and infrared coagulator, ultrasonic cavitron ultrasonic surgical aspirator (CUSA)-type dissector, and water knife (Hydrojet, ERBE), are also occasionally implemented during operations for HB [35].

As mentioned above, it is widely known that there were many discrepancies in terms of the different protocols and approaches followed by SIOPEL, COG, GPOH and JPLT. Their current collaborative initiative, also faced many challenges in terms of extracting and pooling the data thought of being related to prognosis, so as to stratify patients in very low-, low-, intermediate- and high-risk backbone groups [24]. According to this model, very low- and low risk patients are separated only by tumor resectability at diagnosis as per the surgical guidelines for PHITT. Interestingly, older age seems to override low PRETEXT, hence yielding worse prognostic outcomes. Even though at first there were three age groups: a) <3, b) 3-7, and c) ≥ 8 years old, children falling into the 3-7 years' age group with PRETEXT I/II present with resectable HBs at the time of diagnosis, so they should still be perceived as low-risk patients. This decision is reasonable on the basis of resecting potentially chemo-resistant tumors. So, except for the case of PRETEXT IV, in which children between 3 and 7 years old have equally poor prognosis as those ≥ 8 years old, the authors suggest a simplification such that of <8 years and ≥8 years, but yet future trials may determine better age cut-offs [24]. The results of PHITT are awaited in suspense, as they may retrospectively validate the approaches utilized, as well as determine when surgical resection should be implemented.

CHEMOTHERAPY

Over the years, although overall survival (OS) seems to be on the rise, a common pattern observed in all of the study groups was the administration of a more or less modified combination of cisplatin chemotherapy and complete surgical resection. The contribution of chemotherapy in these improved survival outcomes is unquestionable. In fact, up until a few decades ago, only 20-30% of HB patients would usually survive [36], but the introduction of neoadjuvant and adjuvant chemotherapy raised those percentages up to 70-80% [37].

The North American cooperative group studies for the management of pediatric liver malignancies were firstly carried out in the 1970s. Initially, the chemotherapeutic regimens consisted of either vincristine, cyclophosphamide, and actinomycin D or vincristine, cyclophosphamide, doxorubicin, and 5-fluorouracil if a more aggressive approach was necessary [38]. Nevertheless, cisplatin (CDDP) skyrocketed survival rates and, according to the Children's Cancer Study Group (CCCG), when used with continuous infusion doxorubicin (DOXO), a combined therapy named PLADO, for patients with unresectable or metastatic HB (stage III and IV) showed an improved 3-year disease-free survival up to 55 and 30%, respectively [39]. Moreover, when the regimen of CDDP, 5-fluorouracil, and vincristine (C5V) was implemented, the EFS for stage I/II HB patients was 90%, for stage III HB patients 67%, and for those with stage IV HB 12.5% (POG8697 trial) [40]. The INT-0098 trial was carried out in order to compare those two chemotherapeutic schemas [26]. Six courses of PLADO showed lower rates of disease progression, but higher rates of toxicity versus six courses of C5V, and as 5-year EFS was not significantly different between the two regimens, C5V was adopted by the COG trials due to its lower toxicity. The SIOPEL-1 trial (1989-1994) also assessed the PLADO schema by administering it as a 4 triweekly preoperative course, followed by two postoperative courses [37]. The results showed a 66% EFS and a 75% 5-year OS, while it also achieved downstaging in around 28% of the patients. However, the outcomes for patients with PRETEXT-IV or metastatic disease were poor.

In order to improve those disappointing outcomes in patients with metastatic and unresectable HB, as well as to decrease the chemotherapy-associated toxicity, the P9645 trial was carried out [41]. Intensified platinum therapy, specifically alternating cisplatin and carboplatin, was compared to C5V with or without amifostine and the study showed that a 1-year EFS of 37% *vs* 57%, respectively. As a result, the study was discontinued based on the results of the interim analysis and patients were continued on C5V with or without amifostine. Nonetheless, the potential protective role of amifostine could not be elucidated, as patients with stage I or II stage HB showed no reduced hemato- or ototoxicity [42]. Concomitantly, the SIOPEL-2 study was designed in order to evaluate the adequacy of CDDP monotherapy in comparison to the addition of DOXO for standard-risk patients, so as to prevent DOXO's toxicity. On the other hand, high-risk patients were treated with alternating CDDP and carboplatin/DOXO [43]. The investigators reported that CDDP monotherapy is adequate for standard-risk patients, but for high-risk patients the outcomes were not yet promising. Therefore, the SIOPEL group designed the SIOPEL-3 trial, in which they initiated all standard-risk patients on CDDP monotherapy and then randomized them on either continuing with CDDP monotherapy or switching to PLADO [44]. The results showed equal rates of survival and complete surgical resection between the two groups, hence suggesting the safe abandonment of DOXO from the treatment plan of those patients. However, for high-risk patients, they implemented 7 preoperative and 3 postoperative courses of alternating CDDP and carboplatin/DOXO [45], and according to the results 3-year EFS was 65%, and 3-year OS was 69% for all patients, thus indicating that intensification of CDDP therapy may improve survival. Consequently, the single-arm SIOPEL-4 trial [46] was designed and patients were initiated on preoperative treatment with PLADO (cycle A), followed by surgical removal of the remaining malignant lesions if possible. If the tumor was still unresectable, a second cycle of preoperative chemotherapy with carboplatin and DOXO was administered (cycle B), while a postoperative regimen of carboplatin and DOXO (cycle C) was given to those that did not receive cycle B. The investigators reported complete resection in 74% of the patients with a 3-year EFS and OS of 76% and 83%, respectively, therefore reporting the highest survival rates ever even in metastatic HB. However, this was a single-arm study comparing the recruited patients with historical cohorts, and in addition to the high rates of toxicity, such as hematologic complications, ototoxicity and toxic deaths, it is profound that further evaluation with a randomized controlled trial is needed. Hopefully, the ongoing PHITT may come up with more meaningful outcomes.

The JPLT group also designed two trials in order to elucidate the optimal treatment approach for HB. Their first one, JPLT-1 study (1989-1999), used a regimen consisting of CDDP and pirarubicin instead of DOXO (CITA regimen) postoperatively in early-stage HB and both pre- and postoperatively in advanced-stage HB with the CDDP dose in the latter group being double than that of the first one [32]. The outcomes for the first group were acceptable, but the EFS among the patients with advanced disease was less than 50%, thus further proving the challenging management of unresectable and metastatic HB. Therefore, in the same manner as SIOPEL, the group from Japan designed a second multi-institutional trial, JPLT-2 (1999-2008), so as to improve the outcomes in patients with HB [31]. This was by the time that the different groups started coming on the same page as per using the same staging systems, such as the PRETEXT classification. Patients with PRETEXT 1 HB were treated with upfront resection followed by postoperative CITA, while the rest of the cases were treated with preoperative CITA and surgery, followed by postoperative chemotherapy. As the results of JPLT-1 were not promising for advanced HB, they followed two different approaches for that stage in their second trial. To elaborate this, patients without even partial response to CITA received a salvage regimen called ITEC (ifosfamide, pirarubicin, etoposide and carboplatin), while those with metastatic disease received high-dose chemotherapy with autologous hematopoietic stem cell transplantation. Based on the interim analysis, the OS rates for non-metastatic PRETEXT I, II, III, and IV were 100%, 87.1%, 89.7%, and 78.3%, respectively. Unfortunately, the OS for metastatic disease was only 43.9%, even though one-third of them was treated with high-dose chemotherapy and autologous hematopoietic stem cell transplantation. In these cases, intensifying chemotherapy in the neoadjuvant setting may be efficacious, as reported by the SIOPEL-4 trial [46]. The real challenge lays on the fact that the vast majority of these patients can sufficiently be treated with standard instead of intensified CDDP monotherapy, according to the SIOPEL-3 study [47]. Generally, the outcomes for PRETEXT I-III in JPLT-2 were similar to those from other multi-institutional studies, while in comparison to JPLT-1 the survival outcomes in patients with PRETEXT III and IV HB were improved [31]. In those non-metastatic HBs, the intensified regimen

ITEC, partial hepatectomy thereafter transarterial chemoembolization (TACE), and LT played a vital role in these improved results. Another controversy lays on the appropriate intensity for the locally advanced HBs (PRETEXT IV). This is because on the one hand many of those patients will eventually require LT so we should prevent the toxic effects of intensive chemotherapy, while on the other hand preoperative chemotherapy can downstage around 30-50% of the tumors, which will then require partial hepatectomy instead of LT [23].

The rarity of HB poses a great challenge to investigators when it comes to designing and carrying out phase 1 and 2 trials and to date no novel efficacious drugs have come to light [48]. Also, despite the promising results of SIOPEL-4 the toxicities of CDDP and DOXO are significant. So, the need for novel agents has emerged, especially in the context of refractory or recurrent HB. The best way to evaluate response to these drugs are the AFP levels, as well as the Response Evaluation Criteria in Solid Tumors (RECIST). A recent SIOPEL study assessed the monotherapy with irinotecan and reported partial responses as per the two above mentioned methods in about 25% of the patients with recurrent or refractory HB [49]. With the intent of further assessing potential agents for high-risk HB patients, the COG group designed the AHEP0731 study to evaluate the use of irinotecan and vincristine [50]. Specifically, patients with metastatic HB and AFP less than 100 ng/mL received two cycles of vincristine and irinotecan, while response was defined either as 30% decrease in tumor burden based on RECIST criteria or a 90% decrease in AFP levels. If patients responded, they received two additional cycles of vincristine and irinotecan mixed with six cycles of C5V and DOXO (C5VD), while if they did not respond, they received only six cycles of C5VD. It was shown that even though this regimen did not fulfill the predetermined criteria for adequate control of the disease, these agents have substantial activity against high-risk HB. Nevertheless, more studies are required to further assess this combination. Around 33% of the patients with disease progression or recurrence after initial therapy without anthracyclines can still be rescued with DOXO regimens and surgery [42]. Carboplatin, etoposide and ifosfamide, have been used not only as rescue regimens, but as upfront treatment in high-risk patients as well [42, 51, 52]. Small groups of patients with relapse have also been tested on irinotecan and oxaliplatin [49, 52, 53]. In an attempt to decrease the toxicity of CDDP, the SIOPEL-6 study was designed in order to evaluate the potential protective effect of sodium thiosulfate for CDDP-induced ototoxicity. Its result showed that if it is administered 6 hours after CDDP, it can reduce the CDDP-induced hearing loss, while concomitantly preserving the OS and EFS [54]. When it comes to the implementation of chemotherapy in the LT context, it is controversial if there is a potential advantage prior to LT. Specifically, for the management of pulmonary metastases, many surgeons will still request surgical exploration before LT, so it is unclear if chemotherapy has something to add in this setting. As far as administering chemotherapy post-transplantation, although there may be a risk for higher rates of LT-related complications, more and more LT centers seem to adopt this approach. Current data suggest equal outcomes with either administering or not chemotherapeutic regimens in the post-transplant setting [55 - 57].

TRANSARTERIAL CHEMOEMBOLIZATION (TACE) & HIGH-INTENSITY FOCUSED ULTRASOUND (HIFU)

In the cases of relapsed or progressive HB, apart from LT, other non-chemotherapy modalities have been proven to be efficacious. The need for these therapies is immense, as chemotherapy can be associated with numerous side effects, like myelosuppression, cardiotoxicity, and secondary malignancies [54, 58 - 61]. TACE aptly represents this group by efficiently decreasing tumor burden, hence facilitating complete tumor resection after initial management with chemotherapy [62, 63]. The rate of complete surgical resection is around 81% without any morbidity [64]. Its efficiency is based on the higher drug concentrations accumulated, hence destroying tumor cells, a process otherwise impossible with systemic chemotherapy. However, laparotomy is needed, so as to facilitate catheter access to the artery [65, 66]. Data showed an 87.5% 1-year OS, 68.7% 3-year OS and 50% 5-year OS, as well as a 75%, 62.5% and 43.7% 1-, 3- and 5-year EFS, respectively [64]. Regardless if the tumor is resectable or not, TACE can be the initial and sole preoperative treatment in patients with no distant metastases, while for patients with distant metastases, systemic chemotherapy before the implementation of TACE is essential [63]. Additionally, it can facilitate the transition of a tumor from the unresectable status to resectable, especially in patients without distant metastases, without the severe side effects of liver or renal failure, myelosuppression or cardiac damage [67]. On the other hand, a "postembolization syndrome" comprising of fever, abdominal pain, nausea, vomiting, and hepatitis, and increased CRP levels can afflict the vast majority of patients, even though these symptoms are temporary and clinically insignificant [64].

High-intensity focused ultrasound (HIFU) has also been used in combination with TACE and its ability to directly target tumor cells and enhance their death is impressive. In a trial assessing HIFU ablation plus TACE versus C5V chemotherapy reported an increased rate of complete resection and a decreasedrate of serious adverse events in comparison to C5V treatment in advanced pediatric HB [68]. Presuming that HIFU ablation is as efficacious as surgery in the management of HB, it was used after TACE in stage III and IV HBs and achieved complete ablation in all of the cases with the significant percentages of tumor size reduction by 50-60% [69]. At this point, it is essential to highlight the importance of administering HIFU ablation after TACE. This lays on the fact that TACE interferes with tumor blood flow, which may result in heat loss during HIFU, by reducing it. At the same time, TACE leads to iodinated oil deposition in the HB itself, hence not only increasing the acoustic impendence, but also providing synergistic thermogenic effects up to those of HIFU [69]. Further research is warranted before introducing those techniques to first-line treatment protocols.

LIVER TRANSPLANTATION (LT)

LT is supposed to be the last curative treatment resort for unresectable and metastatic HB. In fact, from the low rate of 5% in 1990, LT was performed as frequently as 43% in 2013 [70]. Even though HB's frequency has increased four times over a 32-year period, LT is performed significantly twenty times more frequently [71]. Interestingly, in the 1990s only half of the recipients of primary LT were expected to survive [72], while nowadays the rate is about 80-90% [70, 73]. However, data suggest that surgeons with high expertise may be able to resect otherwise unresectable tumors. As such, many controversies exist as per which is the optimal treatment for very large or critically positioned HBs that impinge on vital vessels or multifocal HBs in all four sectors of the liver before neoadjuvant chemotherapy [37, 74 - 77].

Current indications for LT in HB are the unifocal POST-TEXT IV HBs and/or POST-TEXT III or IV that are multifocal in nature or invade the vasculature [35, 78]. The presence of active extrahepatic HB sites, both regional spread and metastases, that have not been completely treated either surgically or with chemotherapy, poses a contraindication to LT. As mentioned before, pulmonary metastases and their management specifically is a controversial topic. Nevertheless, even partial response by HB size reduction and fall of AFP levels constitute good prognostic factors. Remnants of extrahepatic disease before LT, even if cleared on computed tomography (CT) scan before LT, is a significant risk factor for HB recurrence after LT [79]. Similar outcomes have been observed in terms of disease clearance and recurrence rates between surgery and chemotherapy [35, 70, 80].

There is an ongoing debate regarding the best method for the management of multifocal HB, between LT versus conventional surgical resection after clearance of intrahepatic lesions with neoadjuvant chemotherapy [27, 76, 79, 80]. At least for POST-TEXT IV HBs with multifocal spread that present without metastases post neoadjuvant chemotherapy, the reasonable management is LT [81]. Studies have shown that the exact extent of the disease may be overestimated in about 40% of the patients, if staging is based solely on imaging findings [76, 82]. So many surgeons, especially in liver centers with high expertise in extensive liver cancer resections, suggest exploratory laparotomy upfront prior to listing for LT, so as to determine the actual extent of the disease. However, the vast majority of liver surgeons agree that radiographic findings are enough for listing for LT, before exploratory surgical procedure. If intraoperatively the tumor presents to be unresectable, LT if necessary and usually from a living donor, can be carried out at the same time [77, 78, 83]. On the contrary, the COG guidelines clearly state that referral to LT centers for LT should be timely for unresectable tumors [27, 35]. This was based on the optimal outcomes observed after primary LT for these patients (80% survival) versus rescue LT after failure of primary surgical resection due to recurrence (30-40%) [47, 75, 84, 85]. Actually, on multivariate analysis, it was seen that the only factor affecting OS was macroscopic venous invasion. In general, long-lasting preoperative chemotherapy protocols in HBs that remain unresectable should be avoided, as not only may the effects on treating the tumor decrease with prolonged therapy, but resistance in chemotherapeutic agents can also be seen. In fact, continuing the anticancer regimen for more than four chemotherapy cycles has no impact in increasing the rates of conventional tumor resectability [86, 87]. So, in that context when local control is needed, especially after four cycles of chemotherapy, LT is the best possible option [27]. The ongoing trial by COG (AHEP0731) is about to assess the feasibility and outcomes of early referral for LT versus primary extreme surgical resection [88]. However, the scarcity of liver grafts poses another real therapeutic challenge, which may afflict survival of HB patients (waiting time for LT ranges from 1 to 50 days, with a median of 16 days) [80]. Living donor LT can be a potential solution to this problem by increasing the liver graft pool. Notably, the rates of recurrence were higher in patients waiting for a cadaveric graft (mean 31 versus 15 days in patients with and without recurrence, respectively) [70].

In contrast, it is actively advocated that liver resection can provide similar oncologic outcomes without the disadvantages of post-LT immunosuppression and of the absence of liver donors and cadaveric livers, especially in countries like Egypt where cadaveric livers are not culturally acceptable [89, 90]. Another argument of those vouching for liver resection over LT is that the latter is supposed to carry some serious complications, as it is a significant operation. These include but are not limited to malfunction, hepatic artery and portal vein thrombosis, long-lasting immunosuppression, lymphoproliferative disease and chronic rejection [35], while data from large registries (like the PLUTO registry) indicate lack of hepatic artery thrombosis [91]. Another study reported a 10% hepatic artery or portal vein thrombosis requiring a second LT operation [70]. Post-LT chemotherapy and immunosuppression can also lead to either a secondary malignancy, like Burkitt lymphoma [80], or infection, such as CMV [92].

Overall, a recent study assessing the long-term outcomes in a 14-year period of LT reported a 1-, 3-, and 5-year graft survival rate of 96%, 87%, and 80%, respectively with even 66% of the patients that received salvage LT surviving for a 1.5 year now postoperatively [93]. Generally, it is really difficult to pool the data of previous studies and reach solid conclusions about the actual survival of HB patients receiving LT over the years, because of the discordances in age, staging systems, chemotherapy schemas, the presence of metastatic disease pre-LT and the implementation of chemotherapy post-LT among the individual studies. A worth mentioning review article gathered the data from 292 HB patients who received LT and showed that, at the time of each individual paper's publication, 41% of the patients that underwent a rescue LT were alive, while the percentage was 85% for those that received primary LT [81]. Another recently published study from Japan reported that primary LT is superior to liver resection for advanced HB with an OS of 100% *vs* 91.7%, respectively [94]. Thus, primary LT is the suggested treatment for advanced stage HB, at least until the AHEP0731 trial elucidates those controversies.

THE ROLE OF AFP

Serum AFP levels tend to somehow correlate with HB, thus have been defined as a sensitive prognostic marker. AFP levels are usually increased in children with HB, while in around 5-10% of the cases they can be either normal or low [95]. The actual number is not that significant for prognosis, but there are two other ways that AFP levels can be found useful. Firstly, AFP levels are related to the tumor extent and biologic nature, so they can be helpful at the time of diagnosis. Secondly, they can also be monitored after administering chemotherapy to evaluate response to treatment. Actually, the SIOPEL stratified children with HB into two groups, as standard-risk and high-risk, as per the AFP levels. Levels lower than 100 ng/mL are thought of carrying a higher risk of a worse response to chemotherapy and poorer prognosis [95, 96]. High-risk were the tumors confined in all four liver sectors or even those presenting with distant metastases. Standard-risk were the HBs limited to the liver and not involving more than three liver sectors [96]. However, recently the CHIC is making attempts to re-stratify patients based on more accurate prognostic factors, and AFP plays a vital role in this process [24]. As previously mentioned, they divide patients into five backbone groups and, when it comes to AFP, in the first four backbone groups AFP is defined as over 100 ng/mL, while the level of AFP ≤100 ng/mL is set for the fifth backbone group, while in general groups are defined based on PRETEXT and the presence or not of metastatic disease. In terms of the outcomes of this attempt to pool the data of previous trials, children in the backbone 5 group exhibited a poor prognosis and low AFP did not seem to be as predictive of a poor outcome, because children with PRETEXT I and low AFP (≤100 ng/mL) did not show such a bad prognosis. Consequently, AFP levels are useful prognostic factors, but the resectability of the tumor seems to outweigh AFP in terms of significance. They also introduced a new category as per the AFP levels (≤100, 100–1000 and >1000 ng/mL) based on the notion that infants younger than 6 months of age present with a broader range of normal AFP levels, which does not coalesce with the predetermined "adult" normal values at least until they become 6-12 months old, after reviewing previously published work in this topic [97]. It was shown that patients with AFP >1000 ng/mL exhibited improved survival regardless of being positive for one of the annotation factors. Additionally, patients with AFP ranging between 100 and 1000 ng/mL, even though being PRETEXT III, <8 years of age, and without metastasis, had a relatively worse 5-year EFS. Besides, it is known based on data that patients that not survive of HB tend to have a lower median AFP at presentation [93].

When it comes to response to chemotherapy, previous studies pointed towards the perception that the level of decrease in AFP levels was more predictive for survival than the actual numerical value [98], while more recent data suggest that the actual AFP levels after neoadjuvant chemotherapy and before surgical resection are more predictive [99]. Moreover, AFP levels tend to increase postoperatively when a relapse occurs with less than 1% of relapses thought of being AFP-negative [96]. So instead of utilizing imaging for post-treatment relapse surveillance, it is recommended that AFP levels are routinely monitored and imaging studies are reserved for patients with increased risk of relapse, such as the older ones and those presenting with a low AFP value or a SCU histopathology result [99]. Nevertheless, further trials are needed to solidify the currently available data regarding the prognostic significance of AFP in HB, but the recent collaborative approaches seem promising.

CONCLUSION

HB is a one of the most commonly intraabdominal solid tumors of childhood, and presents occasionally with several genetic associations, such as familial adenomatous polyposis, Beckwith-Wiedemann syndrome, and various genetic mutations. The discrepancies among the grouping systems and treatment approaches among the four study groups dealing with this entity posed a real challenge for many years in terms of determining the best possible risk-stratification system and therapeutic plan that would lead to the most favorable prognosis. The different modalities implemented are neoadjuvant chemotherapy, surgical resection and adjuvant chemotherapy, especially for low-risk tumors, while high-risk patients are mostly favored by pre- and/or postoperative chemotherapy and LT or liver resection. Future studies evaluating TACE and HIFU may drastically alter the current first-line treatment protocols. The ongoing work of the current international collaborative initiative, which consists of the four major HB study groups, seems really promising and the PHITT that is now still recruiting patients may further elucidate foggy areas and result into better survival outcomes for children afflicted by HB.

CONSENT FOR PUBLICATION

Not applicable.

CONFLICT OF INTEREST

The authors declare no conflict of interest, financial or otherwise.

ACKNOWLEDGEMENT

Declare None.

REFERENCES

[1] Aronson DC, Meyers RL. Malignant tumors of the liver in children. Semin Pediatr Surg 2016; 25(5): 265-75.
[http://dx.doi.org/10.1053/j.sempedsurg.2016.09.002] [PMID: 27955729]

[2] Czauderna P, Lopez-Terrada D, Hiyama E, Häberle B, Malogolowkin MH, Meyers RL. Hepatoblastoma state of the art: pathology, genetics, risk stratification, and chemotherapy. Curr Opin Pediatr 2014; 26(1): 19-28.
[http://dx.doi.org/10.1097/MOP.0000000000000046] [PMID: 24322718]

[3] Czauderna P, Haeberle B, Hiyama E, Rangaswami A, Krailo M, Maibach R. The Children's Hepatictumors International Collaboration(CHIC): Novel global rare tumor database yields new prognostic factor sinhepatoblastomaandbecomesaresearch model. Eur J Cancer 2016; 52(1): 92-101.
[http://dx.doi.org/10.1016/j.ejca.2015.09.023] [PMID: 26655560]

[4] Wu JF, Chang HH, Lu MY, *et al.* Prognostic roles of pathology markers immunoexpression and clinical parameters in Hepatoblastoma. J Biomed Sci 2017; 24(1): 62.
[http://dx.doi.org/10.1186/s12929-017-0369-1] [PMID: 28851352]

[5] Spector LG, Birch J. The epidemiology of hepatoblastoma. Pediatr Blood Cancer 2012; 59(5): 776-9.
[http://dx.doi.org/10.1002/pbc.24215] [PMID: 22692949]

[6] Stocker JT. Hepatoblastoma. Semin Diagn Pathol 1994; 11(2): 136-43.
[PMID: 7809507]

[7] Takayasu H, Horie H, Hiyama E, *et al.* Frequent deletions and mutations of the beta-catenin gene are associated with overexpression of cyclin D1 and fibronectin and poorly differentiated histology in childhood hepatoblastoma. Clin Cancer Res 2001; 7(4): 901-8.
[PMID: 11309340]

[8] Sugimachi K, Taguchi K, Aishima S, *et al.* Altered expression of β-catenin without genetic mutation in intrahepatic cholangiocarcinoma. Mod Pathol 2001; 14(9): 900-5.
[http://dx.doi.org/10.1038/modpathol.3880409] [PMID: 11557787]

[9] Hiyama E, Hiyama K, Yokoyama T, Shay JW. Immunohistochemical detection of telomerase (hTERT) protein in human cancer tissues and a subset of cells in normal tissues. Neoplasia 2001; 3(1): 17-26.
[http://dx.doi.org/10.1038/sj.neo.7900134] [PMID: 11326312]

[10] Ueda Y, Hiyama E, Kamimatsuse A, Kamei N, Ogura K, Sueda T. Wnt signaling and telomerase activation of hepatoblastoma: correlation with chemosensitivity and surgical resectability. J Pediatr Surg 2011; 46(12): 2221-7.
[http://dx.doi.org/10.1016/j.jpedsurg.2011.09.003] [PMID: 22152854]

[11] Cairo S, Armengol C, De Reyniès A, et al. Hepatic stem-like phenotype and interplay of Wnt/beta-catenin and Myc signaling in aggressive childhood liver cancer. Cancer Cell 2008; 14(6): 471-84.
[http://dx.doi.org/10.1016/j.ccr.2008.11.002] [PMID: 19061838]

[12] Konsavage WM Jr, Yochum GS. Intersection of Hippo/YAP and Wnt/β-catenin signaling pathways. Acta Biochim Biophys Sin (Shanghai) 2013; 45(2): 71-9.
[http://dx.doi.org/10.1093/abbs/gms084] [PMID: 23027379]

[13] Li H, Wolfe A, Septer S, et al. Deregulation of Hippo kinase signalling in human hepatic malignancies. Liver Int 2012; 32(1): 38-47.
[http://dx.doi.org/10.1111/j.1478-3231.2011.02646.x] [PMID: 22098159]

[14] López-Terrada D, Alaggio R, de Dávila MT, et al. Towards an international pediatric liver tumor consensus classification: proceedings of the Los Angeles COG liver tumors symposium. Mod Pathol 2014; 27(3): 472-91.
[http://dx.doi.org/10.1038/modpathol.2013.80] [PMID: 24008558]

[15] Bell D, Ranganathan S, Tao J, Monga SPS. Novel advances in understanding of molecular pathogenesis of hepatoblastoma: A wnt/β-catenin perspective. Gene Expr 2017 Feb; 17(2): 141-54.
[http://dx.doi.org/10.3727/105221616X693639]

[16] Fuchs J, Rydzynski J, Von Schweinitz D, et al. Pretreatment prognostic factors and treatment results in children with hepatoblastoma: a report from the German Cooperative Pediatric Liver Tumor Study HB 94. Cancer 2002; 95(1): 172-82.
[http://dx.doi.org/10.1002/cncr.10632] [PMID: 12115331]

[17] Haas JE, Muczynski KA, Krailo M, et al. Histopathology and prognosis in childhood hepatoblastoma and hepatocarcinoma. Cancer 1989; 64(5): 1082-95.
[http://dx.doi.org/10.1002/1097-0142(19890901)64:5<1082::AID-CNCR2820640520>3.0.CO;2-G] [PMID: 2547506]

[18] Malogolowkin MH, Katzenstein HM, Meyers RL, et al. Complete surgical resection is curative for children with hepatoblastoma with pure fetal histology: a report from the Children's Oncology Group. J Clin Oncol 2011; 29(24): 3301-6.
[http://dx.doi.org/10.1200/JCO.2010.29.3837] [PMID: 21768450]

[19] Haas JE, Feusner JH, Finegold MJ. Small cell undifferentiated histology in hepatoblastoma may be unfavorable. Cancer 2001; 92(12): 3130-4.
[http://dx.doi.org/10.1002/1097-0142(20011215)92:12<3130::AID-CNCR10115>3.0.CO;2-#] [PMID: 11753992]

[20] Trobaugh-Lotrario AD, Tomlinson GE, Finegold MJ, Gore L, Feusner JH. Small cell undifferentiated variant of hepatoblastoma: adverse clinical and molecular features similar to rhabdoid tumors. Pediatr Blood Cancer 2009; 52(3): 328-34.
[http://dx.doi.org/10.1002/pbc.21834] [PMID: 18985717]

[21] López-Terrada D, Alaggio R, de Dávila MT, et al. Towards an international pediatric liver tumor consensus classification: proceedings of the Los Angeles COG liver tumors symposium. Mod Pathol 2014; 27(3): 472-91.
[http://dx.doi.org/10.1038/modpathol.2013.80] [PMID: 24008558]

[22] Zhou S, Gomulia E, Mascarenhas L, Wang L. Is INI1-retained small cell undifferentiated histology in hepatoblastoma unfavorable? Hum Pathol 2015; 46(4): 620-4.
[http://dx.doi.org/10.1016/j.humpath.2014.12.013] [PMID: 25649007]

[23] Roebuck DJ, Aronson D, Clapuyt P, et al. 2005 PRETEXT: a revised staging system for primary

malignant liver tumours of childhood developed by the SIOPEL group. Pediatr Radiol 2007; 37(2): 123-32.
[http://dx.doi.org/10.1007/s00247-006-0361-5] [PMID: 17186233]

[24] Meyers RL, Maibach R, Hiyama E, *et al.* Risk-stratified staging in paediatric hepatoblastoma: a unified analysis from the Children's Hepatic tumors International Collaboration. Lancet Oncol 2017; 18(1): 122-31.
[http://dx.doi.org/10.1016/S1470-2045(16)30598-8] [PMID: 27884679]

[25] ClinicalTrials.gov [Internet]. Bethesda (MD): National Library of Medicine (US) 2000 Feb 29 - Identifier: NCT03017326, Paediatric Hepatic International Tumour Trial (PHITT) , 2017 Jan 11; [cited 2018 Aug 14]; [about 13 screens]. Available from: https://clinicaltrials.gov/ct2/show/NCT03017326

[26] Ortega JA, Douglass EC, Feusner JH, *et al.* Randomized comparison of cisplatin/vincristin/5-fluorouracil and cisplatin/doxorubicin for the treatment of pediatric hepatoblastoma (HB): A report from the Children's Cancer Group and the Pediatric Oncology Group. J Clin Oncol 2000; 18(14): 2665-75.
[http://dx.doi.org/10.1200/JCO.2000.18.14.2665] [PMID: 10894865]

[27] Meyers RL, Tiao G, de Ville de Goyet J, Superina R, Aronson DC. Hepatoblastoma state of the art: pre-treatment extent of disease, surgical resection guidelines and the role of liver transplantation. Curr Opin Pediatr 2014; 26(1): 29-36.
[http://dx.doi.org/10.1097/MOP.0000000000000042] [PMID: 24362406]

[28] Malogolowkin MH, Katzenstein HM, Krailo M, Meyers RL. Treatment of hepatoblastoma: the North American cooperative group experience. Front Biosci (Elite Ed) 2012; 4: 1717-23.
[http://dx.doi.org/10.2741/e492] [PMID: 22201987]

[29] Trobaugh-Lotrario AD, Katzenstein HM. Chemotherapeutic approaches for newly diagnosed hepatoblastoma: past, present, and future strategies. Pediatr Blood Cancer 2012; 59(5): 809-12.
[http://dx.doi.org/10.1002/pbc.24219] [PMID: 22648979]

[30] Perilongo G, Malogolowkin M, Feusner J. Hepatoblastoma clinical research: lessons learned and future challenges. Pediatr Blood Cancer 2012; 59(5): 818-21.
[http://dx.doi.org/10.1002/pbc.24217] [PMID: 22678761]

[31] Hishiki T, Matsunaga T, Sasaki F, *et al.* Outcome of hepatoblastomas treated using the Japanese Study Group for Pediatric Liver Tumor (JPLT) protocol-2: report from the JPLT. Pediatr Surg Int 2011; 27(1): 1-8.
[http://dx.doi.org/10.1007/s00383-010-2708-0] [PMID: 20922397]

[32] Sasaki F, Matsunaga T, Iwafuchi M, *et al.* Outcome of hepatoblastoma treated with the JPLT-1 (Japanese Study Group for Pediatric Liver Tumor) Protocol-1: A report from the Japanese Study Group for Pediatric Liver Tumor. J Pediatr Surg 2002; 37(6): 851-6.
[http://dx.doi.org/10.1053/jpsu.2002.32886] [PMID: 12037748]

[33] Hiyama E, Hishiki T, Watanabe K, *et al.* Mortality and morbidity in primarily resected hepatoblastomas in Japan: Experience of the JPLT (Japanese Study Group for Pediatric Liver Tumor) trials. J Pediatr Surg 2015; 50(12): 2098-101.
[http://dx.doi.org/10.1016/j.jpedsurg.2015.08.035] [PMID: 26388131]

[34] Grotegut S, Kappler R, Tarimoradi S, Lehembre F, Christofori G, Von Schweinitz D. Hepatocyte growth factor protects hepatoblastoma cells from chemotherapy-induced apoptosis by AKT activation. Int J Oncol 2010; 36(5): 1261-7.
[PMID: 20372801]

[35] Meyers RL, Czauderna P, Otte JB. Surgical treatment of hepatoblastoma. Pediatr Blood Cancer 2012; 59(5): 800-8.
[http://dx.doi.org/10.1002/pbc.24220] [PMID: 22887704]

[36] Exelby PR, Filler RM, Grosfeld JL. Liver tumors in children in the particular reference to hepatoblastoma and hepatocellular carcinoma: American Academy of Pediatrics Surgical Section

Survey--1974. J Pediatr Surg 1975; 10(3): 329-37.
[http://dx.doi.org/10.1016/0022-3468(75)90095-0] [PMID: 49416]

[37] Brown J, Perilongo G, Shafford E, *et al.* Pretreatment prognostic factors for children with hepatoblastoma-- results from the International Society of Paediatric Oncology (SIOP) study SIOPEL 1. Eur J Cancer 2000; 36(11): 1418-25.
[http://dx.doi.org/10.1016/S0959-8049(00)00074-5] [PMID: 10899656]

[38] Holton CP, Burrington JD, Hatch EI. A multiple chemotherapeutic approach to the management of hepatoblastoma. A preliminary report. Cancer 1975; 35(4): 1083-7.
[http://dx.doi.org/10.1002/1097-0142(197504)35:4<1083::AID-CNCR2820350410>3.0.CO;2-K] [PMID: 163673]

[39] Ortega JA, Krailo MD, Haas JE, *et al.* Effective treatment of unresectable or metastatic hepatoblastoma with cisplatin and continuous infusion doxorubicin chemotherapy: a report from the Childrens Cancer Study Group. J Clin Oncol 1991; 9(12): 2167-76.
[http://dx.doi.org/10.1200/JCO.1991.9.12.2167] [PMID: 1720452]

[40] Douglass EC, Reynolds M, Finegold M, Cantor AB, Glicksman A. Cisplatin, vincristine, and fluorouracil therapy for hepatoblastoma: a Pediatric Oncology Group study. J Clin Oncol 1993; 11(1): 96-9.
[http://dx.doi.org/10.1200/JCO.1993.11.1.96] [PMID: 8380296]

[41] Malogolowkin MH, Katzenstein H, Krailo MD, *et al.* Intensified platinum therapy is an ineffective strategy for improving outcome in pediatric patients with advanced hepatoblastoma. J Clin Oncol 2006 Jun; 24(18): 2879-84.
[http://dx.doi.org/10.1200/JCO. 2005.02.6013]

[42] Malogolowkin MH, Katzenstein HM, Krailo M, *et al.* Redefining the role of doxorubicin for the treatment of children with hepatoblastoma. J Clin Oncol 2008 May; 26(14): 2379-83.
[http://dx.doi.org/10. 1200/JCO.2006.09.7204]

[43] Perilongo G, Shafford E, Maibach R, *et al.* Risk-adapted treatment for childhood hepatoblastoma. final report of the second study of the International Society of Paediatric Oncology--SIOPEL 2. Eur J Cancer 2004; 40(3): 411-21.
[http://dx.doi.org/10.1016/j.ejca.2003.06.003] [PMID: 14746860]

[44] Perilongo G, Maibach R, Shafford E, *et al.* Cisplatin versus cisplatin plus doxorubicin for standard-risk hepatoblastoma. N Engl J Med 2009; 361(17): 1662-70.
[http://dx.doi.org/10.1056/NEJMoa0810613] [PMID: 19846851]

[45] Zsiros J, Maibach R, Shafford E, *et al.* Successful treatment of childhood high-risk hepatoblastoma with dose-intensive multiagent chemotherapy and surgery: final results of the SIOPEL- 3HR study. J Clin Oncol 2010 May; 28(15): 2584-90.
[http://dx.doi.org/10.1200/JCO.2009.22.4857]

[46] Zsiros J, Brugieres L, Brock P, *et al.* Dose-dense cisplatin-based chemotherapy and surgery for children with high-risk hepatoblastoma (SIOPEL-4): a prospective, single-arm, feasibility study. Lancet Oncol 2013; 14(9): 834-42.
[http://dx.doi.org/10.1016/S1470-2045(13)70272-9] [PMID: 23831416]

[47] Otte JB, Pritchard J, Aronson DC, *et al.* Liver transplantation for hepatoblastoma: results from the International Society of Pediatric Oncology (SIOP) study SIOPEL-1 and review of the world experience. Pediatr Blood Cancer 2004; 42(1): 74-83.
[http://dx.doi.org/10.1002/pbc.10376] [PMID: 14752798]

[48] Beaty O III, Berg S, Blaney S, *et al.* A phase II trial and pharmacokinetic study of oxaliplatin in children with refractory solid tumors: a Children's Oncology Group study. Pediatr Blood Cancer 2010; 55(3): 440-5.
[http://dx.doi.org/10.1002/pbc.22544] [PMID: 20658614]

[49] Zsíros J, Brugières L, Brock P, *et al.* Efficacy of irinotecan single drug treatment in children with

[50] refractory or recurrent hepatoblastoma--a phase II trial of the childhood liver tumour strategy group (SIOPEL). Eur J Cancer 2012; 48(18): 3456-64.
[http://dx.doi.org/10.1016/j.ejca.2012.06.023] [PMID: 22835780]

[50] Katzenstein H, Furman W, Malogolowkin M, *et al.* Vincristine/Irinotecan Upfront Window Treatment of High-risk Hepatoblastoma: A Report from the Children's Oncology Group (COG) AHEP0731 Study Committee. Cancer 2017; 123(12): 2360-7.
[http://dx.doi.org/10.1002/cncr.30591] [PMID: 28211941]

[51] Katzenstein HM, London WB, Douglass EC, *et al.* Treatment of unresectable and metastatic hepatoblastoma: a pediatric oncology group phase II study. J Clin Oncol 2002; 20(16): 3438-44.
[http://dx.doi.org/10.1200/JCO.2002.07.400] [PMID: 12177104]

[52] Qayed M, Powell C, Morgan ER, Haugen M, Katzenstein HM. Irinotecan as maintenance therapy in high-risk hepatoblastoma. Pediatr Blood Cancer 2010; 54(5): 761-3.
[http://dx.doi.org/10.1002/pbc.22408] [PMID: 20063426]

[53] Ijichi O, Ishikawa S, Shinkoda Y, *et al.* Response of heavily treated and relapsed hepatoblastoma in the transplanted liver to single-agent therapy with irinotecan. Pediatr Transplant 2006; 10(5): 635-8.
[http://dx.doi.org/10.1111/j.1399-3046.2006.00517.x] [PMID: 16857004]

[54] Brock PR, Maibach R, Childs M, *et al.* Sodium Thiosulfate for Protection from Cisplatin-Induced Hearing Loss. N Engl J Med 2018; 378(25): 2376-85.
[http://dx.doi.org/10.1056/NEJMoa1801109] [PMID: 29924955]

[55] Liu C, Tsai HL, Chin T, Wei C. Experience of surgical treatment for hepatoblastoma. Formosan Journal of Surgery 2016; 49(2): 56-62.
[http://dx.doi.org/10.1016/j.fjs.2015.10.001]

[56] Kubota M, Yagi M, Kanada S, *et al.* Effect of postoperative chemotherapy on the serum alpha-fetoprotein level in hepatoblastoma. J Pediatr Surg 2004; 39(12): 1775-8.
[http://dx.doi.org/10.1016/j.jpedsurg.2004.08.038] [PMID: 15616926]

[57] Moon SB, Shin HB, Seo JM, Lee SK. Hepatoblastoma: 15-year experience and role of surgical treatment. J Korean Surg Soc 2011; 81(2): 134-40.
[http://dx.doi.org/10.4174/jkss.2011.81.2.134] [PMID: 22066113]

[58] Pritchard J, Brown J, Shafford E, *et al.* Cisplatin, doxorubicin, and delayed surgery for childhood hepatoblastoma: a successful approach--results of the first prospective study of the International Society of Pediatric Oncology. J Clin Oncol 2000; 18(22): 3819-28.
[http://dx.doi.org/10.1200/JCO.2000.18.22.3819] [PMID: 11078495]

[59] Evans AE, Land VJ, Newton WA, Randolph JG, Sather HN, Tefft M. Combination chemotherapy (vincristine, adriamycin, cyclophosphamide, and 5-fluorouracil) in the treatment of children with malignant hepatoma. Cancer 1982; 50(5): 821-6.
[http://dx.doi.org/10.1002/1097-0142(19820901)50:5<821::AID-CNCR2820500502>3.0.CO;2-K]
[PMID: 6284345]

[60] Farhi DC, Odell CA, Shurin SB. Myelodysplastic syndrome and acute myeloid leukemia after treatment for solid tumors of childhood. Am J Clin Pathol 1993; 100(3): 270-5.
[http://dx.doi.org/10.1093/ajcp/100.3.270] [PMID: 8379535]

[61] Moppett J, Oakhill A, Duncan AW. Second malignancies in children: the usual suspects? Eur J Radiol 2001; 38(3): 235-48.
[http://dx.doi.org/10.1016/S0720-048X(08)00291-X] [PMID: 11399379]

[62] Malogolowkin MH, Stanley P, Steele DA, Ortega JA. Feasibility and toxicity of chemoembolization for children with liver tumors. J Clin Oncol 2000; 18(6): 1279-84.
[http://dx.doi.org/10.1200/JCO.2000.18.6.1279] [PMID: 10715298]

[63] Ohtsuka Y, Matsunaga T, Yoshida H, Kouchi K, Okada T, Ohnuma N. Optimal strategy of preoperative transcatheter arterial chemoembolization for hepatoblastoma. Surg Today 2004; 34(2):

127-33.
[http://dx.doi.org/10.1007/s00595-003-2663-7] [PMID: 14745612]

[64] Li JP, Chu JP, Yang JY, Chen W, Wang Y, Huang YH. Preoperative transcatheter selective arterial chemoembolization in treatment of unresectable hepatoblastoma in infants and children. Cardiovasc Intervent Radiol 2008; 31(6): 1117-23.
[http://dx.doi.org/10.1007/s00270-008-9373-x] [PMID: 18560935]

[65] Takayama T, Makuuchi M, Takayasu K, et al. Resection after intraarterial chemotherapy of a hepatoblastoma originating in the caudate lobe. Surgery 1990; 107(2): 231-5.
[PMID: 2154056]

[66] Yokomori K, Hori T, Asoh S, Tuji A, Takemura T. Complete disappearance of unresectable hepatoblastoma by continuous infusion therapy through hepatic artery. J Pediatr Surg 1991; 26(7): 844-6.
[http://dx.doi.org/10.1016/0022-3468(91)90152-J] [PMID: 1654408]

[67] Zhang J, Xu F, Chen K, et al. An effective approach for treating unresectable hepatoblastoma in infants and children: Pre-operative transcatheter arterial chemoembolization. Oncol Lett 2013; 6(3): 850-4.
[http://dx.doi.org/10.3892/ol.2013.1444] [PMID: 24137424]

[68] Chen B, Chen J, Luo Q, Guo C. Effective strategy of the combination of high-intensity focused ultrasound and transarterial chemoembolization for improving outcome of unresectable and metastatic hepatoblastoma: a retrospective cohort study. Transl Oncol 2014; 7(6): 788-94.
[http://dx.doi.org/10.1016/j.tranon.2014.09.006] [PMID: 25500089]

[69] Wang S, Yang C, Zhang J, et al. First experience of high-intensity focused ultrasound combined with transcatheter arterial embolization as local control for hepatoblastoma. Hepatology 2014; 59(1): 170-7.
[http://dx.doi.org/10.1002/hep.26595] [PMID: 23813416]

[70] Pham TA, Gallo AM, Concepcion W, Esquivel CO, Bonham CA. Effect of liver transplant on long-term disease-free survival in children with hepatoblastoma and hepatocellular cancer. JAMA Surg 2015; 150(12): 1150-8.
[http://dx.doi.org/10.1001/jamasurg.2015.1847] [PMID: 26308249]

[71] Khaderi S, Guiteau J, Cotton RT, O'Mahony C, Rana A, Goss JA. Role of liver transplantation in the management of hepatoblastoma in the pediatric population. World J Transplant 2014; 4(4): 294-8.
[http://dx.doi.org/10.5500/wjt.v4.i4.294] [PMID: 25540737]

[72] Koneru B, Flye MW, Busuttil RW, et al. Liver transplantation for hepatoblastoma. The American experience. Ann Surg 1991; 213(2): 118-21.
[http://dx.doi.org/10.1097/00000658-199102000-00004] [PMID: 1847033]

[73] Tiao GM, Bobey N, Allen S, et al. The current management of hepatoblastoma: a combination of chemotherapy, conventional resection, and liver transplantation. J Pediatr 2005; 146(2): 204-11.
[http://dx.doi.org/10.1016/j.jpeds.2004.09.011] [PMID: 15689909]

[74] Pimpalwar AP, Sharif K, Ramani P, et al. Strategy for hepatoblastoma management: Transplant versus nontransplant surgery. J Pediatr Surg 2002; 37(2): 240-5.
[http://dx.doi.org/10.1053/jpsu.2002.30264] [PMID: 11819207]

[75] Otte JB, de Ville de Goyet J, Reding R. Liver transplantation for hepatoblastoma: indications and contraindications in the modern era. Pediatr Transplant 2005; 9(5): 557-65.
[http://dx.doi.org/10.1111/j.1399-3046.2005.00354.x] [PMID: 16176410]

[76] Lautz TB, Ben-Ami T, Tantemsapya N, Gosiengfiao Y, Superina RA. Successful nontransplant resection of POST-TEXT III and IV hepatoblastoma. Cancer 2011; 117(9): 1976-83.
[http://dx.doi.org/10.1002/cncr.25722] [PMID: 21509775]

[77] Meyers RL, Tiao GM, Dunn SP, McGahren ED III, Langham MR Jr. Surgical management of children with locally advanced hepatoblastoma. Cancer 2012; 118(16): 4090-1.

[http://dx.doi.org/10.1002/cncr.26715] [PMID: 22760520]

[78] Otte JB. Progress in the surgical treatment of malignant liver tumors in children. Cancer Treat Rev 2010; 36(4): 360-71.
[http://dx.doi.org/10.1016/j.ctrv.2010.02.013] [PMID: 20227190]

[79] Cruz RJ Jr, Ranganathan S, Mazariegos G, *et al.* Analysis of national and single-center incidence and survival after liver transplantation for hepatoblastoma: new trends and future opportunities. Surgery 2013; 153(2): 150-9.
[http://dx.doi.org/10.1016/j.surg.2012.11.006] [PMID: 23331862]

[80] Héry G, Franchi-Abella S, Habes D, *et al.* Initial liver transplantation for unresectable hepatoblastoma after chemotherapy. Pediatr Blood Cancer 2011; 57(7): 1270-5.
[http://dx.doi.org/10.1002/pbc.23301] [PMID: 21910210]

[81] Trobaugh-Lotrario AD, Meyers RL, Tiao GM, Feusner JH. Pediatric liver transplantation for hepatoblastoma. Transl Gastroenterol Hepatol 2016; 1: 44.
[http://dx.doi.org/10.21037/tgh.2016.04.01] [PMID: 28138611]

[82] Aronson DC, Schnater JM, Staalman CR, *et al.* Predictive value of the pretreatment extent of disease system in hepatoblastoma: results from the International Society of Pediatric Oncology Liver Tumor Study Group SIOPEL-1 study. J Clin Oncol 2005; 23(6): 1245-52.
[http://dx.doi.org/10.1200/JCO.2005.07.145] [PMID: 15718322]

[83] Millar AJ, Hartley P, Khan D, Spearman W, Andronikou S, Rode H. Extended hepatic resection with transplantation back-up for an "unresectable" tumour. Pediatr Surg Int 2001; 17(5-6): 378-81.
[http://dx.doi.org/10.1007/s003830000531] [PMID: 11527170]

[84] Otte JB, Meyers RL, de Ville de Goyet J. Transplantation for liver tumors in children: time to (re)set the guidelines? Pediatr Transplant 2013; 17(8): 710-2.
[http://dx.doi.org/10.1111/petr.12160] [PMID: 24164822]

[85] McAteer JP, Goldin AB, Healy PJ, Gow KW. Surgical treatment of primary liver tumors in children: time to reconsider the role of liver transplantation? Pediatr Transplant 2013; 17: 744-50.
[http://dx.doi.org/10.1111/petr.12144] [PMID: 23992390]

[86] von Schweinitz D, Hecker H, Harms D, *et al.* Complete resection before development of drug resistance is essential for survival from advanced hepatoblastoma--a report from the German Cooperative Pediatric Liver Tumor Study HB-89. J Pediatr Surg 1995; 30(6): 845-52.
[http://dx.doi.org/10.1016/0022-3468(95)90762-9] [PMID: 7545228]

[87] Warmann SW, Fuchs J. Drug resistance in hepatoblastoma. Curr Pharm Biotechnol 2007; 8(2): 93-7.
[http://dx.doi.org/10.2174/138920107780487456] [PMID: 17430157]

[88] ClinicalTrials.gov. 2000. https://clinicaltrials.gov/ct2/show/NCT00980460

[89] El-Gendi A, Fadel S, El-Shafei M, Shawky A. Avoiding liver transplantation in post-treatment extent of disease III and IV hepatoblastoma. Pediatr Int (Roma) 2018; 60(9): 862-8.
[http://dx.doi.org/10.1111/ped.13634] [PMID: 29906299]

[90] Fuchs J, Cavdar S, Blumenstock G, *et al.* POST□TEXT III and IV hepatoblastoma: Extended hepatic resection avoids liver transplantation in selected cases. Ann Surg 2017; 266(2): 318-23.
[http://dx.doi.org/10.1097/SLA.0000000000001936] [PMID: 27501172]

[91] Otte JB, Meyers R. PLUTO first report. Pediatr Transplant 2010; 14(7): 830-5.
[http://dx.doi.org/10.1111/j.1399-3046.2010.01395.x] [PMID: 20946516]

[92] Nodomi S, Umeda K, Kato I, *et al.* Cytomegalovirus infection in pediatric patients with hepatoblastoma after liver transplantation. Pediatr Transplant 2018; 22(7): e13273.
[http://dx.doi.org/10.1111/petr.13273] [PMID: 30051556]

[93] Ramos-Gonzalez G, LaQuaglia M, O'Neill AF, *et al.* Long-term outcomes of liver transplantation for hepatoblastoma: A single-center 14-year experience. Pediatr Transplant 2018; e13250: e13250.

[http://dx.doi.org/10.1111/petr.13250] [PMID: 29888545]

[94] Uchida H, Sakamoto S, Sasaki K, *et al.* Surgical treatment strategy for advanced hepatoblastoma: Resection versus transplantation. Pediatr Blood Cancer 2018; 65(12): e27383.
[http://dx.doi.org/10.1002/pbc.27383] [PMID: 30084209]

[95] De Ioris M, Brugieres L, Zimmermann A, *et al.* Hepatoblastoma with a low serum alpha-fetoprotein level at diagnosis: the SIOPEL group experience. Eur J Cancer 2008; 44(4): 545-50.
[http://dx.doi.org/10.1016/j.ejca.2007.11.022] [PMID: 18166449]

[96] Semeraro M, Branchereau S, Maibach R, *et al.* Relapses in hepatoblastoma patients: clinical characteristics and outcome--experience of the International Childhood Liver Tumour Strategy Group (SIOPEL). Eur J Cancer 2013; 49(4): 915-22.
[http://dx.doi.org/10.1016/j.ejca.2012.10.003] [PMID: 23146961]

[97] Blohm MEG, Vesterling-Hörner D, Calaminus G, Göbel U. Alpha 1-fetoprotein (AFP) reference values in infants up to 2 years of age. Pediatr Hematol Oncol 1998; 15(2): 135-42.
[http://dx.doi.org/10.3109/08880019809167228] [PMID: 9592840]

[98] Van Tornout JM, Buckley JD, Quinn JJ, *et al.* Timing and magnitude of decline in alpha-fetoprotein levels in treated children with unresectable or metastatic hepatoblastoma are predictors of outcome: a report from the Children's Cancer Group. J Clin Oncol 1997; 15(3): 1190-7.
[http://dx.doi.org/10.1200/JCO.1997.15.3.1190] [PMID: 9060563]

[99] Koh KN, Park M, Kim BE, *et al.* Prognostic implications of serum alpha-fetoprotein response during treatment of hepatoblastoma. Pediatr Blood Cancer 2011; 57(4): 554-60.
[http://dx.doi.org/10.1002/pbc.23069] [PMID: 21370433]

CHAPTER 2

The Emerging Role of Monocarboxylate Transporter-1 in Cancer: Overview and Therapeutic Opportunities

Gouthami Thumma[1], Kiran Gangarapu[2,*], Anvesh Jallapally[3] and Anil Kumar Mondru[4]

[1] *Department of Pharmaceutics, Mother Theresa College of Pharmacy, Hyderabad, 500 088, Telangana, India*

[2] *School of Pharmacy, Anurag Group of Institutions, Hyderabad-500 088, Telangana, India*

[3] *Department of Pharmaceutical Sciences, University of Antwerp, Antwerp, Belgium*

[4] *Department of Molecular and Clinical Cancer Medicine, Institute of Translational Medicine, University of Liverpool, Liverpool, L69 3GE, United Kingdom*

Abstract: Cancer has become a global pandemic that accounts for almost 13% more deaths than any other infectious diseases. According to the World Health Organization (WHO), projections of cancer prevalence is expected to raise to 21.7 million cases and 13 million deaths by 2030. Over the last 10 years, considerable improvements have been achieved in the management of cancer, and yet the disease remains incurable. There is an urgent need to develop therapeutic agents with novel drug combinations to achieve better efficacy, and reduce the possibility of relapse and drug resistance.

Cancer progression, development of metastases represents the major characteristic feature for solid tumours in the presence of hypoxia. Under hypoxic conditions, cancer cells consume glucose that is metabolized to lactate, and then exported into the extracellular milieu, contributing to the acidic microenvironment. In this context, monocarboxylate transporters (MCTs) will play a significant role in maintaining the hyper-glycolytic acid resistant phenotype of cancer, allowing the maintenance of the high glycolytic rates by performing lactate efflux, and pH regulation by the co-transport of protons. Hence, MCTs constitute attractive adjuvant targets for cancer therapy.

In this chapter, we review cancer biology from the perspective of the lactate shuttle concept which mainly focuses on the development of MCT inhibitors and highlights current and potential future therapeutic approaches that supports the notion of targeting lactate metabolism with novel anticancer agents.

---

* **Corresponding author Kiran Gangarapu:** School of Pharmacy, Anurag Group of Institutions, Venkatapur, Ghatkesar (M), Medchal (D), Hyderabad-500 088, Telangana, India; Tel: +919912345280; E-mail: gangakiran1905@gmail.com

Atta-ur-Rahman and M. Iqbal Choudhary (Eds.)
All rights reserved-© 2019 Bentham Science Publishers

Keywords: Cancer, Flavanoids, Glycolysis, Hypoxia, Lactate Shuttle, Monocarboxylic Transporters, Natural and Synthetic MCT Inhibitors, Warburg.

INTRODUCTION

Cancer has become global pandemic, it is projected that there will be approximately 21.7 million new cancer cases and 13 million cancer deaths by 2030 [1 - 3]. Toll of cancer is greater in economically low- and middle-income countries. Population growth and aging are the largest contributors to the increasing total number of cancer cases [4]. Over the last 10 years, considerable improvements have been achieved in the management of cancer, and yet the disease remains incurable. There is a clear need to develop therapeutic agents with novel drug combinations to achieve better efficacy, and reduce the possibility of relapse and drug resistance.

Glycolysis is a physiological response to hypoxia in normal tissues, the energy produced through glycolysis process is needed for cancer cell proliferation. The differences in the metabolism of normal and cancerous cells were described more than a century ago.

According to Warburg's hypothesis, cancer cells choose aerobic glycolysis as the main mode of glucose metabolism instead of efficient oxidative phosphorylation. Dysfunction of mitochondrial function, loss or reduction of tumour suppressor gene function (TP53) expression, the hypoxic microenvironment, and oncogene-driven metabolic reprogramming are initiating events of the abnormal energy metabolism of cancer cells [5 - 7]. Therefore, understanding the biological differences between normal and cancer cells is essential for the design and development of new anticancer drugs. Several studies suggests that the activation of aerobic glycolysis in tumour cells is the major hallmark of cancer development [8, 9]. In anaerobic glycolysis, glucose is preferentially catabolized to lactate, rather than fully metabolized to carbon dioxide *via* mitochondrial oxidative phosphorylation (OXPHOS) [10, 11].

The lactate, (2-hydroxypropanoic acid) is synthesized from pyruvate which emerged as a critical regulator for cancer progression. Malignant tumours are heterogeneous in nature and the microenvironment contains aerobic and hypoxic regions. Under hypoxic conditions, cancer cells consume glucose and produce lactate. High-lactate levels are often associated with worse prognosis [12, 13]. Therefore, lactate acts as both a potent fuel (oxidative) and signalling molecule (angiogenesis). Indeed, this phenomenon resembles the processes that involve cell-cell and intracellular lactate shuttles. Two control points exists for regulating lactate shuttles: the lactate dehydrogenase (LDH)-dependent conversion of lactate into pyruvate (and back) as well as the transport of lactate into and out of tumour cells by MCTs to regulate these processes (Fig. **1**).

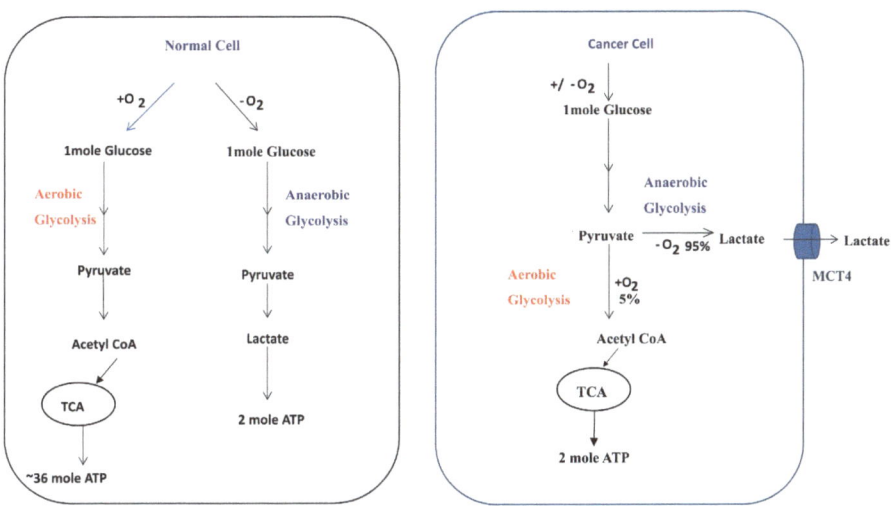

Fig. (1). Metabolic difference between normal and cancer cells. Normal cells undergo metabolism of glucose by aerobic and anaerobic processes and produces 36 and 2 Adenosine triphosphates (ATP) per mole of glucose respectively. However, cancer cells convert glucose to lactate (Warburg effect) regardless of O_2 in order to accelerate cell proliferation and produces only 2 ATPs per mole of glucose.

MCTs and their Isoforms

MCTs are membrane-bound, bidirectional symports belonging to the solute carrier 16 (SLC16) gene family and there are 14 known MCT isoforms (MCT 1-14). Among them MCT1-4 isoform transporter proteins are proton-dependent facilitative carriers and have 12 transmembrane domains with both intracellular N- and C- terminals(14). MCTs and their isoforms are summarized in Table **1**. Two partner chaperone glycoproteins basigin and embigin were found to be necessary for the proper insertion of MCT1-4 transporter proteins in the plasma membrane. Previous studies reported that several MCTs were overexpressed in variety of cancers and often associated with poor prognosis and high mortality. Also MCTs exhibit different selectivity and affinity for their substrates [14 - 17]. Notably, MCT1 and MCT4 isoforms were highly expressed in different tumour types and are commonly believed to promote growth and survival of cancer cells by regenerating pyruvate that can be extruded to refuel the cancer cells or can be used for OXPHOS [18]. Hence, these cancer cells engage in metabolic pathways, thus recycling products of anaerobic metabolism to sustain cancer cell survival and growth. Several systems are adapted for the transport of protons among which MCT1, MCT2, MCT3, and MCT4 are passive lactate–proton symporters [19].

MCT1 or MCT2 takes up lactate and ketone bodies for oxidation or lactate for gluconeogenesis depending on the tissue and the species [20]. MCT3 is expressed uniquely in the retinal pigment epithelium. Under hypoxia, MCT4 is primarily expressed in highly glycolytic cells, which facilitates lactic acid effuse out of the tissue. Then nearby aerobic cancer cells take up the lactate *via* MCT1 (influx transporter) involving lactate oxidation into pyruvate to fuel the Krebs cycle [21]. In recent studies, it was shown that over expression of MCTs correlates with invasiveness and poor prognosis in several solid tumours including colorectal, cervical, breast cancers and glioblastoma. Therefore, this incites the development of MCT inhibitors with potential clinical applications. The substrate and inhibitor specificity have been extensively studied for MCT1. MCT isoforms 1-3 are expressed in brains of rodents. MCT2 expressed in neurons while MCT1 and MCT4 are expressed in glial cells. Masaya Ideno *et al.*, has demonstrated that MCT1 is highly expressed in human astrocytes which are the most abundant glial cells in the CNS and helps neurons survive. MCTs are transporter for L-lactate and are important for CNS physiology and cognitive function.

Table 1. MCTs and their isoforms.

S.No.	MCT Subtype	Primary Name	Disease States
01	MCT 1	SLC16A1	All Tissue cancers
02	MCT 2	SLC16A7	Hypoglycaemia
03	MCT 3	SLC16A8	Atypical depressive disorder
04	MCT 4	SLC16A3	Retinopathy of prematurity
05	MCT 4	SLC16A4	Pseudomyxoma peritonei
06	MCT 5	SLC16A5	Multiple endocrine neoplasia type 2A
07	MCT 6	SLC16A6	Multiple endocrine neoplasia type 2A
08	MCT 7	SLC16A2	Allan-Herndon-Dudley syndrome
09	MCT 9	SLC16A9	Gout
10	MCT 10	SLC16A10	Allan-Herndon-Dudley syndrome
11	MCT 11	SLC16A11	Diabetes mellitus
12	MCT 12	SLC16A12	Multiple acyl-CoA dehydrogenase deficiency
13	MCT 13	SLC16A13	Diabetes mellitus
14	MCT14	SLC16A14	Corneal edema

MCT1 Inhibitors

MCT1 is expressed in a multitude of cancers including human colon, breast, head, neck, lung, *etc* [22]. MCT1 catalyses the rapid transport of many monocarboxylates (such as lactate, pyruvate, branched chain keto acids derived from leucine, valine and isoleucine, and the ketone bodies like acetoacetate, β-hydroxybutyrate and acetate) across the plasma membrane for mitochondrial oxidative phosphorylation and further proliferation [23]. It plays an important role in cellular responses by modulating the lactate and pyruvate cellular levels, that contributes to the regulation of central metabolic pathways and glucose homeostasis. MCT1 expression has been associated with not only cancer progression and but also responsible for poor prognosis. Hence, MCT1 has become an attractive therapeutic target for cancer. MCT1 inhibition action has been hypothesized by interfering with this metabolic coupling, by inhibiting lactate uptake into oxygenated tumour cells, increasing glucose uptake, and indirectly starving hypoxic tumour cells of glucose (Fig. **2**).

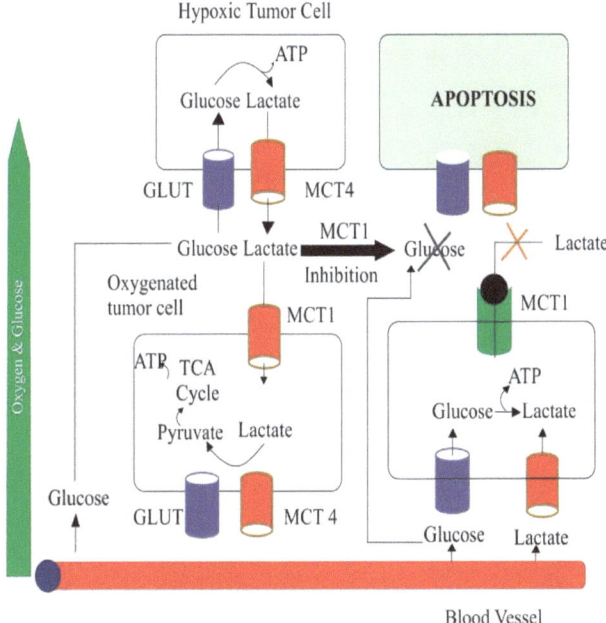

Fig. (2). Mechanism of action of MCT1 Inhibitors.

Other MCT's

MCT8 facilitates cellular uptake and efflux of thyroid hormone [24]. MCT10 transports aromatic amino acids and iodothyronines and these two are not proton-linked transporter. The energy utilized to transport through these important metabolites are by using hydrogen ion and substrate gradient and not by ATP [25].

SYNTHETIC MCT 1 INHIBITORS

Murray et al. [26], identified MCT1 target, using a strategy of photo affinity labelling and proteomic characterization for extended series of immuno-modulatory analogues. They discovered MCT1 as an immunosuppressive therapy target and have uncovered an unsuspected role for MCT1 immune biology. They showed that inhibition of MCT1 during T lymphocyte activation results in selective and profound inhibition of the extremely rapid phase of T cell division essential for an effective immune response.

Wang et al. [27], has established SAR studies for newly designed pteridinones (**1-5**) that impair cell proliferation in Raji cell lines at sub micromolar doses and their potency correlates with their ability to inhibit lactate transport. Their SAR studies reveal that side chains bearing hydroxyl group at either C5 or C6 and in alkyl and thioether-containing tethers are essential for MCT1 inhibition. In contrast, related sulfones, amides and triazoles are weakly active or inactive. These studies showed that SAR trends in [6, 5] and [6, 6] systems diverge, and these altered substituents effects provide new opportunities in MCT inhibitor design.

X = SCH$_2$; CH$_2$CH$_2$; cis CH=CH

α–χψ ano-4-hydroxy cinnamic acid (CHC, **6**) is a novel MCT1 inhibitor with a low affinity (IC$_{50}$>100 μM). Venkataram.R. Mereddy et al. [28], have modified the CHC and have developed more potent MCT1 inhibitors. According to them, on suitable modification on nitrogen group increases activity, CN and –COOH group provides better activity and double bond and – OMe is essential for activity. The variations could be possible on the 4-OH group with N-substituted or N-disubstituted groups. SAR studies have shown that N-dialkyl with O-Me groups into cyanocinnamic acid has maximal MCT activity. The compound with N,N-diphenyl CHC (**7**) have exhibited 29 nM IC_{50} inhibitor activity and has also shown excellent tumour growth reduction in *In vivo* MCT1 expressions colorectal cancer (WiDr). These studies could suggest MCT1 inhibitors have potential to develop as a novel strategy to treat cancer.

CHC (6)   **7**

Deitmer *et al.* [29], have demonstrated N-cyanosulphonamide (S0859, **8**) is an inhibitor of MCT 1, 2 and 4 which transport lactate, pyruvate and ketone bodies and are widely expressed in *Xenopus oocytes* and reversible inhibited with IC_{50} values ranges between 4-10μM. Earlier, N-cyanosulphonamide was a selective inhibitor of NBC SLC4 (sodium-bicarbonate cotransporter) in mammalian heart and also alter the cellular uptake or release.

S0859 (8)

Recently, AZD3965 (**9**) has been advanced into phase I/II clinical trials for treating some solid tumours [30, 31]. MCT1 inhibitors may also be useful for treating auto-immune diseases and preventing organ transplant rejection. Ar-C117977 (**20**) has been developed as MCT 1 inhibitor for mild immunosuppression [32]. There is an urgency for agents that are useful for diagnosis, treating or preventing cancer or preventing transplant rejection.

AZD 3965 (9)

Thomas *et al.* [33], described about the compounds which inhibit monocarboxylate transporters such as MCT1 and MCT4. These compounds can be used for treatment of a condition in a patient with cancer or type II diabetes wherein the condition is characterized by the heightened activity or by the high prevalence of MCT1 and/or MCT4. This study concluded that, treatment with SR-11105 (**10**) led to a significant reduction of tumor growth rate over time and treatment with SR-13779 (**11**) effectively blocked tumor growth over time.

SR-11105 (10)   **SR-13779 (11)**

Schönrogge *et al.* [33], have demonstrated that combination of CHC and metformin has a strong anticancer effect. The combination therapy disrupts the cancer cell metabolism in which metformin blocks the oxidative phosphorylation and CHC inhibit the efflux of lactate from cytosol. This study has given the scope for combination therapy in treatment of pancreatic cancers. They have also illustrated that CHC inhibits the ERK signaling pathway and strongly activates the p38 protein expression which in turn suppresses Ras induced activity, results in inhibiting cell proliferation and promoting apoptosis. Some of the potent MCT inhibitors are illustrated in Table **2**.

Targeting MCTs in Cancer

Typically, MCT 1-4 consists of either basigin or embigin for the translocation into plasma membrane and have major metabolic adaptations. Inhibition of MCTs, will directly influence on pH regulation which in turn significant effect on cancer

Table 2. Potent MCT inhibitors.

S.No.	Agent	Action	Target	Status	Reference
01	SR-13779 (11)	Inhibition of lactate uptake	MCT1 and MCT4	US 2018/0002343 A1 Jan 4, 2018	[34]
02	SR-11431 (12)	Immunomodulator, Type II diabetic agent	MCT1 and MCT4	US 2018/008605 A1 11th Jan 2018	[35]
03	(13)	Inhibition of Lactate Efflux	MCT1	US 2018/0009792 A1 11th Jan 2018	[36]
04	(14)	Inhibition of Lactate uptake	MCT1	US 9,573,888 B2 21st Feb 2017	[37]
05	(15)	Inhibition of lactate efflux	MCT4	WO2016201426A1 15th Dec 2016	[38]

(Table 2) cont.....

S.No.	Agent	Action	Target	Status	Reference
06	(16)	Inhibits Lactate Uptake	Nonspecific MCT Inhibitor	WO 2016/081464 A1 26th May 2016	[39]
07	(17)	Immunomodulator	Non-specific MCT inhibitor	US 2004/0072746A1 15th April 2004	[40]
08	(18)	Blocking Lactate Transport	MCT1	Phase I/II clinical trial	[30]
09	AR-C155858 (19)	Blocks uptake of Lactate	MCT1 and MCT2	Phase I	[41]
10	AR-C117977 (20)	Immunosuppressive activity	MCT1	Phase-I	[42, 43]

cell existence [14]. As described above, contribution of lactate to the malignant phenotype results in upregulation of two major proteins MCT1 and MCT4 in variety of tumour cell lines and represent favourable therapeutic targets in cancer

[44]. The inhibition of MCTs could be a possible mechanism for treating cancer, however recent evidences suggests that *in vitro* MCT inhibition reduces intracellular pH which then lead to apoptosis [22]. In order to monitor MCT1 dependent lactate uptake in tumour cells, a positron emission tomography (PET) tracer studies have reported by which *in vitro* (±)-[18F]-3-fluoro-2-hydroxypropionate ([^{18}F]-FLac) has actively retained and taken up by aerobic cancer cells that consume lactate and *in vivo* lactate accumulates in tumour cells and also in tissues. [^{18}F]-FLac tracer could be an ideal diagnostic tool to assess the lactate metabolism in tumours [45]. Recently in the oncology imaging field the upregulation of nutrient transporters has gained significant in the validation of tumours. Tumour upregulation of amino acid transporters could be exploited for the targeted delivery of imaging agents. The imaging agents which highly upregulated in tumours are ^{18}F-Fluorodeoxyglucose *via* glucose transporter; ^{18}F-FBPA *via* LAT1 transporter and these principles could be applied to the targeted delivery for MCT1 inhibitors rather than imaging agent. The drug conjugates of Phe-MCT1 (**21**) inhibitor and Gln-MCT1 (**22**) inhibitor are widely upregulated in tumours and displayed higher efficacy in Burkitt lymphoma (Raji) cells. These amino acid conjugate MCT inhibitors has leads to high tumour intracellular levels and also increased the duration of action.

NATURAL MCT1 INHIBITORS

A wide range of MCT inhibitors such as flavonoids, polyphenol, monoterpenes are largely found in many fruits, vegetables and plants derived foods as secondary metabolites and have showed a prominent activity on MCT's.

Flavonoid Analogues [46]

Among the naturally occurring polyphenols phytochemicals flavonoids have shown a wide range of pharmacological and biological activities. Flavonoids have shown wide applications in numerous diseases such as diabetes, CVS, obesity and cancer. It has been widely reported that flavanoids have modulated a wide variety of transporters such as glucose transporters (GLUT, SGLT), P-glycoprotein transporters *etc.*, Natural MCT1 inhibitors are illustrated in Fig. (3). Natural flavonoids that could modulate MCT's are apigenin (23), biochanin A (24), chyrsin (25), fisetin (26), genistein (27), hesperidin (28), kaempferol (29), diosemin (30), luteolin (31), morin (32), narigenin (33) quercetin (34), Silybin (35) and Naringin (36)

Naringenin (33) is a flavanone found in citrus fruits such as grape fruits, oranges & tomatoes. It is predominant in African medicinal plants such as *Catharanthus roseus* (Apocynaceae). *Acalypha Wilkesiana* (Euphorbiaceae) and *Elaeodeudron croceum* (Celastraceae) [47].

Naringenin (33) is known to possess various pharmacological activities such as antitumor, antidiabetic, CNS effect viz., antidepressant, memory enhancers, antihyperlipidemic, scavenging of oxidants, DNA protective, cardiac activities and peroxisome proliferator-activated receptors(PPARs).

Shim *et al.* [48], have reported that flavonoids morin (32), naringenin (32) quercetin (34) and Silybin (35) could modulate MCT1 and are competitive inhibitors and there is potential for diet-drug interactions between flavonoids and MCT1 substrates in $CaCO_2$ cells. Naringin (36) has not exhibited significant activity among the other flavonoids in cellular uptake of [^{14}C] benzoic acid. Naringenin (33) & silybin (35) have shown strong MCT1 activity with IC_{50} value of 23 μM & 30.2 μM, respectively and K_i value 15-20 μM and these are not modulated by genetic expression.

Morris *et al.* [49], demonstrated in human MCT6 gene transfected *Xenopus laevis* oocytes that uptake of bumetanide was significantly decreased in presence of aglycone flavonoids such as quercetin (34), phloretin (37) and morin(32) but not affected by glycone flavonoids naringin (36), phlorizin (38), rutin (39), and Phloretin (37) have shown K_i value 22.8 μM and is reversible and competitive inhibitor. MCT6 could be considered as a distinct class as the substrates of MCT1, 2, 4, 8 &10 did not significantly decrease the bumetanide uptake.

Phloretin (37) is a phytochemical derived natural dihydrochalcone found in apples, peas and tomatoes and many other fruits. It is the aglucone of phlorizin (38) and inhibit the growth and induce apoptosis of several cancer (B16 melanoma, H260 leukemia and H-29) cell lines. Phloretin (37) has significantly decreased the uptake of bumetanide which was demonstrated in human MCT 6 gene transferred *Xenopus laevis* oocytes. Phloretin have shown K_i value (22.8 μM) and is reversible competitive inhibitors on MCT 6.

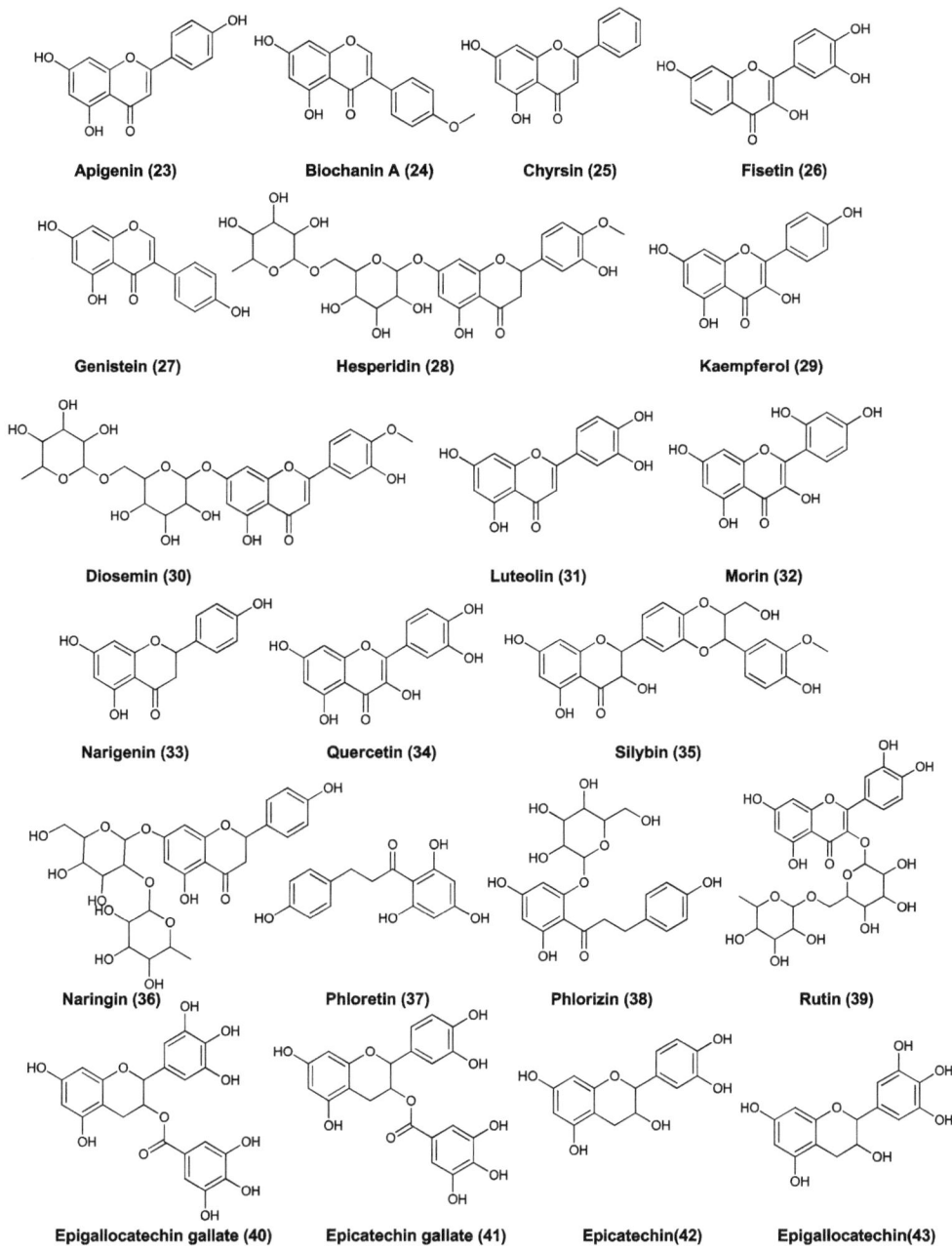

Fig. (3). Natural MCT1 Inhibitors.

Quercetin (**34**) is present in apples, peppers, red wine, tomatoes, leafy green vegetables, and cruciferous veggies. It is a polyphenol from a flavonoid group and has many therapeutics uses the diabetes, schizophrenia, inflammation, asthma, cancer, antioxidant and chemo preventive and anti-proliferative activity. It reversibly inhibits L-lactate transport by red blood cells (RBC) and tumour cells [50]. No study has been reported on quercetin binding to MCT transporters.

There are many derivatives of catechins available in nature such as epigallocatechin gallate (EGCG **40**), epicatechin gallate (ECG **41**), epicatechin (**42**), catechin, and epigallocatechin (EGC **32**). Catechin is a natural antioxidant which belongs to the flavonoid class. Catechin, epicatechin and their gallic acid conjugates are found in Chinese medicinal plant *Uncaria rhynchophylla*. These compounds are found mostly in cacao and tea which acts as a very good antioxidant.

Patrick reported that the tea catechins could inhibit lactate uptake by inhibiting MCT1 [51]. The study was conducted by BCECF assay to access the lactate uptake in adherent cell lines. It demonstrated that these catechins inhibiting the lactate uptake compared to standard MCT1 inhibitor phloretin (**37**). The above mentioned MCT1 inhibitors could potentially target cancer cells by attacking proteins or enzymes responsible for their abnormal growth. Targeted therapy not only effect on tumour growth but also has little effect on normal or healthy cells.

Mechanism of MCT1 Inhibition

There are several reports for competitive inhibitors are described that inhibits the functions of MCTs and these may be categorised into specific and non-specific inhibitors. The inhibitors which inhibit MCTs with higher affinity for MCT1 and 2, and also ability to inhibit other transporters depending on the binding on different MCT isoforms are categorised as non-specific. Non-specific inhibitors are aromatic compounds such as CHC (**6**) and phenylpyruvate, stilbenes are 4'-dibenzamidostilbene-2,2'-disulfonate (DBDS) and 4,4'-diisothiocyanostilben--2,2'-disulfonate (DIDS) [52]. Bioflavonoids such as phloretin and quercetin and thiol reagents as p-chloromercuribenzenesulfonic acid (p-CMBS) are non-specific inhibitors [53]. Specific inhibitors which are high-affinity inhibitors of MCT1 or 2. Recently AstraZeneca have developed numerous specific inhibitors such as AR-C155858 (**19**), AR-C11797 (**20**), AZD3965 (**9**).

MCTs structure contains 12 transmembrane domain (TM) with intracellular C- and N- termini and large intracellular loop between 7 and 8 TMs. By means of homology modelling MCT 1 probable structure has generated with "closed" and "open" conformations. In open conformation the substrate binding site have identified the key lysine residues which are involved in binding of DIDS. The key residues involved in binding of DIDS with MCT1 are found to be Lys38, Lys45, Lys282 and Lys413 in which isothiocyanate is in close contact with Lys38 and two sulfonates are bound to Lys45, Lys282 and Lys413 [52] (Fig. **4**). AR-C155858 binds to MCT1 open conformation and interacts with residues Asn147, Arg306, Ser364 in intracellular and extracellular with Lys38, Asp302, Phe360, Lys274 and Ser278 residues [54].

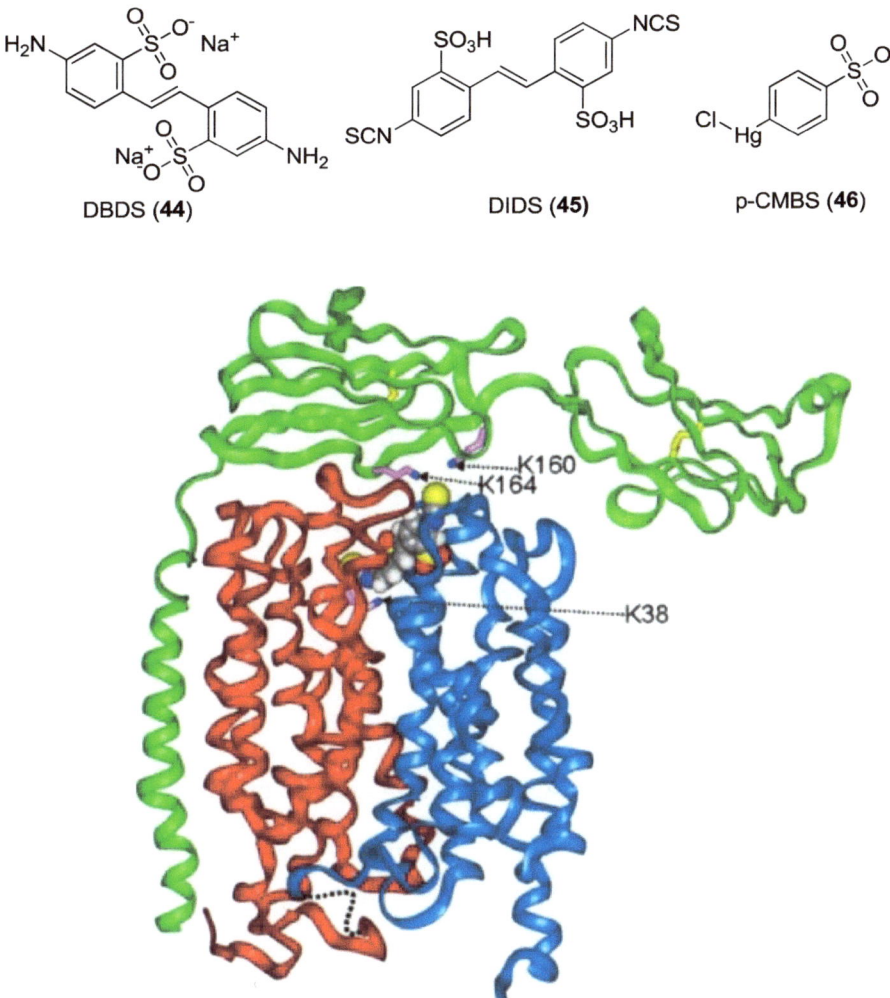

Fig. (4). Binding Structure of MCT1 in complex with embigin and DIDS complex.
(Diagram from Marieangela C. Wilson *et al.*, *The Journal of Biological Chemistry* Vol. 284, No. 30, pp. 20011–20021)

CONCLUSION AND FUTURE DIRECTIONS

The purpose of this chapter is to highlight the need for further research to assess whether targeting MCT1 may be an appropriate option for the treatment of cancer. In recent years, glycolytic phenotype has been identified as a renewed interest in cancer metabolism, a continuous and efficient oxygen-consuming metabolism seems to be the key to this phenomenon. This describes preferential usage of glycolytic pathway by tumor cell to generate lactate under anaerobic conditions. The metabolic profile of cancer cells within tumours is quite complex and is represented by a highly heterogeneous situation in which various metabolic sections collaborate with each other to guarantee cancer progression. Depending on the specific site of metastasis, the metabolic plasticity of tumour cells allows them to differentially engage in distinct metabolic programs (*i.e.*, tissue invasion, angiogenesis and immune escape) to ensure their survival. MCTs plays a major role in removing excess of lactate in cells which contribute in several ways to understand lactate transport inhibition and provide a basis for understanding complex cellular signalling. One of the future challenges is to understand the mechanisms underlying regulatory roles by metastatic cancer cells and defining key metabolic co-dependencies between cancer cells and the surrounding stroma may afford new approaches to clinically manage metastatic diseases. Lastly, MCT-1 inhibition as a potential target which could ultimately improve therapeutic strategies used in the management of cancer.

AREA OF INTEREST

Drug design and discovery of anticancer agents.

KEY FEATURES

This chapter provides the latest information in a clear and concise on Monocarboxylate transporters in the context of cancer biology. Provides overview on novel Monocarboxylate transporters inhibitors against cancer.

READERSHIP

Undergraduates and postgraduates' students in medicinal chemistry and pharmacology, also for academia and industry researchers, scientists in medicinal chemistry, organic chemistry and pharmacology departments.

CONSENT FOR PUBLICATION

Not applicable.

CONFLICT OF INTEREST

The authors declare no conflict of interest, financial or otherwise.

ACKNOWLEDGEMENTS

The corresponding author is thankful to Prof. Ramaiah Muthyala, University of Minnesota College of Pharmacy for the support and suggestions.

REFERENCES

[1] Fidler MM, Bray F, Soerjomataram I. The global cancer burden and human development: A review. Scand J Public Health 2018; 46(1): 27-36.
[http://dx.doi.org/10.1177/1403494817715400] [PMID: 28669281]

[2] Vineis P, Wild CP. Global cancer patterns: causes and prevention. Lancet 2014; 383(9916): 549-57.
[http://dx.doi.org/10.1016/S0140-6736(13)62224-2] [PMID: 24351322]

[3] Zoorob RJ. The global burden of preventable cancer mortality. Family Medicine and Community Health 2017; 5(1): 1-2.
[http://dx.doi.org/10.15212/FMCH.2017.0101]

[4] Thun MJ, DeLancey JO, Center MM, Jemal A, Ward EM. The global burden of cancer: priorities for prevention. Carcinogenesis 2010; 31(1): 100-10.
[http://dx.doi.org/10.1093/carcin/bgp263] [PMID: 19934210]

[5] Kim JW, Dang CV. Cancer's molecular sweet tooth and the Warburg effect. Cancer Res 2006; 66(18): 8927-30.
[http://dx.doi.org/10.1158/0008-5472.CAN-06-1501] [PMID: 16982728]

[6] Warburg O, Wind F, Negelein E. The metabolism of tumors in the body. J Gen Physiol 1927; 8(6): 519-30.
[http://dx.doi.org/10.1085/jgp.8.6.519] [PMID: 19872213]

[7] Marín-Hernández A, Gallardo-Pérez JC, Rodríguez-Enríquez S, Encalada R, Moreno-Sánchez R, Saavedra E. Modeling cancer glycolysis. Biochimica et Biophysica Acta (BBA) -. Bioenergetics 2011; 1807(6): 755-67.
[http://dx.doi.org/10.1016/j.bbabio.2010.11.006]

[8] Icard P, Shulman S, Farhat D, Steyaert J-M, Alifano M, Lincet H. How the Warburg effect supports aggressiveness and drug resistance of cancer cells? Drug Resist Updat 2018; 38: 1-11.
[http://dx.doi.org/10.1016/j.drup.2018.03.001] [PMID: 29857814]

[9] Allen AE, Locasale JW. Glucose metabolism in cancer: The saga of pyruvate kinase continues. Cancer Cell 2018; 33(3): 337-9.
[http://dx.doi.org/10.1016/j.ccell.2018.02.008] [PMID: 29533776]

[10] Vander Heiden MG, Cantley LC, Thompson CB. Understanding the Warburg effect: the metabolic requirements of cell proliferation. Science 2009; 324(5930): 1029-33.
[http://dx.doi.org/10.1126/science.1160809] [PMID: 19460998]

[11] Martinez-Outschoorn UE, Peiris-Pagés M, Pestell RG, Sotgia F, Lisanti MP. Cancer metabolism: a therapeutic perspective. Nat Rev Clin Oncol 2017; 14(1): 11-31.
[http://dx.doi.org/10.1038/nrclinonc.2016.60] [PMID: 27141887]

[12] Brooks GA. Cell-cell and intracellular lactate shuttles. J Physiol 2009; 587(Pt 23): 5591-600.
[http://dx.doi.org/10.1113/jphysiol.2009.178350] [PMID: 19805739]

[13] Anastasiou D. Tumour microenvironment factors shaping the cancer metabolism landscape. Br J Cancer 2017; 116(3): 277-86.

[http://dx.doi.org/10.1038/bjc.2016.412] [PMID: 28006817]

[14] Halestrap AP, Wilson MC. The monocarboxylate transporter family role and regulation. IUBMB Life 2012; 64(2): 109-19.
[http://dx.doi.org/10.1002/iub.572] [PMID: 22162139]

[15] Pérez-Escuredo J, Van Hée VF, Sboarina M, et al. Monocarboxylate transporters in the brain and in cancer. Biochimica et Biophysica Acta (BBA)-. Molecular Cell Research 2016; 1863(10): 2481-97.

[16] Payen VL, Hsu MY, Rädecke KS, et al. Monocarboxylate Transporter MCT1 Promotes Tumor Metastasis Independently of Its Activity as a Lactate Transporter. Cancer Res 2017; 77(20): 5591-601.
[http://dx.doi.org/10.1158/0008-5472.CAN-17-0764] [PMID: 28827372]

[17] Pinheiro C, Longatto-Filho A, Azevedo-Silva J, Casal M, Schmitt FC, Baltazar F. Role of monocarboxylate transporters in human cancers: state of the art. J Bioenerg Biomembr 2012; 44(1): 127-39.
[http://dx.doi.org/10.1007/s10863-012-9428-1] [PMID: 22407107]

[18] Kroemer G, Pouyssegur J. Tumor cell metabolism: cancer's Achilles' heel. Cancer Cell 2008; 13(6): 472-82.
[http://dx.doi.org/10.1016/j.ccr.2008.05.005] [PMID: 18538731]

[19] Porporato PE, Dhup S, Dadhich RK, Copetti T, Sonveaux P. Anticancer targets in the glycolytic metabolism of tumors: a comprehensive review. Front Pharmacol 2011; 2: 49.
[http://dx.doi.org/10.3389/fphar.2011.00049] [PMID: 21904528]

[20] Martin PM, Gopal E, Ananth S, et al. Identity of SMCT1 (SLC5A8) as a neuron-specific Na+-coupled transporter for active uptake of L-lactate and ketone bodies in the brain. J Neurochem 2006; 98(1): 279-88.
[http://dx.doi.org/10.1111/j.1471-4159.2006.03878.x] [PMID: 16805814]

[21] Iwanaga T, Kishimoto A. Cellular distributions of monocarboxylate transporters: a review. Biomed Res 2015; 36(5): 279-301.
[http://dx.doi.org/10.2220/biomedres.36.279] [PMID: 26522146]

[22] Sonveaux P, Végran F, Schroeder T, et al. Targeting lactate-fueled respiration selectively kills hypoxic tumor cells in mice. J Clin Invest 2008; 118(12): 3930-42.
[PMID: 19033663]

[23] Halestrap AP. Monocarboxylic acid transport. Compr Physiol 2013; 3(4): 1611-43.
[http://dx.doi.org/10.1002/cphy.c130008] [PMID: 24265240]

[24] Friesema EC, Jansen J, Jachtenberg JW, Visser WE, Kester MH, Visser TJ. Effective cellular uptake and efflux of thyroid hormone by human monocarboxylate transporter 10. Mol Endocrinol 2008; 22(6): 1357-69.
[http://dx.doi.org/10.1210/me.2007-0112] [PMID: 18337592]

[25] Visser WE, van Mullem AA, Jansen J, Visser TJ. The thyroid hormone transporters MCT8 and MCT10 transport the affinity-label N-bromoacetyl-[(125)I]T3 but are not modified by it. Mol Cell Endocrinol 2011; 337(1-2): 96-100.
[http://dx.doi.org/10.1016/j.mce.2011.02.003] [PMID: 21315799]

[26] Murray CM, Hutchinson R, Bantick JR, et al. Monocarboxylate transporter MCT1 is a target for immunosuppression. Nat Chem Biol 2005; 1(7): 371-6.
[http://dx.doi.org/10.1038/nchembio744] [PMID: 16370372]

[27] Wang H, Yang C, Doherty JR, Roush WR, Cleveland JL, Bannister TD. Synthesis and structure-activity relationships of pteridine dione and trione monocarboxylate transporter 1 inhibitors. J Med Chem 2014; 57(17): 7317-24.
[http://dx.doi.org/10.1021/jm500640x] [PMID: 25068893]

[28] Gurrapu S, Jonnalagadda SK, Alam MA, et al. Monocarboxylate transporter 1 inhibitors as potential anticancer agents. ACS Med Chem Lett 2015; 6(5): 558-61.

[http://dx.doi.org/10.1021/acsmedchemlett.5b00049] [PMID: 26005533]

[29]   Kazokaitė J, Ames S, Becker HM, Deitmer JW, Matulis D. Selective inhibition of human carbonic anhydrase IX in Xenopus oocytes and MDA-MB-231 breast cancer cells Journal of enzyme inhibition and medicinal chemistry 2016; 31 (sup4): 38-44.

[30]   Sborov DW, Haverkos BM, Harris PJ. Investigational cancer drugs targeting cell metabolism in clinical development. Expert Opin Investig Drugs 2015; 24(1): 79-94.
[http://dx.doi.org/10.1517/13543784.2015.960077] [PMID: 25224845]

[31]   Dhup S, Dadhich RK, Porporato PE, Sonveaux P. Multiple biological activities of lactic acid in cancer: influences on tumor growth, angiogenesis and metastasis. Curr Pharm Des 2012; 18(10): 1319-30.
[http://dx.doi.org/10.2174/138161212799504902] [PMID: 22360558]

[32]   Påhlman C, Malm H, Qi Z, et al. Operational tolerance in nonvascularized transplant models induced by AR-C117977, a monocarboxylate transporter inhibitor. Transplantation 2008; 86(8): 1135-8.
[http://dx.doi.org/10.1097/TP.0b013e318186b978] [PMID: 18946353]

[33]   Schönrogge M, Kerndl H, Zhang X, Kumstel S, Vollmar B, Zechner D. α-cyano-4-hydroxycinnamate impairs pancreatic cancer cells by stimulating the p38 signaling pathway. Cell Signal 2018; 47: 101-8.
[http://dx.doi.org/10.1016/j.cellsig.2018.03.015] [PMID: 29609037]

[34]   Bannister TD, Roush WR, Choi JY, et al. Heterocyclic inhibitors of monocarboxylate transporters. Google Patents 2018.

[35]   Bannister TD, Wang H, Wang C, Cleveland JL. Pteridine dione monocarboxylate transporter inhibitors. Google Patents 2018.

[36]   Bannister TD, Wang H, Wang C, Cleveland JL. Chromenone inhibitors of monocarboxylate transporters. Google Patents 2018.

[37]   Mereddy VR, Drewes LR, Alam MA, Jonnalagadda SK, Gurrapu S. Therapeutic compounds. Google Patents 2017.

[38]   Parnell KM, McCall J. Mct4 inhibitors for treating disease. Google Patents 2016.

[39]   DeMattei J, Looker AR, Neubert-Langille B, et al. Process for making modulators of cystic fibrosis transmembrane conductance regulator. Google Patents 2017.

[40]   Sullivan M, Murray C, Hutchinson R, et al. Inhibitors of monocarboxylate transport. Google Patents 2004.

[41]   Ovens MJ, Manoharan C, Wilson MC, Murray CM, Halestrap AP. The inhibition of monocarboxylate transporter 2 (MCT2) by AR-C155858 is modulated by the associated ancillary protein. Biochem J 2010; 431(2): 217-25.
[http://dx.doi.org/10.1042/BJ20100890] [PMID: 20695846]

[42]   Bueno V, Binet I, Steger U, et al. The specific monocarboxylate transporter (MCT1) inhibitor, AR-C117977, a novel immunosuppressant, prolongs allograft survival in the mouse. Transplantation 2007; 84(9): 1204-7.
[http://dx.doi.org/10.1097/01.tp.0000287543.91765.41] [PMID: 17998878]

[43]   Witkiewicz AK, Whitaker-Menezes D, Dasgupta A, et al. Using the "reverse Warburg effect" to identify high-risk breast cancer patients: stromal MCT4 predicts poor clinical outcome in triple-negative breast cancers. Cell Cycle 2012; 11(6): 1108-17.
[http://dx.doi.org/10.4161/cc.11.6.19530] [PMID: 22313602]

[44]   Draoui N, Feron O. Lactate shuttles at a glance: from physiological paradigms to anti-cancer treatments. Dis Model Mech 2011; 4(6): 727-32.
[http://dx.doi.org/10.1242/dmm.007724] [PMID: 22065843]

[45]   Van Hée VF, Labar D, Dehon G, et al. Radiosynthesis and validation of (±)-[18F]-3-fluoro-2-hydroxypropionate ([18F]-FLac) as a PET tracer of lactate to monitor MCT1-dependent lactate

uptake in tumors. Oncotarget 2017; 8(15): 24415-28.
[http://dx.doi.org/10.18632/oncotarget.14705] [PMID: 28107190]

[46] Li Y, Lu J, Paxton JW. The role of ABC and SLC transporters in the pharmacokinetics of dietary and herbal phytochemicals and their interactions with xenobiotics. Curr Drug Metab 2012; 13(5): 624-39.
[http://dx.doi.org/10.2174/1389200211209050624] [PMID: 22475331]

[47] Tomás□Barberán FA, Clifford MN. Flavanones, chalcones and dihydrochalcones–nature, occurrence and dietary burden. J Sci Food Agric 2000; 80(7): 1073-80.
[http://dx.doi.org/10.1002/(SICI)1097-0010(20000515)80:7<1073::AID-JSFA568>3.0.CO;2-B]

[48] Shim CK, Cheon EP, Kang KW, Seo KS, Han HK. Inhibition effect of flavonoids on monocarboxylate transporter 1 (MCT1) in Caco-2 cells. J Pharm Pharmacol 2007; 59(11): 1515-9.
[http://dx.doi.org/10.1211/jpp.59.11.0008] [PMID: 17976262]

[49] Jones RS, Parker MD, Morris ME. Quercetin, Morin, Luteolin, and Phloretin Are Dietary Flavonoid Inhibitors of Monocarboxylate Transporter 6. Mol Pharm 2017; 14(9): 2930-6.
[http://dx.doi.org/10.1021/acs.molpharmaceut.7b00264] [PMID: 28513167]

[50] Belt JA, Thomas JA, Buchsbaum RN, Racker E. Inhibition of lactate transport and glycolysis in Ehrlich ascites tumor cells by bioflavonoids. Biochemistry 1979; 18(16): 3506-11.
[http://dx.doi.org/10.1021/bi00583a011] [PMID: 38832]

[51] Talbott P. Inhibition of Monocarboxylate Transporter-1-Mediated Lactate Uptake by Tea Catechins. The Ohio State University 2012.

[52] Wilson MC, Meredith D, Bunnun C, Sessions RB, Halestrap AP. Studies on the DIDS binding site of monocarboxylate transporter 1 suggest a homology model of the open conformation and a plausible translocation cycle Journal of Biological Chemistry 2009. jbc. M109. 014217
[http://dx.doi.org/10.1074/jbc.M109.014217]

[53] Halestrap AP. Monocarboxylic acid transport. Compr Physiol 2013; 3(4): 1611-43.
[http://dx.doi.org/10.1002/cphy.c130008] [PMID: 24265240]

[54] Nancolas B, Sessions RB, Halestrap AP. Identification of key binding site residues of MCT1 for AR-C155858 reveals the molecular basis of its isoform selectivity. Biochem J 2015; 466(1): 177-88.
[http://dx.doi.org/10.1042/BJ20141223] [PMID: 25437897]

CHAPTER 3

In-vitro Anti-Proliferative Assays and Techniques Used in Pre-Clinical Anti-Cancer Drug Discovery

Meran Keshawa Ediriweera*, Kamani Hemamala Tennekoon and **Sameera Ranganath Samarakoon**

Institute of Biochemistry, Molecular Biology and Biotechnology, University of Colombo, 90, Cumaratunga Munidasa Mawatha, Colombo 03, Sri Lanka

Abstract: The hallmark features of cancer emphasize essential biological characteristics associated with malignant transformation. Anti-cancer drug discovery is a strenuous task, requiring a number of pre-clinical and clinical investigations. Pre-clinical investigations offer a foundation for anti-cancer drug discovery. A number of cell based *in-vitro* assays have been introduced to investigate each major hallmark feature of cancer. Selection of the most suitable *in-vitro* assay for pre-clinical investigations mainly depends on the researcher's objective(s) to be investigated. A wide range of cell based *in-vitro* anti-proliferative assays/techniques have been developed based on different assay principles and chemistries to evaluate the effects of testing agent (s) on cancer cell proliferation. In this chapter, we have outlined commonly utilized cell based anti-proliferative assays in pre-clinical anti-cancer drug discovery approaches.

Keywords: Cell based anti-proliferative assays, Cellular techniques, Anti-cancer drug discovery, Hallmarks of cancer.

INTRODUCTION

Cancer is a serious health issue among the non-communicable diseases, reporting as one of the key obstacles in improving life expectancy in almost all the countries in the world. Despite the availability of modern diagnosis methods and cancer treatment options, cancer remains as one of the main causes of deaths worldwide. According to the latest cancer statistics, breast, lung, cervical, endometrial, colorectal, uterine and thyroid cancers have been identified as most common cancer types in females, while most common cancer types in men are prostate, lung, colorectal, head and neck, kidney, bladder and leukemia [1]. Low cancer survival rates have been reported in economically developing countries

---

* **Corresponding author Meran Keshawa Ediriweera:** Institute of Biochemistry, Molecular Biology and Biotechnology, University of Colombo, 90, Cumaratunga Munidasa Mawatha, Colombo 03, Sri Lanka; Tel: +94(0)779960397; E-mail: mk.ediriweera@gmaail.com

Atta-ur-Rahman and M. Iqbal Choudhary (Eds.)
All rights reserved-© 2019 Bentham Science Publishers

over economically developed countries [2]. Lack of early diagnosis and awareness have been recognized as major causes for low cancer survival rates in economically developing countries [3]. Genetic mutations have been identified as the main risk factor for cancer. In addition to genetic factors, diet, age, chemicals, obesity, use of alcohol and physical inactivity are associated with an increased risk of developing cancer [4, 5]. Chemotherapy, radiotherapy, immunotherapy, hormone therapy and surgery are the available treatment options to control cancer. Cancer treatment options or plans are mainly determined based on the types and stages of cancer. Although primary tumors are treatable with available chemo and radio therapies, metastatic tumors are difficult to treat with chemo and radio therapies [6]. A number of adverse side effects such as hair loss, bone marrow suppression, anemia, diarrhea and kidney damage are associated with chemo and radio therapy treatments. Moreover, surgical removal of metastatic tumors results in functional loss in patients.

Bench to bedside anti-cancer drug development is always a challenging task with uncertain positive outcomes. Many anti-cancer drugs with desirable pre-clinical efficacies do not exhibit anticipated clinical outcomes in clinical trials. It has been reported that, for every 5000 anti-cancer drugs investigated pre-clinically, only one or two drugs are clinically approved [7]. Recently, much attention has been paid to identify naturally derived or chemically synthesized anti-cancer drug leads [8]. Sophisticated high-throughput drug screening techniques in modern science accelerate modern drug discovery approaches by permitting swift screening of a large number drug candidates in a short period of time [9].

In pre-clinical anti-cancer drug development strategies, a range of *in-vitro* techniques/assays is being utilized [10]. *In-vitro* assays are conducted outside the living systems under a controlled environment. Most of the *in-vitro* assays utilized in pre-clinical anti-cancer drug development studies are designed to investigate each hallmark feature of cancer (sustaining proliferative signaling, evading growth suppressors, enabling replicative immortality, resisting cell death, activating invasion and metastasis, genomic instability, avoiding immune destruction and deregulating cellular energetics) [10. 11]. As tumorigenesis is a complex process with the association of eight major hallmark features, selection of a perfect *in-vitro* assay to investigate a single hallmark feature is always challenging. Therefore, to answer the exact research need, it is important to choose the most suitable *in-vitro* assay or combined assays (multiplexing). Assay multiplexing gives more detailed information over a single assay. However, assay multiplexing needs compatible endpoint detection methods for parallel measurements. Additionally, assay cost, equipment required for end-point detections and assay duration should be considered before choosing a suitable *in-vitro* assay [10].

Mainly, a range of *in-vitro* assays/techniques necessary to evaluate cancer cell proliferation cancer cell migration and invasion, apoptosis, angiogenesis, energy metabolism, cellular senescence, oxidative stress markers and gene mutations in cancer cells *etc.* are widely employed in pre-clinical in anti-cancer drug discovery and development studies. In addition to these assays/techniques, modern techniques such as, High content screening (HCS), reporter gene assays and High throughput screening (HTS) are also being utilized in modern anti-cancer drug discovery approaches [12 - 14]. Cell based *in-vitro* anti-proliferative assays are primarily manufactured based on some viable cell markers such as intracellular enzymes or proteins in metabolically active cells, intracellular ATP levels, DNA synthesis, impedance and cell membrane integrity [15 - 17] (Fig. **1**).

In this chapter, we describe commonly used cell based *in-vitro* anti-proliferative assays/techniques used in anti-cancer drug discovery and we have managed to include recent anti-cancer drug discovery related pre-clinical investigations which utilized respective anti-proliferative assays. Detailed assay procedures and protocols of respective assays are not described here as this chapter is mainly focused to provide information on anti-proliferative assays based on their assay chemistries and principles.

Assays Based on Cellular Enzymes and Proteins

Uncontrolled cell proliferation and resisting cell death are two main biological features of cancer cells [18]. In cell-based *in-vitro* anti-proliferative assays, cytotoxic/anti-proliferative effects of the testing agents on the above mentioned viable cell markers are evaluated under controlled conditions. Commonly used testing agents in cell-based investigations include natural or synthetic drugs, organic extracts, small inhibitory RNAs, some peptides, hormones and nano-molecules, *etc.* A wide range of colorimetric and fluorometric anti-proliferative assays with distinct assay chemistries have been manufactured for *in-vitro* drug discovery approaches [19]. Before selecting a colorimetric or fluorometric assay, it is advisable to choose the correct assay depending on cancer cell type used, physical nature of the testing agent and the availability of instruments for end-point detection.

In cell based *in-vitro* colorimetric anti-proliferative assays, the assay principle includes conversion of a substrate to a coloured substance by cellular enzymes present in metabolically active cells, and the colour generated is measured with the help of spectrophotometric techniques [19]. The colour intensity developed is proportional to the degree of viable cells [19]. The MTT (3-(4,5-dimethylthiaz-l-2-yl)-2,5-diphenyltetrazolium bromide) assay is a commonly used *in-vitro* anti-proliferative assay in pre-clinical studies [20, 21]. In the MTT assay, NAD(P)H dependent dehydrogenases present in viable cell mitochondria reduce MTT to insoluble formazan (purple coloured). Insoluble formazan can be solubilized using isopropanol for spectrophotometric measurements [20, 21]. A recent study conducted by Rekha and Anila [22] used the MTT assay to evaluate *in-vitro* cytotoxic effects of CaS nano-particles in L929 fibroblasts cells. In another study Aboubakr *et al.* [23] demonstrated cytotoxic effects of a drug combination comprising vincristine and combretastatin A-4 in hepatocellular carcinoma (Hep G2) cells using the MTT assay. Ahamed *et al.* [24] utilized the MTT assay to determine cytotoxic effects of bismuth oxide (Bi_2O_3) nanoparticles in MCF-7 breast cancer cells.

In addition to MTT tetrazolium, other MTT related-tetrazolium based anti-proliferative assays are also available. For example, WST (water-soluble tetrazolium salts), XTT (2,3-bis(2-methoxy-4-nitro-5-sulfophenyl)-2H-tetrazolium-5-carboxanilide) and MTS (3-(4,5-dimethylthiazol-2-yl)-5-(3-carboxymethoxyphenyl)-2-(4-sulfophenyl)-2H-tetrazolium) can also react with viable cell dehydrogenases to generate formazan [19]. Nevertheless, in contrast to MTT, formazan generated in WST, MTS and XTT assays is water soluble, and therefore evades solubilization steps with isopropanol [19]. As a result of this, WST, MTS and XTT assay reagents can be directly added to the medium, permitting these reagents to be used for anti-proliferative assays with cells grown in suspension. The MTS assay was used by Wu *et al.* [25] to investigate anti-proliferative effects of Pinicolol B in nasopharyngeal carcinoma cells. Murayyan *et al.* [26] also used the MTS assay to determine anti-proliferative effects of Ontario grown onions in colorectal adenocarcinoma cells. Abdelmageed *et al.* [27] have utilized the XTT assay to evaluate anti-proliferative effects of oleanolic acid methyl ester in prostate cancer cells. Cytotoxic efficacy of novel triazole derivatives has been evaluated using the XTT assay in a study reported by Özdemir *et al.* [28]. In a recent study conducted in our laboratory, the WST assay was used to examine the anti-proliferative effects of different plants extracts of Sri Lankan endemic plants in breast cancer stem cells (bCSCs) [29]. Chen *et al.* [30] used the same assay to evaluate anti-proliferative effects of hinokitiol, a monoterpenoid, in bCSCs.

Resazurin (7-hydroxy-10-oxidophenoxazin-10-ium-3-one, sodium) is a fluorogenic blue dye. In viable cells, resazurin is reduced by viable cell oxidoreductases to generate resorufin (red fluorescent) [31, 32]. Resazurin assay was used by Goto *et al.* [33] to examine cytotoxic effects of dihydropyridine derivative (VdiE-2N) in normal human oral healthy mucosa, human embryonic kidney cells and head and neck squamous cell carcinoma.

Calcein AM is another example for a viable cell permeable dye. In viable cells Calcein AM is hydrolyzed by the intracellular esterases to produce fluorescent compound calcein [34]. In a recent study conducted by Zhou *et al.* [35], the effect of monofunctional platinum complex on A2780 human ovarian cancer cell viability was determined using the Calcein AM dye. Calcein Red-Orange AM, Calcein Blue AM, Calcein Green AM and Calcein Violet AM are other examples of viable cell permeable dyes, which possess a similar chemistry to Calcein AM [36].

The sulforhodamine B (SRB) assay is another commonly used simple cell viability/anti-proliferative assay in anti-cancer drug screening. The SRB dye can bind with basic amino acids present in viable cells under mild acidic conditions. Bound SRB dye can be removed from proteins and solubilized for spectroscopy readings in mild basic conditions [37]. The SRB assay is one of the commonly used assays for cytotoxicity screening in our laboratory [38 - 41]. Interaction of testing substances with assay reagents has been reported as a major disadvantage associated with the SRB, MTT, WST, MTS and XTT assays. In contrast to the MTT, WST, MTS and XTT assays, SRB assay is a time consuming assay as it requires several incubation steps [42].

In addition to tetrazolium-based anti-proliferative assays, assays based on viable cell Adenosine triphosphate (ATP) and Lactate dehydrogenase (LDH) contents have been developed. In the ATP assay, cellular ATP content is measured by colorimetrically, fluorometrically or luminometrically [43]. A sensitive assay called CellTiter-Glo assay, manufactured by the Promega Corporation (Madison, WI) uses bioluminescence based technique to monitor cellular ATP content in viable cells [44]. A study conducted by Cusimano *et al.* [45] has used the CellTiter-Glo assay to evaluate the effects of a natural drug on T-cell acute lymphoblastic leukemia cells. Cells with damaged cell membranes efflux LDH to the external medium and the LDH present in the external medium is measured in the LDH assay [16, 46]. The LDH assay has been recently used to investigate cervical cancer cells (HeLa) viability upon photodynamic treatments [47]. Another study has also used the LDH assay to assess cell viability of HEC-1-A and HEC-1-B endometrial cancer cells exposed to verteporfin [48]. The Promega Corporation (Madison, WI) has introduced new cell viability assays based on viable/dead cell marker substrates called GF-AFC and bis-AAF-R110. Proteases present in live cells can cleave the substrate GF-AFC, while dead cell proteases can cleave the substrate bis-AAF-R110 [49]. The assays such as ATP, LSH and GF-AFC and bis-AAF-R110 markers based assays are more sensitive over conventional anti-proliferative. High cost associated with these assays has been identified as a major disadvantage.

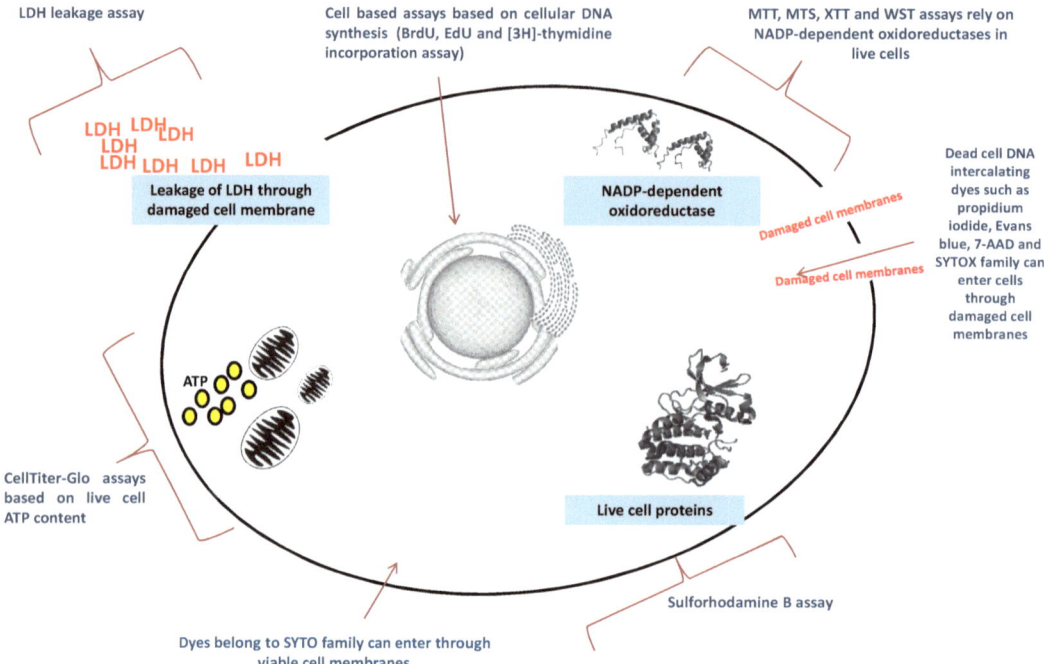

Fig. (1). Schematic demonstration of commonly utilized cell-based anti-proliferative assays based on live cell enzyme activity, live/dead cell protein content, DNA synthesis/DNA content, ATP content and membrane integrity.

General Assay Procedures for Tetrazolium-Based Anti-proliferative Assays

1. Cancer cells are grown in 96-well cell culture plates at a density of 5×10^3 cells/well and incubated for 24 h.
2. Following incubation, cells are treated with different concentrations of test compound/s and incubated for a desired period (24-72 h). Positive and negative controls should also be kept along with test compounds.
3. After incubation, all the wells are washed with PBS three times. Wells are then replaced with 180 μL of fresh medium and 20 μL of MTT solution (1mg/mL).
4. Plates are again incubated at 37°C for 4 h and medium is removed by aspiration.
5. 100 μL of isopropanol/HCL is added to each well and plates are shaken for 30 min at room temperature.
6. Finally, absorbance is measured at 540 nm using a micro-plate reader.
   - Formazan generated in WST, MTS and XTT assays is water soluble, and therefore solubilization step with isopropanol/HCL is not requited. WST, MTS and XTT assays can be used with cells grown in suspension.

General Assay Procedure for the sulforhodamine B (SRB)

1. Cancer cells are grown in 96-well cell culture plates at a density of 5×10^3 cells/well and incubated for 24 h.
2. Following incubation, cells are treated with different concentrations of test compound/s and incubated for a desired period (24-72 h). Positive and negative controls should also be kept along with test compounds.
3. After incubation, all the wells are washed with PBS three times. Cells are then fixed with 25 μL of ice-cold 50% trichloroacetic acid (TCA) solution and incubated for 1 h at 4 °C. Wells are then rinsed with tap water five times.
4. 0.4% SRB solution (100 μL) is added to each well and incubated for 15 min at room temperature. Acetic acid (1%) is used to remove unbound dye.
5. Bound SRB dye is solubilized by adding Tris-base solution (200 μL/well).
6. Finally, absorbance is measured at 540 nm using a micro-plate reader.

Electric Cell-substrate Impedance Sensing (ECIS)

ECIS involves an impedance-based experimental technique, which can be used to monitor cell proliferation, migration and different behaviors associated with cytoskeleton [50, 51]. In this technique, cells are cultured in special cell culture chambers comprising gold electrodes. When cells grow on gold electrodes, cells behave as insulators and thereby raising the impedance. Variation in the impedance is measured against the alterative current (AC) during the experiment [50 - 52]. The three dimensional shape of a cell and dielectric behavior of cell membrane have been reported as the major factors responsible for the deviations in impedance. As the three dimensional shape of cells and cell attachment alter upon exposing to cytotoxic agents, resulting in reduction of the impedance, the ESIC technique can be used to evaluate the effects of cytotoxic agents on the alterations in cell shape [52]. The unit Cell Index (CI) is used to express the relationship between viable cell count and the impedance [53]. xCELLigence (ACEA Biosciences, USA) is an example for an instrument, which uses the technique ECIS [54]. A recent study has utilized the xCELLigence to investigate the effects of interleukin 11 on endometrial epithelial cancer cells proliferation [55]. Although this technique is informative and sophisticated, high cost associated with these kinds of instruments is one of the major disadvantages.

Assays Based on DNA Synthesis

^{3}H-thymidine incorporation assay is one of the commonly used anti-proliferative assays, which is used to identify newly synthesized DNA using the radioactive ^{3}H-thymidine [56]. In this assay, radioactive ^{3}H-thymidine is incorporated with newly synthesized DNA of cells and incorporated ^{3}H-thymidine is measured using a scintillation counter at the endpoint [56]. Use of a radioactive material is the main disadvantage associated with this assay [56, 57]. Studies reported by Lagler *et al.* [58] and Vale *et al.* [59] have used the ^{3}H-thymidine incorporation assay as an anti-proliferative assay. Assays such as 5-bromo-2'-deoxyuridine (BrdU) and 5-ethynyl-2'-deoxyuridine (EdU) do not use radioactive substances as in the ^{3}H-thymidine incorporation assay [60, 61]. In the BrdU assay, BrdU binds with DNA and, primary and secondary antibodies are used to detect bound BrdU with DNA [60]. Unlike the BrdU assay, EdU doses not use primary antibodies, making the EdU assay as a sensitive and rapid anti-proliferative assay [61]. Dai *et al.* [62] and Lu *et al.* [63] utilized the BrdU assay to investigate the anti-proliferative effects of isocostunolide and cryptotanshinone against glioma stem cells. Ruan *et al.* [64] used the EdU assay to evaluate the anti-proliferative effects of berberine in KM12C colon cancer cells. Moreover, another recent study .conducted by Nan *et al.* [65] reported anti-proliferative effects of C-terminal binding protein 2 (CtBP2) in SHSY5Y neuroblastoma cell using the EdU assay.

General Assay Procedure for the ^{3}H-thymidine incorporation assay

1. Cancer cells are grown in 24-well cell culture plates at a density of 5×10^5 cells/well and incubated for 24 h.
2. Following incubation, cells are treated with different concentrations of test compound/s and incubated for a desired period (24-72 h). Positive and negative controls should also be kept along with test compounds.
3. After incubation, all the wells are washed with PBS three times. Cells are then treated with ^{3}H-thymidine with an optimized concentration (mixed with cell culture medium).
4. Plates are incubated at 37°C for 8 h.
5. Medium is removed from each well and each well is washed with PBS.
6. Cells are then fixed with ice-cold 5% TCA and incubated at 4°C for 1 h.
7. TCA solution is removed and again cells are washed with PBS.
8. 0.5 ml of 0.5 M NaOH/0.5% SDS solution is added to each well to lyse cells.
9. Finally, radioactive nucleotide incorporation is measured using a scintillation counter.

General Assay Procedure for the BrdU assay

1. Cancer cells are grown in 24-well cell culture plates at a density of 5×10^4 cells/well and incubated for 24 h.
2. Following incubation, cells are treated with different concentrations of test compound/s and incubated for a desired period (24-72 h). Positive and negative controls should also be kept along with test compounds.
3. After incubation, all the wells are washed with PBS three times and incubated with BrdU solution (3 µg/mL.) at 37°C for 4 h.
4. Following incubation, cells are fixed with 4% paraformaldehyde.

5. Cells are washed with PBS for three times.
6. Cells are treated with 2N HCL to spate DNA into single stranded DNA.
7. Cells are again washed with PBS three times.
8. Treatment with 5% normal horse serum to block nonspecific epitopes.
9. Overnight incubation with anti-BrdU primary antibody.
10. Cells are washed with PBS for three times.
11. Incubation with secondary antibody.
12. Absorbance is measured at 450 nm.
    o Unlike the BrdU assay, EdU doses not use primary antibodies, making the EdU assay as a sensitive and rapid anti-proliferative assay

Dye Exclusion Assays

Dye exclusion assays are frequently employed as cell viability assays as these assays are easy to conduct in a short period of time. Most of the dyes used in dye exclusion assays can penetrate through damaged cell membranes [66, 67]. The Trypan blue cell viability assay is one of such simple dye exclusion assays, which has been widely used in preclinical investigations. The dye Trypan blue can only penetrate through damaged cell membranes, while cells with undamaged cell membranes reject this dye [66, 67]. In a recent investigation, the Trypan blue cell viability assay has been used to evaluate the effects of polyvinyl alcohol (PVA) capped silver nanoparticles in breast cancer and human glioblastoma cells [68] Cytotoxic effects of carob leaf polyphenols against colon cancer cell viability were examined using the trypan blue dye exclusion assay by Ghanemi *et al.* [69]. The dye Propidium iodide (PI) can also be used to differentiate viable and non-viable cells [70]. PI can enter through damaged cell membranes and bind with DNA. Fluorescent dye 7-Aminoactinomycin D (7-AAD) can also be utilized to distinguish viable/non-viable cell populations [71]. Moreover, dead cell penetrating dyes such as Evans blue, ethidium homodimer, TOTO, TO-PRO and SYTOX can also be used in cell based experiments to differentiate viable and non-viable cells [72]. In contrast to SYTOX family, dyes in SYTO family can penetrate through viable cell membranes [73, 74]. When performing dye exclusion assays, it is necessary to use appropriate dye concentrations and cell number, as high concentration of dyes can cause overstating of samples [75]. Although these dye exclusion assays are simple and inexpensive, care must be taken when counting cells as cell counting errors can affect the overall results of the experiments.

General Assay Procedure for the Trypan Blue Cell Viability Assay

1. Cell suspension is placed on a microscopic slide.
2. Equal volume of 0.4% trypan blue dye is mixed with the cell suspension.
3. Mixture is incubated for 2-3 minutes at room temperature.

4. Cell suspension (10-20 µL) is placed on a hemocytometer and viable cells are observed under a light microscope.
5. Non-viable cells are appeared in blue.

Colony Formation Assay

Colony formation assay is another simple cell based assay, which is used to evaluate the effects of testing agents on clonogenic ability of cancer cells grown as a monolayer or in suspension [76]. Prior to the colony formation assay, self-aggregation of cancer cells should be avoided by a suitable cell detaching technique to prevent initial cell colonization. Normally, colony formation assays are initiated with 50 single cells [76]. Following incubation at a desired period, cell colonies can be manually counted using a light microscope. In contrast to the colony formation assay, soft agar colony formation assay is used to assess the effects of testing agents on the clonogenic ability of cancer cells which are grown in suspension [77]. In this assay, cancer cells are grown as colonies embedded in agar and the cell culture medium present over the agar layer is mixed with the testing agent. A recent investigation conducted by Bisht *et al.* [78] utilized the colony formation assay to investigate the anti-clonogenic ability of a nano-formulation comprising curcumin analog (EF 24) in pancreatic cancer cells. The soft agar colony formation assay has been used in recent study to investigate the anti-clonogenic effects of 15α-methoxypuupehenol in breast and glioblastoma cells [79]. Although these assays are easy to perform, some disadvantages are associated with these colony formation assays. For example, a soft-agar colony formation assay takes about a week to complete and, care must be taken during drug incubations as all the assay procedures have to be repeated from initial steps if there is a microbial contamination is detected [80].

General Assay Procedure for the Colony Formation Assay

1. 50-60 cancer cells are seeded in 24-well cell culture plates and incubated with desired concentrations of test compound/s.
2. Following incubations, cell colonies are fixed with TCA and stained with crystal violet (0.5% *w/v*).
3. Stained cell colonies are counted manually using a phase contrast microscopy.
    - In soft-agar colony formation assay, cancer cells are grown as colonies embedded in agar and the cell culture medium present over the agar layer is mixed with the testing agent.

Real-time Monitoring and Live Cell Imaging Techniques

Over the past decade, sophisticated scientific instruments have been introduced by several reputed biotech companies for *in-vitro* live cell imaging applications.

Instruments such as IncuCyte™ (Essen BioScience, Michigan, USA and XCELLigence), xCELLigence™ (ACEA Biosciences, USA), Cytation 5™ (Biotek, Winooski, VT), ZEISS Cell discoverer 7™ (Carl Zeiss Microscopy GmbH, Jena, Germany), EVOS™ (EVOS FL Auto, Thermo Fisher Scientific, USA) and Cell-IQ 2™ (Chip-Man Technologies, Tampere, Finland) have widely been used to assess detailed physiological information, real-time monitoring of cancer cell proliferation, apoptosis and necrosis, *etc* [81, 82]. Although these instruments are employed to obtain detailed physiological information about cancer cells in anti-cancer drug discovery approaches, high maintenance cost associated with these instruments is a major disadvantage [83]. Several recent pre-clinical investigations have utilized IncuCyte™ and Cell-IQ™ platforms for live cell imaging [81 - 85]. Although this technique is informative and sophisticated, high cost associated with these kinds of instruments is one of the major disadvantages. A summary of cell-based *in-vitro* assay used in pre-clinical anti-cancer drug discovery approaches has been mentioned in Table **1**.

Table 1. Summary of *in-vitro* cell based assays or techniques available to evaluate cell proliferation.

Assay Feature	Name of the Assay	Major Assay Constituent/Substance(s)	Assay Principle or Assay Chemistry	Method(s) of Endpoint Detection
Live cell enzymes and proteins (metabolic activity)	MTT assay	Tetrazolium dye MTT	Reduction of MTT to formazan	Colorimetric
	MTS assay	Tetrazolium dye MTS	Reduction of MTS to formazan	Colorimetric
	XTT assay	Tetrazolium dye XTT	Reduction of XTT to formazan	Colorimetric
	WST assay	Tetrazolium dye WST	Reduction of WST to formazan	Colorimetric
	SRB assay	SRB dye	SRB dye binds with basic amino acids in viable cells	Colorimetric
	Cellular ATP assay	Intracellular ATP	Measurement of cellular ATP levels in viable cells	Colorimetric/ fluorometric
	LDH leakage assay	Intracellular LDH	Measurement of cellular LDH levels in viable cells	Colorimetric/ fluorometric
	Resazurin assay	Resazurin	In the viable cells resazurin is reduced by viable cell oxidoreductases to generate resorufin	Fluorometric

(Table 1) cont.....

Assay Feature	Name of the Assay	Major Assay Constituent/Substance(s)	Assay Principle or Assay Chemistry	Method(s) of Endpoint Detection
Live cell enzymes and proteins (metabolic activity)	Calcein AM viability assay	Calcein	In viable cells Calcein AM is hydrolyzed by intracellular esterases to produce fluorescent compound calcein	Fluorometric
DNA synthesis	[^{3}H]-Thymidine incorporation assay		Radioactive 3H-thymidine incorporate with the newly synthesized DNA	Scintillation counter
	BrdU assay	BrdU	BrdU binds with cellular DNA	Colorimetric/ fluorometric
	EdU assay	EdU	EdU binds with cellular DNA	Colorimetric/ fluorometric
Membrane integrity	Trypan blue cell viability assay	Dye trypan blue	Trypan blue can penetrate through damaged cell membranes, while cells with undamaged cell membranes reject this dye	Colorimetric
	Propidium iodide uptake assay	Dye propidium iodide	Propidium iodide can enter through damaged cell membranes and bind with DNA	Fluorometric
	7-aminoactinomycin D (7-AAD) staining	Dye 7-AAD	7-AAD binds with DNA	Fluorometric
	Ethidium homodimer assay	Dye ethidium homodimer	Dye ethidium homodimer binds with DNA and emits red fluorescence	Fluorometric
Formation of cell colonies	Colony formation assay	-	Cell colonies formed are counted	Manual counting
Impedance of cells	Electric cell-substrate impedance sensing (ECIS)- a technique	-	Impedance of living cells	Impedance is measured using electrodes attached to wells

CONCLUDING REMARKS

Uncontrolled cell proliferation is a hallmark feature of cancer. *In-vitro* anti-proliferative assays are employed to evaluate whether the testing agent(s) exert direct anti-proliferative properties in cancer cells. Anti-proliferative assays not only provide information on anti-proliferative efficacy of testing agent(s) but also offer evidence about some physiological processes in living cells (For example dye exclusion or LDH release assays provide information on cell membrane integrity upon exposure to cytotoxic agents). In this chapter, we have outlined commonly used cell based *in-vitro* anti-proliferative assays utilized in pre-clinical anti-cancer drug discovery approaches. Although the content of this chapter is not exhaustive, our aim is to provide information on widely used cell based anti-proliferative assays/techniques in pre-clinical investigations and to encourage researcher or scientist to select the most suitable *in-vitro* assay/technique for anti-cancer drug discovery strategies.

CONSENT FOR PUBLICATION

Not applicable.

CONFLICT OF INTEREST

The authors confirm that this chapter contents have no conflict of interest.

ACKNOWLEDGEMENT

Declared none.

REFERENCES

[1] Bray F, Ferlay J, Soerjomataram I, Siegel RL, Torre LA, Jemal A. Global cancer statistics 2018: GLOBOCAN estimates of incidence and mortality worldwide for 36 cancers in 185 countries. CA Cancer J Clin 2018; 68(6): 394-424.
[http://dx.doi.org/10.3322/caac.21492] [PMID: 30207593]

[2] Jemal A, Bray F, Center MM, Ferlay J, Ward E, Forman D. Global cancer statistics. CA Cancer J Clin 2011; 61(2): 69-90.
[http://dx.doi.org/10.3322/caac.20107] [PMID: 21296855]

[3] Sankaranarayanan R. Screening for cancer in low- and middle-income countries. Ann Glob Health 2014; 80(5): 412-7.
[http://dx.doi.org/10.1016/j.aogh.2014.09.014] [PMID: 25512156]

[4] Islami F, Goding Sauer A, Miller KD, *et al.* Proportion and number of cancer cases and deaths attributable to potentially modifiable risk factors in the United States. CA Cancer J Clin 2018; 68(1): 31-54.
[http://dx.doi.org/10.3322/caac.21440] [PMID: 29160902]

[5] Loeb LA, Loeb KR, Anderson JP. Multiple mutations and cancer. Proc Natl Acad Sci USA 2003; 100(3): 776-81.
[http://dx.doi.org/10.1073/pnas.0334858100] [PMID: 12552134]

[6] Schnipper LE, Davidson NE, Wollins DS, *et al.* American Society of Clinical Oncology statement: a conceptual framework to assess the value of cancer treatment options. J Clin Oncol 2015; 33(23): 2563-77.

[http://dx.doi.org/10.1200/JCO.2015.61.6706] [PMID: 26101248]

[7]   USITC. Pharmaceutical Products and Chemical Intermediates, Fourth Review¬: Advice Concerning the Addition of Certain Products to the Pharmaceutical Appendix to the HTS 2010.

[8]   Newman DJ, Cragg GM. Natural products as sources of new drugs from 1981 to 2014. J Nat Prod 2016; 79(3): 629-61.
[http://dx.doi.org/10.1021/acs.jnatprod.5b01055] [PMID: 26852623]

[9]   Roy A, McDonald PR, Sittampalam S, Chaguturu R. Open access high throughput drug discovery in the public domain: a Mount Everest in the making. Curr Pharm Biotechnol 2010; 11(7): 764-78.
[http://dx.doi.org/10.2174/138920110792927757] [PMID: 20809896]

[10] Rahman AU, Choudhary MI, Thomsen WJ. Bioassay techniques for drug development. British library, UK: Harwood academic 2001.

[11] Lord CJ, Ashworth A. Biology-driven cancer drug development: back to the future. BMC Biol 2010; 8: 38.
[http://dx.doi.org/10.1186/1741-7007-8-38] [PMID: 20385032]

[12] Abraham VC, Taylor DL, Haskins JR. High content screening applied to large-scale cell biology. Trends Biotechnol 2004; 22(1): 15-22.
[http://dx.doi.org/10.1016/j.tibtech.2003.10.012] [PMID: 14690618]

[13] Bronstein I, Fortin J, Stanley PE, Stewart GS, Kricka LJ. Chemiluminescent and bioluminescent reporter gene assays. Anal Biochem 1994; 219(2): 169-81.
[http://dx.doi.org/10.1006/abio.1994.1254] [PMID: 8080073]

[14] Fox S, Farr-Jones S, Sopchak L, *et al.* High-throughput screening: update on practices and success. J Biomol Screen 2006; 11(7): 864-9.
[http://dx.doi.org/10.1177/1087057106292473] [PMID: 16973922]

[15] Eisenbrand G, Pool-Zobel B, Baker V, *et al.* Methods of *in vitro* toxicology. Food Chem Toxicol 2002; 40(2-3): 193-236.
[http://dx.doi.org/10.1016/S0278-6915(01)00118-1] [PMID: 11893398]

[16] Fotakis G, Timbrell JA. *in vitro* cytotoxicity assays: comparison of LDH, neutral red, MTT and protein assay in hepatoma cell lines following exposure to cadmium chloride. Toxicol Lett 2006; 160(2): 171-7.
[http://dx.doi.org/10.1016/j.toxlet.2005.07.001] [PMID: 16111842]

[17] Mahto SK, Chandra P, Rhee SW. In-vitro models, endpoints and assessment methods for the measurement of cytotoxicity. J Toxicol Environ Health 2010; 2: 87-93.

[18] Hanahan D, Weinberg RA. The hallmarks of cancer. Cell 2000; 100(1): 57-70.
[http://dx.doi.org/10.1016/S0092-8674(00)81683-9] [PMID: 10647931]

[19] Riss TL, Moravec RA, Niles AL, Duellman S, Benink HA, Worzella TJ. Cell Viability Assays. Assay Guidance Manual. Bethesda, MD, USA: Eli Lilly & Co and National Centre for Advancing Translational Sciences 2004.

[20] Berridge MV, Tan AS. Characterization of the cellular reduction of 3-(4,5-dimethylthiazol-2-yl--2,5-diphenyltetrazolium bromide (MTT): subcellular localization, substrate dependence, and involvement of mitochondrial electron transport in MTT reduction. Arch Biochem Biophys 1993; 303(2): 474-82.
[http://dx.doi.org/10.1006/abbi.1993.1311] [PMID: 8390225]

[21] Gerlier D, Thomasset N. Use of MTT colorimetric assay to measure cell activation. J Immunol Methods 1986; 94(1-2): 57-63.
[http://dx.doi.org/10.1016/0022-1759(86)90215-2] [PMID: 3782817]

[22] Rekha S, Anila EI. *in vitro* cytotoxicity studies of surface modified CaS nanoparticles on L929 cell lines using MTT assay. Mater Lett 2019; 236: 637-9.

[http://dx.doi.org/10.1016/j.matlet.2018.11.009]

[23] Aboubakr EM, Taye A, Aly OM, Gamal-Eldeen AM, El-Moselhy MA. Enhanced anticancer effect of Combretastatin A-4 phosphate when combined with vincristine in the treatment of hepatocellular carcinoma. Biomed Pharmacother 2017; 89: 36-46.
[http://dx.doi.org/10.1016/j.biopha.2017.02.019] [PMID: 28214686]

[24] Ahamed M, Akhtar MJ, Khan MAM, Alrokayan SA, Alhadlaq HA. Oxidative stress mediated cytotoxicity and apoptosis response of bismuth oxide (Bi_2O_3) nanoparticles in human breast cancer (MCF-7) cells. Chemosphere 2019; 216: 823-31.
[http://dx.doi.org/10.1016/j.chemosphere.2018.10.214] [PMID: 30399561]

[25] Wu TR, Huang TT, Martel J, *et al.* Pinicolol B from *Antrodia cinnamomea* induces apoptosis of nasopharyngeal carcinoma cells. J Ethnopharmacol 2017; 201: 117-22.
[http://dx.doi.org/10.1016/j.jep.2017.02.008] [PMID: 28167294]

[26] Murayyan AI, Manohar CM, Hayward G, Neethirajan S. Antiproliferative activity of Ontario grown onions against colorectal adenocarcinoma cells. Food Res Int 2017; 96: 12-8.
[http://dx.doi.org/10.1016/j.foodres.2017.03.017] [PMID: 28528091]

[27] Abdelmageed N, Morad SAF, Elghoneimy AA, *et al.* Oleanolic acid methyl ester, a novel cytotoxic mitocan, induces cell cycle arrest and ROS-Mediated cell death in castration-resistant prostate cancer PC-3 cells. Biomed Pharmacother 2017; 96: 417-25.
[http://dx.doi.org/10.1016/j.biopha.2017.10.027] [PMID: 29031200]

[28] Özdemir A, Sever B, Altıntop MD, *et al.* Synthesis and evaluation of new oxadiazole, thiadiazole, and triazole derivatives as potential anticancer agents targeting MMP-9. Molecules 2017; 22(7): 1109.
[http://dx.doi.org/10.3390/molecules22071109] [PMID: 28677624]

[29] Rajagopalan U, Samarakoon SR, Tennekoon KH, Malavige N, de Silva ED. Screening of five Sri Lankan endemic plants for anti-cancer effects on breast cancer stem cells isolated from MCF-7 and MDA-MB-231 cell lines. Trop J Pharm Res 2018; 1: 1825-32.
[http://dx.doi.org/10.4314/tjpr.v17i9.21]

[30] Chen SM, Wang BY, Lee CH, *et al.* Hinokitiol up-regulates miR-494-3p to suppress BMI1 expression and inhibits self-renewal of breast cancer stem/progenitor cells. Oncotarget 2017; 8(44): 76057-68.
[http://dx.doi.org/10.18632/oncotarget.18648] [PMID: 29100291]

[31] Anoopkumar-Dukie S, Carey JB, Conere T, O'sullivan E, van Pelt FN, Allshire A. Resazurin assay of radiation response in cultured cells. Br J Radiol 2005; 78(934): 945-7.
[http://dx.doi.org/10.1259/bjr/54004230] [PMID: 16177019]

[32] Candeias L, MacFarlane DS, McWhinnie SW, Maidwell N, Roeschlaub C, Sammes P. The catalysed NADH reduction of resazurin to resorufin. J Chem Soc Perkin Trans 2 1998; 0: 2333-4.

[33] Goto RN, Sobral LM, Sousa LO, *et al.* Anti-cancer activity of a new dihydropyridine derivative, VdiE-2N, in head and neck squamous cell carcinoma. Eur J Pharmacol 2018; 819: 198-206.
[http://dx.doi.org/10.1016/j.ejphar.2017.12.009] [PMID: 29221949]

[34] Bratosin D, Mitrofan L, Palii C, Estaquier J, Montreuil J. Novel fluorescence assay using calcein-AM for the determination of human erythrocyte viability and aging. Cytometry A 2005; 66(1): 78-84.
[http://dx.doi.org/10.1002/cyto.a.20152] [PMID: 15915509]

[35] Zhou W, Almeqdadi M, Xifaras ME, Riddell IA, Yilmaz ÖH, Lippard SJ. The effect of geometric isomerism on the anticancer activity of the monofunctional platinum complex trans-[Pt(NH_3)$_2$(phenanthridine)Cl]NO_3. Chem Commun (Camb) 2018; 54(22): 2788-91.
[http://dx.doi.org/10.1039/C8CC00393A] [PMID: 29484327]

[36] Smith PJ, Falconer RA, Errington RJ. Micro-community cytometry: sensing changes in cell health and glycoconjugate expression by imaging and flow cytometry. J Microsc 2013; 251(2): 113-22.
[http://dx.doi.org/10.1111/jmi.12060] [PMID: 23763384]

[37] Skehan P, Storeng R, Scudiero D, *et al.* New colorimetric cytotoxicity assay for anticancer-drug

screening. J Natl Cancer Inst 1990; 82(13): 1107-12.
[http://dx.doi.org/10.1093/jnci/82.13.1107] [PMID: 2359136]

[38] Ediriweera MK, Tennekoon KH, Samarakoon SR, Thabrew I, Dilip DE Silva E. A study of the potential anticancer activity of *Mangifera zeylanica* bark: Evaluation of cytotoxic and apoptotic effects of the hexane extract and bioassay-guided fractionation to identify phytochemical constituents. Oncol Lett 2016; 11(2): 1335-44.
[http://dx.doi.org/10.3892/ol.2016.4087] [PMID: 26893740]

[39] Ediriweera MK, Tennekoon KH, Adhikari A, Samarakoon SR, Thabrew I, de Silva ED. New halogenated constituents from *Mangifera zeylanica* Hook.f. and their potential anti-cancer effects in breast and ovarian cancer cells. J Ethnopharmacol 2016; 189: 165-74.
[http://dx.doi.org/10.1016/j.jep.2016.05.047] [PMID: 27224244]

[40] Ediriweera MK, Tennekoon KH, Samarakoon SR, Adhikari A, Thabrew I, Dilip de Silva E. Isolation of a new resorcinolic lipid from *Mangifera zeylanica* Hook.f. bark and its cytotoxic and apoptotic potential. Biomed Pharmacother 2017; 89: 194-200.
[http://dx.doi.org/10.1016/j.biopha.2017.01.176] [PMID: 28222398]

[41] Ediriweera MK, Tennekoon KH, Samarakoon SR, Thabrew I, De Silva ED. Induction of Apoptosis in MCF-7 Breast Cancer Cells by Sri Lankan Endemic Mango (*Mangifera zeylanica*) Fruit Peel through Oxidative Stress and Analysis of its Phytochemical Constituents. J Food Biochem 2017; 41e12294
[http://dx.doi.org/10.1111/jfbc.12294]

[42] Wang P, Henning SM, Heber D. Limitations of MTT and MTS-based assays for measurement of antiproliferative activity of green tea polyphenols. PLoS One 2010; 5(4)e10202
[http://dx.doi.org/10.1371/journal.pone.0010202] [PMID: 20419137]

[43] Strehler BL, McElroy WD. Assay of adenosine triphosphate. Methods Enzymol 1957; 3: 871-3.
[http://dx.doi.org/10.1016/S0076-6879(57)03466-7]

[44] Hannah R, Beck M, Moravec R, Riss T. CellTiter-Glo™ Luminescent cell viability assay: a sensitive and rapid method for determining cell viability. Promega Cell Notes 2001; 2: 11-3.

[45] Cusimano A, Balasus D, Azzolina A, *et al.* Oleocanthal exerts antitumor effects on human liver and colon cancer cells through ROS generation. Int J Oncol 2017; 51(2): 533-44.
[http://dx.doi.org/10.3892/ijo.2017.4049] [PMID: 28656311]

[46] Smith SM, Wunder MB, Norris DA, Shellman YG. A simple protocol for using a LDH-based cytotoxicity assay to assess the effects of death and growth inhibition at the same time. PLoS One 2011; 6(11)e26908
[http://dx.doi.org/10.1371/journal.pone.0026908] [PMID: 22125603]

[47] Hodgkinson N, Kruger CA, Mokwena M, Abrahamse H. Cervical cancer cells (HeLa) response to photodynamic therapy using a zinc phthalocyanine photosensitizer. J Photochem Photobiol B 2017; 177: 32-8.
[http://dx.doi.org/10.1016/j.jphotobiol.2017.10.004] [PMID: 29045918]

[48] Dasari VR, Mazack V, Feng W, Nash J, Carey DJ, Gogoi R. Verteporfin exhibits YAP-independent anti-proliferative and cytotoxic effects in endometrial cancer cells. Oncotarget 2017; 8(17): 28628-40.
[http://dx.doi.org/10.18632/oncotarget.15614] [PMID: 28404908]

[49] Niles AL, Moravec RA, Eric Hesselberth P, Scurria MA, Daily WJ, Riss TL. A homogeneous assay to measure live and dead cells in the same sample by detecting different protease markers. Anal Biochem 2007; 366(2): 197-206.
[http://dx.doi.org/10.1016/j.ab.2007.04.007] [PMID: 17512890]

[50] Wegener J, Keese CR, Giaever I. Electric cell-substrate impedance sensing (ECIS) as a noninvasive means to monitor the kinetics of cell spreading to artificial surfaces. Exp Cell Res 2000; 259(1): 158-66.
[http://dx.doi.org/10.1006/excr.2000.4919] [PMID: 10942588]

[51] Xiao C, Luong JH. On-line monitoring of cell growth and cytotoxicity using electric cell-substrate impedance sensing (ECIS). Biotechnol Prog 2003; 19(3): 1000-5.
[http://dx.doi.org/10.1021/bp025733x] [PMID: 12790667]

[52] Xiao C, Lachance B, Sunahara G, Luong JH. Assessment of cytotoxicity using electric cell-substrate impedance sensing: concentration and time response function approach. Anal Chem 2002; 74(22): 5748-53.
[http://dx.doi.org/10.1021/ac025848f] [PMID: 12463358]

[53] Rahim S, Üdren A. A real-time electrical impedance based technique to measure invasion of endothelial cell monolayer by cancer cells. J Vis Exp 2011; (50): 2792.
[http://dx.doi.org/10.3791/2792] [PMID: 21490581]

[54] Hong J, Kandasamy K, Marimuthu M, Choi CS, Kim S. Electrical cell-substrate impedance sensing as a non-invasive tool for cancer cell study. Analyst (Lond) 2011; 136(2): 237-45.
[http://dx.doi.org/10.1039/C0AN00560F] [PMID: 20963234]

[55] Winship AL, Van Sinderen M, Donoghue J, Rainczuk K, Dimitriadis E. Targeting interleukin-11 receptor-α impairs human endometrial cancer cell proliferation and invasion *in vitro* and reduces tumor growth and metastasis *in vivo*. Mol Cancer Ther 2016; 15(4): 720-30.
[http://dx.doi.org/10.1158/1535-7163.MCT-15-0677] [PMID: 26846819]

[56] Sidman RL, Miale IL, Feder N. Cell proliferation and migration in the primitive ependymal zone: an autoradiographic study of histogenesis in the nervous system. Exp Neurol 1959; 1: 322-33.
[http://dx.doi.org/10.1016/0014-4886(59)90024-X] [PMID: 14446424]

[57] Duque A, Rakic P. Different effects of bromodeoxyuridine and [3H]thymidine incorporation into DNA on cell proliferation, position, and fate. J Neurosci 2011; 31(42): 15205-17.
[http://dx.doi.org/10.1523/JNEUROSCI.3092-11.2011] [PMID: 22016554]

[58] Lagler C, El-Mesery M, Kübler AC, *et al*. The anti-myeloma activity of bone morphogenetic protein 2 predominantly relies on the induction of growth arrest and is apoptosis-independent. PLoS One 2017; 12(10)e0185720
[http://dx.doi.org/10.1371/journal.pone.0185720] [PMID: 29028819]

[59] Vale N, Correia-Branco A, Patrício B, Duarte D, Martel F. *in vitro* studies on the inhibition of colon cancer by amino acid derivatives of bromothiazole. Bioorg Med Chem Lett 2017; 27(15): 3507-10.
[http://dx.doi.org/10.1016/j.bmcl.2017.05.073] [PMID: 28601526]

[60] Miller MW, Nowakowski RS. Use of bromodeoxyuridine-immunohistochemistry to examine the proliferation, migration and time of origin of cells in the central nervous system. Brain Res 1988; 457(1): 44-52.
[http://dx.doi.org/10.1016/0006-8993(88)90055-8] [PMID: 3167568]

[61] Salic A, Mitchison TJ. A chemical method for fast and sensitive detection of DNA synthesis *in vivo*. Proc Natl Acad Sci USA 2008; 105(7): 2415-20.
[http://dx.doi.org/10.1073/pnas.0712168105] [PMID: 18272492]

[62] Dai Z, Li SR, Zhu PF, *et al*. Isocostunolide inhibited glioma stem cell by suppression proliferation and inducing caspase dependent apoptosis. Bioorg Med Chem Lett 2017; 27(13): 2863-7.
[http://dx.doi.org/10.1016/j.bmcl.2017.04.075] [PMID: 28487072]

[63] Lu L, Zhang S, Li C, *et al*. Cryptotanshinone inhibits human glioma cell proliferation *in vitro* and *in vivo* through SHP-2-dependent inhibition of STAT3 activation. Cell Death Dis 2017; 8(5)e2767
[http://dx.doi.org/10.1038/cddis.2017.174] [PMID: 28492557]

[64] Ruan H, Zhan YY, Hou J, *et al*. Berberine binds RXRα to suppress β-catenin signaling in colon cancer cells. Oncogene 2017; 36(50): 6906-18.
[http://dx.doi.org/10.1038/onc.2017.296] [PMID: 28846104]

[65] Nan J, Guan S, Jin X, Jian Z, Linshan F, Jun G. Down-regulation of C-terminal binding protein 2 (CtBP2) inhibits proliferation, migration, and invasion of human SHSY5Y cells *in vitro*. Neurosci Lett

2017; 647: 104-9.
[http://dx.doi.org/10.1016/j.neulet.2017.02.006] [PMID: 28179207]

[66] Altman SA, Randers L, Rao G. Comparison of trypan blue dye exclusion and fluorometric assays for mammalian cell viability determinations. Biotechnol Prog 1993; 9(6): 671-4.
[http://dx.doi.org/10.1021/bp00024a017] [PMID: 7764357]

[67] Strober W. Trypan blue exclusion test of cell viability. Curr Protoc Immunol 1997; 21: A-3B.

[68] Lim HK, Gurung RL, Hande MP. DNA-dependent protein kinase modulates the anti-cancer properties of silver nanoparticles in human cancer cells. Mutat Res 2017; 824: 32-41.
[http://dx.doi.org/10.1016/j.mrgentox.2017.10.001] [PMID: 29150048]

[69] Ghanemi FZ, Belarbi M, Fluckiger A, *et al.* Carob leaf polyphenols trigger intrinsic apoptotic pathway and induce cell cycle arrest in colon cancer cells. J Funct Foods 2017; 33: 112-21.
[http://dx.doi.org/10.1016/j.jff.2017.03.032]

[70] Sasaki DT, Dumas SE, Engleman EG. Discrimination of viable and non-viable cells using propidium iodide in two color immunofluorescence. Cytometry 1987; 8(4): 413-20.
[http://dx.doi.org/10.1002/cyto.990080411] [PMID: 3113897]

[71] Zembruski NC, Stache V, Haefeli WE, Weiss J. 7-Aminoactinomycin D for apoptosis staining in flow cytometry. Anal Biochem 2012; 429(1): 79-81.
[http://dx.doi.org/10.1016/j.ab.2012.07.005] [PMID: 22796502]

[72] King MA. Detection of dead cells and measurement of cell killing by flow cytometry. J Immunol Methods 2000; 243(1-2): 155-66.
[http://dx.doi.org/10.1016/S0022-1759(00)00232-5] [PMID: 10986413]

[73] Baker CJ, Mock NM. An improved method for monitoring cell death in cell suspension and leaf disc assays using Evans blue. Plant Cell Tiss Org 1994; 39: 7-12.
[http://dx.doi.org/10.1007/BF00037585]

[74] Wlodkowic D, Skommer J, Pelkonen J. Towards an understanding of apoptosis detection by SYTO dyes. Cytometry A 2007; 71(2): 61-72.
[http://dx.doi.org/10.1002/cyto.a.20366] [PMID: 17200958]

[75] Cadena-Herrera D, Esparza-De Lara JE, Ramírez-Ibañez ND, *et al.* Validation of three viable-cell counting methods: Manual, semi-automated, and automated. Biotechnol Rep (Amst) 2015; 7: 9-16.
[http://dx.doi.org/10.1016/j.btre.2015.04.004] [PMID: 28626709]

[76] Franken NA, Rodermond HM, Stap J, Haveman J, van Bree C. Clonogenic assay of cells *in vitro*. Nat Protoc 2006; 1(5): 2315-9.
[http://dx.doi.org/10.1038/nprot.2006.339] [PMID: 17406473]

[77] Alley MC, Uhl CB, Lieber MM. Improved detection of drug cytotoxicity in the soft agar colony formation assay through use of a metabolizable tetrazolium salt. Life Sci 1982; 31(26): 3071-8.
[http://dx.doi.org/10.1016/0024-3205(82)90077-7] [PMID: 7162367]

[78] Bisht S, Schlesinger M, Rupp A, *et al.* A liposomal formulation of the synthetic curcumin analog EF24 (Lipo-EF24) inhibits pancreatic cancer progression: towards future combination therapies. J Nanobiotechnology 2016; 14(1): 57.
[http://dx.doi.org/10.1186/s12951-016-0209-6] [PMID: 27401816]

[79] Hilliard TS, Miklossy G, Chock C, Yue P, Williams P, Turkson J. 15□-methoxypuupehenol induces antitumor effects *in vitro* and *in vivo* against human glioblastoma and breast cancer models. Mol Cancer Ther 2017; 16(4): 601-13.
[http://dx.doi.org/10.1158/1535-7163.MCT-16-0291] [PMID: 28069875]

[80] Dong GW, Preisler HD, Priore R. Potential limitations of *in vitro* clonogenic drug sensitivity assays. Cancer Chemother Pharmacol 1984; 13(3): 206-10.
[http://dx.doi.org/10.1007/BF00269030] [PMID: 6488440]

[81] Ke N, Wang X, Xu X, Abassi YA. The xCELLigence system for real-time and label-free monitoring of cell viability. Methods Mol Biol 2011; 740: 33-43.
[http://dx.doi.org/10.1007/978-1-61779-108-6_6] [PMID: 21468966]

[82] Xi B, Yu N, Wang X, Xu X, Abassi YA. The application of cell-based label-free technology in drug discovery. Biotechnol J 2008; 3(4): 484-95.
[http://dx.doi.org/10.1002/biot.200800020] [PMID: 18412175]

[83] Cole R. Live-cell imaging: The cell's perspective. Cell Adhes Migr 2014; 8: 452-9.
[http://dx.doi.org/10.4161/cam.28348]

[84] Kamal MM, Nazzal S. Novel sulforaphane-enabled self-microemulsifying delivery systems (SFN-SMEDDS) of taxanes: Formulation development and *in vitro* cytotoxicity against breast cancer cells. Int J Pharm 2018; 536(1): 187-98.
[http://dx.doi.org/10.1016/j.ijpharm.2017.11.063] [PMID: 29195916]

[85] Wang B, Shi L, Sun X, Wang L, Wang X, Chen C. Production of CCL20 from lung cancer cells induces the cell migration and proliferation through PI3K pathway. J Cell Mol Med 2016; 20(5): 920-9.
[http://dx.doi.org/10.1111/jcmm.12781] [PMID: 26968871]

CHAPTER 4

Polyphenols and Cancer

Peramaiyan Rajendran[1,*], Abdullah M. Alzahrani[1], Thamaraiselvan Rengarajan[2], Ravi Kaushik[3], Palanisamy Arulselvan[2,4] and Arthanari Umamaheswari[5]

[1] *Department of Biological Sciences, College of Science, King Faisal University, Hufouf, Al Hassa, 31982, Saudi Arabia*

[2] *Scigen Research & Innovation, Periyar Technology Business Incubator, Periyar Nagar, Vallam, Thanjavur, Tamilnadu 613403, India*

[3] *ICMR-National Institute of Cancer Prevention and Research, Noida, Uttar Pradesh 201301, India*

[4] *Muthayammal Centre for Advanced Research, Muthayammal College of Arts and Science, Rasipuram, Namakkal, Tamilnadu, 637408, India*

[5] *Department of Plant Biology and Plant Biotechnology, Presidency College, Chennai, Tamilnadu, 600005, India*

Abstract: A solid and useful connection exists among eating regimen and malignancy. An inaccurate diet may increase the incidence of all types of cancer from 10% to 70%. Polyphenols are found in more than 700 foods, particularly foods grown on the ground (such as herbs), flavorings, and even nuts and cocoa items. Many food items considered superfoods; top superfoods include blueberries, apricots, grapes, olives and olive oil, artichoke, herbs (*e.g.,* oregano, peppermint, and cloves), nuts and seeds (*e.g.,* walnuts, almonds and flaxseeds), and green tea. Polyphenolic compounds can lead to epigenetic modification of chromatin and modulation of membrane organization; they can also interfere with interaction of the various macromolecules and regulation of the telomerase activity. They play crucial roles in modulating the multiple cellular pathways individually. Pure polyphenolic agents may be used as therapeutic agents, in combination with conventional therapy for improved cancer treatment. This chapter summarizes the anticancer efficacy of major polyphenolic compounds and discusses the potential mechanisms of action based on epidemiological studies.

Keywords: Cancer, Chemoprevention, Curcumin, Epithelial Mesenchymal Transition, Epigenetics, Epigallocatechin-3-Gallate, Genistein, Histones, Inflammation, Lycopene, Metastasis, Methylation, Polyphenol, Resveratrol, Sulforaphane, Transcription Factors.

---

* Corresponding author Peramaiyan Rajendran: Department of Biological Sciences, College of Science, King Faisal University, Hufouf, Al Hassa, 31982, Saudi Arabia; Tel: +9660135899543; Fax: +9660135899556; E-mails: prajendran@kfu.edu.sa, peramaiyanrajendran@gmail.com

Atta-ur-Rahman and M. Iqbal Choudhary (Eds.)
All rights reserved-© 2019 Bentham Science Publishers

INTRODUCTION

Generally, active components from natural products have been major medicinal sources for humans. Polyphenols, a unique group od compomds present in vegetables, medicinal plants, and fruits, have potentially more beneficial effect in human diseases and have been studied extensively. Polyphenols are compounds with something like one aromatic ring, joined with at least one hydroxyl practical gatherings. natural polyphenols allude to a substantial gathering of plant optional metabolites extending from small molecules to profoundly polymerized mixes [1]. Based on their compound structures, characteristic polyphenols can be partitioned into five classes: flavonoids, phenolic acids, lignans, stilbenes, and different polyphenols. Flavonoids and phenolic acids are the most widely recognized classes, representing around 60% and 30% of all common polyphenols, individually Fig. (**1**). The anticancer adequacy of regular polyphenols is to a great extent inferable from their strong cancer prevention agent and anti-inflammatory exercises and their capacities to regulate atomic targets and signaling pathways, related with cell survival, expansion, separation, and movement; angiogenesis; hormonal exercises; detoxification catalyst action and immune responses [2]. The epigenetic control of DNA-templated forms has been strongly contemplated in the course of the most recent 20 years. DNA methylation, histone adjustment, nucleosome rebuilding, and RNA-intervened focusing on control numerous biological procedures basic to malignancy beginning. This chapter presents the biological effects of plant polyphenols in the context relevant to human cancer, along with the basic principles underlying the epigenetic pathways, the dysregulation of which can culminate in cancer. This data, alongside the promising clinical and preclinical epigenetic effects of polyphenol on chromatin regulators, signifies the time to embrace the central role of epigenetics in cancer.

Types of Polyphenol

In excess of 8000 phenolic structures are presently known; of these, more than 4000 are flavonoids. The expression "polyphenols" alludes to a wide assortment of molecules that can be isolated into numerous subclasses and subdivisions that can be made based on their origin, biological capacity, or compound structure. Chemically, they are mixes with structural phenolic highlights, which can be related with various organic acids and carbohydrates. In plants, the greater part of these compounds are connected to sugars, and consequently, are as glycosides. Carbohydrates and organic acids can be bound in various positions on polyphenol skeletons [3]. They can be arranged into various classes, as per the quantity of phenolic rings in their structure, the auxiliary components that dilemma these rings to each other, and the substituents connected to the rings. Polyphenols include simple molecules (e.g., phenolic acids) and complex, highly polymerized molecules (*e.g.*, condensed tannins). Thusly, two fundamental groups can be distinguished: flavonoids and nonflavonoids. Flavonoids share a structure framed by two aromatic rings, demonstrated as A and B, connected together by three carbon molecules shaping an oxygenated heterocycle, the C ring; they can be additionally subdivided into six primary subclasses, as a component of the sort of heterocycle (the C ring; Table **1**) [4].

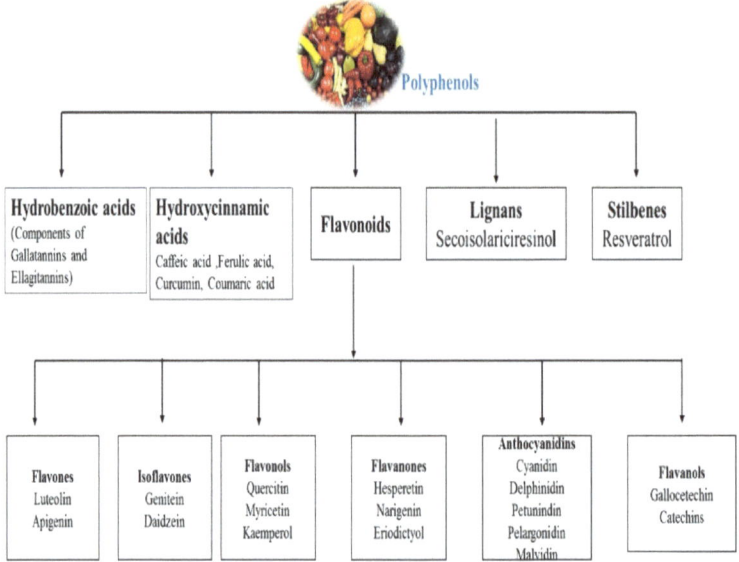

Fig. (1). Types of Polyphenol.

Table 1. Typical phenolic acids.

Hydroxycinnamic Acids					
	Name	R1	R2	R3	R4
	Cinnamic acid	H	H	H	H
	o-Coumaric acid	OH	H	H	H
	m-Coumaric acid	H	OH	H	H
	p-Coumaric acid Ferulic acid	H	H	OH	H
	Sinapic acid Caffeic acid	H	OCH3	OH	H
		H	OCH3	OH	OCH3
		H	OH	OH	H

(Table 1) cont.....

Hydroxycinnamic Acids	Name	R1	R2	R3	R4
	Benzoic acid	H	H	H	H
	p-Hydroxybenzoic acid	H	H	OH	H
	Vanillic acid	H	OCH3	OH	H
	Gallic acid	H	OH	OH	OH
	Protocatechuic acid	H	OH	OH	H
	Syringic acid	H	OCH3	OH	OCH3
	Gentisic acid	OH	H	H	OH
	Veratric acid	H	OCH3	OCH3	H
	Salicylic acid	OH	H	H	H

Polyphenols are isolated into four unique classes in view of the nearness of the number of phenolic groups and structural components. Sustenance, for the most part, contains complex polyphenols, dominatingly found in the external layers of the plants.

Flavonoids

Have a potential effect on radical scavenging and inflammatory responses. They are prevalently found in organic products, vegetables, legumes, red wine, and green tea. They are additionally separated into various subgroups to be specific, flavones, flavonols, flavanones, isoflavones, anthocyanidins, chalcones, and catechins.

Stilbenes

Found in product of graphs, red wine, and peanuts. Resveratrol is the most well-known compound among the group.

Lignans

Found in seeds like flax, linseed, legumes, cereals, grains, fruits, algae, and certain vegetables.

Phenolic Acids

Found in coffee, tea, cinnamon, blueberries, kiwis, plums, apples, and cherries and have two subgroups, namely hydroxybenzoic acids, and hydroxycinnamic acids (Fig. **1**).

Other Polyphenols

Notwithstanding the phenolic acids, flavonoids and phenolic amides, there are a few non-flavonoid polyphenols found in nourishments that are viewed as imperative to human wellbeing. Among these, resveratrol is one of a kind to the grapes and red wine; ellagic corrosive and its subordinates are found in berry fruits, *e.g.*, strawberries and raspberries, and in the skins of various tree nuts. Lignans exist in the bound structures in flax, sesame and numerous grains; structures appeared beneath are hydrolysis items. Curcumin is a solid cancer prevention agent from turmeric. Rosmarinic corrosive is a dimer of caffeic acid, and ellagic acid is a dimer of gallic acid. While both gallic acid and ellagic acid are found in the free structures, their glucose esters, a gathering known as hydrolysable tannins, likewise exist in various plants.

Bioavailability of Polyphenol

Bioavailability studies are not easy to perform because of the following potential factors:

- Outside elements: Ecological variables (*e.g.*, sun exposure and level of readiness) and nourishment accessibility;
- Food handling related variables: Thermal treatments, homogenization, lyophilization, cooking techniques, and capacity;
- Food-related variables: Sustenance grid and nearness of positive or negative effectors of retention (*e.g.*, fat and fiber);
- Interaction with different mixes: Connection with proteins (*e.g.*, egg whites) or polyphenols with similar mechanism of absorption;
- Polyphenol-related elements: Compound structure, fixation in nourishment, and sum presented;
- Host-related elements: Intestinal elements (*e.g.*, protein movement, intestinal travel time, and colonic microflora) and fundamental components (*e.g.*, sex, age, issue, pathology, hereditary genes, and physiological condition).

These variables may influence bioavailability specifically or by decreasing polyphenol content in sustenance. The technique for the most part misused to think about the bioavailability of the polyphenols must be considered. In the *in vivo* approach, the single-measurements configuration is generally utilized. It includes the admission of one portion of sustenance containing the tried polyphenol to take note of the expansion in blood concentration, which is transitional and for the most reflect the capacity of the living being to expend the polyphenol from the food matrix.

Subsequently, the watched addition can simply have a minor repercussions for tissue take-up and bioactivity. On the other hand, under normal admission conditions without a doubt, even low proportions of polyphenols can be on and on acclimatized to through and through grow the obsessions at both plasma and cell levels. Finish ends on the bioavailability and bioactivity of a lone phenolic compound are difficult to get in perspective of the synergistic effects of polyphenol mixes show in each nourishment network tried. This condition may improve later on, for instance, by using isogenic lines of onions contrasting just in their quercetin content, in this manner empowering correlations between gatherings expending a similar nourishment however with various polyphenol substance [5 - 7].

Polyphenol and Inflammation

Chronic inflammatory mediators exert pleiotropic effects during cancer development. Although inflammation favors carcinogenesis, malignant transformation, tumor growth, invasion, and metastatic spread, inflammation can also stimulate immune effector mechanisms that might limit tumor growth [8]. The immune-inflammatory signaling and metabolic impacts are the fundamental columns that physiologically associate the polyphenols and diverse chronic diseases [9]. An inside and out comprehension of the ramifications of dietary polyphenols in directing these impacts is an essential to creating successful dietary mediation for inflammatory disease prevention strategies. The capacity of dietary polyphenols to diminish inflammation is thought to be from the accompanying capacities: (1) acting as antioxidants, (2) interfering with oxidative stress signaling, and (3) suppressing the pro-inflammatory signaling transduction. The biological implication of phenolic compounds is based not only on directly reacting with reactive oxygen species (ROS) but also on agonistically activating cellular signaling pathways.

Polyphenol on Cytokines

Cytokines are the real mediators of neighborhood intercellular interchanges required for a coordinated reaction to an assortment of stimuli in immune and inflammatory processes [10]. Various cytokines have been recognized in tissues over a scope of immuno-intervened inflammatory diseases. In addition, a harmony between the impacts of pro-inflammatory (*i.e.* IL-1β, IL-2, TNFα, Il-6, IL-8, and IFNγ) and anti-inflammatory (*i.e.* IL-10, IL-4, and TGFβcytokines are thought to decide the outcome of ailment, regardless of whether in the short or long term [11].

Henceforth, the cytokine system is a remarkable focus for the advancement of clinically important anti-inflammatory drugs. Distinguishing proof of plant-derived compounds, for example, phenolic compounds that can specifically meddle with cytokine production and capacity could be an essential option for the treatment of numerous inflammatory diseases [12]. To this end, contemplates have demonstrated that few flavonoids can diminish the outflow of various pro-inflammatory cytokines and chemokines, in particular TNFα, IL-1β, IL-6, IL-8, and MCP-1, in many cell types, such as LPS-activated mouse primary macrophages and PMA- or phytohemagglutinin [13, 14]. These examinations firmly bolster that flavonoids have the ability to regulate the insusceptible reaction and have a potential anti-inflammatory activity. Be that as it may, their consequences for the pro-inflammatory and anti-inflammatory cytokine articulation have been appeared to be particular for a few cytokines and to be impacted by polyphenol structures featuring the complex action exerted by these mixes [15]. Indeed, polyphenols, for example, quercetin and catechins, coupled their inhibitory activity on TNFα and IL-1β to the upgrade of IL-10 discharge. Phenolic compounds from EVOO have been appeared to adjust the outflow of a few cytokines. In fact, in actuated human entire blood cultures, oleuropein glycoside and caffeic acid diminished the generation of IL1β without influencing IL-6 focus, while kaempferol decreased IFNγ production [16]. A portion subordinate hindrance of IFNγ age by kaempferol has been found in murine spleen cells and T-cell lines as well. In a model course of action of irritation, LPS-treated BALB/c mice, and furthermore in the human monocyte cell line THP-1, the treatment with olive vegetation water, particularly rich in polyphenols, diminished TNFα creation. At long last, an ongoing clinical trial, performed in stable coronary illness patients, gave intriguing proof that the utilization of polyphenol-enhanced additional virgin olive oil is related with diminished IL-6 and C-responsive protein articulation [17, 18].

Polyphenols Modulate Nitric Oxide Synthase Family

Nitric oxide (NO), a cellular mediator of physiological and obsessive procedures, is integrated from L-arginine by NO synthase family, including endothelial (eNOS), neuronal (nNOS) and inducible isoforms. eNOS and nNOS are constitutively communicated in the body, while iNOS is an inducible protein exceedingly communicated by inflammation stimuli. In spite of the fact that the little measure of NO blended by eNOS and nNOS is fundamental to keep up typical body function (*i.e.*, homeostasis), a noteworthy increment of NO combination by iNOS takes part in the inflammatory process and acts synergistically with other inflammatory mediators. Along these lines, intensifies that can decrease iNOS-interceded NO generation might be alluring as anti-inflammatory agents; consequently, the impacts of polyphenols on iNOS action have been seriously contemplated. Catechin, EGC, naringenin, and fisetin stifled NO generation in RAW 264.7 macrophages and LPS-or PMA-empowered human fringe blood mononuclear cells [19]. The outcomes acquired up to this point propose that polyphenols restrain NO discharge by stifling NOS articulation or potentially action (Fig. **2**). Specifically, an assortment of flavonoids, including apigenin, luteolin, kaempferol, myricetin, and genistein, downregulate NO generation as well as iNOS articulation and movement in inflammatory cells [20].

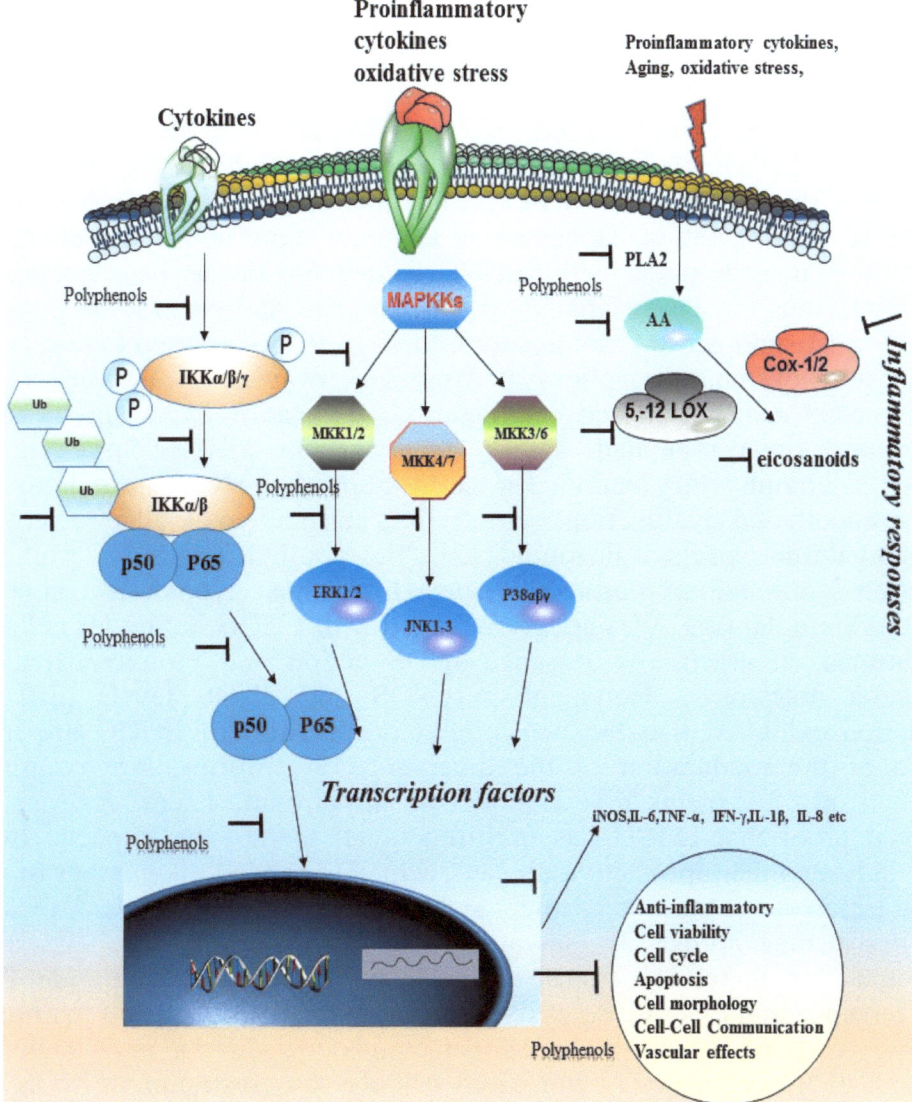

Fig. (2). Possible facts of exploit of polyphenols within inflammatory cascade.

Quercetin has been appeared to upset NO age in LPS/cytokine-treated macrophages or macrophage-like cells by coordinating iNOS protein explanation and mRNA translation. The anti-inflammatory impacts of tea catechins could be connected by differential change of the three particular NOS isoforms. Undoubtedly, epigallocatechin-3-gallate (EGCG) and distinctive catechins stifled the acknowledgment of iNOS mRNA and activity in rodent cell lines after treatment with LPS or IFNγ [10]. The hindrance of iNOS interpretation appears to happen by counteracting binding of NFκB to the promoter of the iNOS expression, accordingly inactivating it. Quite, EGCG applied its impact on iNOS articulation and action by lessening their movement through focused restraint of the binding of arginine and tetrahydrobiopterin. What's more, the gallate structure of this catechin has been appeared to be imperative for its activity. By differentiate, the organization of EGCG to rodent aortic rings incited a dosage subordinate vasorelaxation happening at the same time with the enlistment of eNOS action in endothelial cells. EGCG-incited eNOS has been proposed to create NO, thus to enact guanylate cyclase and deliver cyclic guanosine monophosphate and cause vasorelaxation through PI3K-, protein kinase A-, and Akt-subordinate signaling pathways. Moreover, cyanidin-3-glucoside (Cy3G) initiates eNOS articulation and heightens NO generation by means of an Src-extracellular signal-regulated kinase 1/2-Sp1 (Src-ERK1/2-Sp1) signaling pathway in bovine-artery endothelial cells. Expanded eNOS articulation may enhance endothelial dysfunction, settle pulse, and anticipate atherosclerosis as long haul gainful impacts of flavonoids [21]. Besides, EGCG is a powerful cancer prevention agent and neuroprotective specialist against hypoxia-ischemia (HI)-instigated brain damage. Westar rats managed with EGCG before HI enlistment demonstrated an essentially lessened iNOS action and protein articulation, however a noteworthy increment in eNOS and nNOS levels [22]. This information exhibited that the neuroprotective impacts of EGCG are in part because of the modulation of the diverse NOS isoforms. An examination performed in a transgenic mouse model of amyotrophic lateral sclerosis gave additional proof that EGCG has multifunctional therapeutic impacts. In fact, EGCG indicated neuroprotective impacts, which expanded the number of motor neurons lessened microglial enactment and diminished protein levels of iNOS and NFκB in the spinal cords [23]. Flavonoids might be restorative specialists against type-1 and -2 diabetes process. Specifically, quercetin, epicatechin, and EGCG have been appeared to apply defensive impact on β-cells by various instruments, including hindering the streptozotocin-actuated NO production and checking the IL1β-and IFNγ-intervened cytotoxicity likely by restraining iNOS gene expression [24].

Procyanidin crude extract, a blend of polyphenols acquired from grape seeds, essentially repressed the overproduction of NO in a dosage and a time-subordinate way by decreasing iNOS mRNA and protein levels [25]. Prominently, trimeric and longer oligomeric-rich procyanidin divisions from the concentrate hindered iNOS production, while the monomeric structures, catechin and epicatechin, did not; this demonstrated the level of polymerization is essential in deciding procyanidin impacts [26]. So also, a few reports have exhibited that EVOO phenolics, for example, oleuropein, hydroxytyrosol, caffeic corrosive, and tyrosol, can distinctively adjust the creation of NO in actuated cell lines, contingent upon the fixation and concoction structure. In an intriguing *in vivo* study, mice were treated with a hydroxytyrosol-rich concentrate arranged from olive factory wastewater. The outcomes showed that hydroxytyrosol upgraded the protection from oxidative stress and weaken NO-prompted cytotoxicity in separated cerebrum cells. This information fortify the promising biologic impacts of EVOO, recommending that the neuroprotective impacts of oral hydroxytyrosol admission may add to the lower rate of neurodegenerative diseases, as saw in the Mediterranean zone [27].

Polyphenols Interact with The Mitogen-Activated Protein Kinase Pathway

Regardless of its central part in the inflammation-related gene articulation, NFκB, a translation factor, requires help from other arrangement particular interpretation factors, among which are the mitogen-initiated protein kinases (MAPKs). MAPKs constitute a group of Ser/Thr kinases, which manage essential cell forms, including cell development, multiplication, passing, and separation by balancing genes translation in light of changes in the cell condition and constitute upstream controllers of interpretation factor exercises. The MAPK signaling is a three-tiered cascade. Mammals express at least four distinctly regulated groups of MAPKs: ERK-1/2, c-Jun amino-terminal kinase (JNK) 1/2/3, p38-MAPK α/β/δ/γ, and ERK5, which are activated by specific MAPK kinases (MKK), such as MEK1/2 for ERK1/2, MKK3/6 for p38, MKK4/7 (JNKK1/2) for JNKs, and MEK5 for ERK5. Each MKK, however, can be activated, in turn, by more than one MKK kinases, increasing the complexity and diversity of MAPK signaling [28 - 30]. The signaling specificity is likewise controlled by control of scaffolding proteins, which can sequester and protect signaling parts and direct them to particular subcellular limitations, improving the signal flux and intervening crosstalk with different pathways. Among the MAPK families, mitogens and development factors oftentimes actuate the ERK1/2 course, though stress and inflammation comprise key triggers for the JNK and p38 course, a portion of the time implied as pressure actuated protein kinases. Expanding action of MAPKs and their relationship in the control of the union of aggravation center individuals, at both understanding and elucidation levels, make them potential concentrations for novel anti-inflammatory therapeutics. To this end, preliminary preclinical data suggests that inhibitors that objective JNK and p38 falls and inhibitor κB (IκB) kinase β show anti-inflammatory action, demonstrating an unpredictable collaboration amongst MAPK and NFκB in the control of the inflammatory reaction. As of late, phenolic mixes have been appeared to balance MAPK pathway by following up on a few stages of the initiation course and thus on downstream effectors (Fig. 2) [10, 31]. Polyphenols, for example, kaempferol, chrysin, apigenin, and luteolin, by restraining every one of the three mitogen-enacted protein kinase, ERK, JNK and p38, exercises have been appeared to be dynamic inhibitors of TNFα-animated ICAM-1 articulation in respiratory epithelial cells [32, 33]. By differentiating, in LPS-enacted mouse macrophages, the pretreatment with luteolin obstructed the TNF-α discharge by restraining ERK1/2 and p38, yet not JNK1/2 phosphorylation, recommending a specificity of the polyphenol movement likely relying upon cell composes, phenolic chemical structure and fixation. Reliable with this theory, in actuated THP-1 human monocytes cell line, quercetin and catechin diminished oxidative stress and repressed an extensive variety of proinflammatory genes by applying diverse administrative consequences for the MAPK pathways. In particular, quercetin demonstrated an inhibitory impact on ERK, JNK, and their phosphorylated forms, while catechin hindered p38, JNK, and their phosphorylated forms. In addition, in LPS-treated murine macrophages, quercetin smothered the interpretation of TNFα by restraining the phosphorylation and initiation of JNK/SAPK, however hindered the generation of TNFα by repressing ERK1/2 phosphorylation and p38 MAPK action. An *in vitro* consider exhibited that cyanidin-3-O-glucoside hindered both ERK-1/2 initiation and IκBα debasement and along these lines iNOS expression in a fixation subordinate way. Besides, the examination gave prove that cyanidin-3-O-glucoside could apply its inhibitory impact by attenuating IκBα debasement through ERK-1/2, by straightforwardly hindering ERK-1/2 actuation, or by the two components in the meantime. Delphinidin and cyanidin could square vascular endothelial development factor (VEGF) discharge invigorated by the platelet inferred development factor (PDGF(AB)), by forestalling actuation of p38 and JNK MAPKs in human aortic vascular smooth muscle cells [10].

The broadly considered EGCG has been appeared to inspire a hostile to MAPK action ready to smother the production of a few pro-inflammatory cytokines in various cell writes. In LPS-initiated murine macrophages, EGCG kept the IL-12 production by hindering phosphorylation of p38 MAPK, enlarging phosphorylation of p44/p42 ERK, and nuclear protein authoritative to the NFκB site. In osteoblast-like MC3T3-E1 cells and additionally in essential refined mouse osteoblasts, EGCG fundamentally decreased the endothelin1-incited amalgamation of IL-6 by stifling p44/p42 MAPK and MEK1/2 phosphorylation [10, 34]. In addition, through particular phosphorylation of p38 MAPK, EGCG shielded ordinary human salivary acinar cells from TNFα-actuated cytotoxicity. EGCG may likewise give a level of security, mostly interceded through the enactment of MAPK components, against immune system incited tissue damage in Sjogren's disorder, a lymphocytic invasion of the salivary and lachrymal organs related with the destruction of the secretory capacities. At last, an intriguing *in vivo* mouse study exhibited that organization of EGCG restrained the statement of COX-2 incited by the tumor promotor 12-O-tetradecanoylphorbol-13-acetic acid derivation in the skin by hindering the initiation of p38 MAPK and DNA-authoritative of NFκB. Both catechin and quercetin take an interest to the restraint of plasminogen activator inhibitor 1 (PAI-1) genes articulation by actuating the MAPKs, p38, ERK1/2, and JNK, in a time- and dose-dependent, in human coronary artery endothelial cells. In general, the modulator impacts of polyphenols on signaling pathways are affected by their fixation as showed for quercetin, which could restrain the arrival of recently combined IL-6 by lessening p38 and PKC-θ phosphorylation in a measurements subordinate way in IL--stimulated human leukemic cells and human umbilical cord blood-derived refined mast cells. All in all, phenolic mixes ready to hinder MAPK pathways could be viewed as potential therapeutic agents against inflammatory processes [4, 35].

Polyphenols Modulate NFκB Pathway

Since their disclosure, NFκB/Rel interpretation factors have been suspected to assume a key part in chronic and acute inflammatory diseases. In fact, NFκB assumes a significant part in immune, inflammatory, stress, proliferative, and apoptotic reactions of a cell to countless. NFκB organize the enlistment of an extensive variety of genes encoding pro-inflammatory cytokines, chemokines, adhesion molecule, acute-phase proteins, immunoreceptors, growth factors, and inducible enzymes *e.g.*, VEGF, COX-2, MMPs, iNOS, and all molecules involved in inflammation, but not in angiogenesis and cell proliferation, adhesion, migration, and invasion [36, 37]. The hindrance of NFκB is by and large idea a helpful methodology for treatment of the inflammatory disorder, and this pathway is a vital and appealing remedial focus for compounds selectively interfering with it. Ongoing information recommend that dietary polyphenols can adjust signal transduction pathways to move their profitable effects. The NFκB/Rel family comprises of five individuals, in particular p65, RelB, c-Rel, NFκB1, and NFκB2, all made out of individuals from the Rel group of DNA-restricting proteins that perceive a typical sequined theme. NFκB is a dimer, traditionally including a p50 subunit and a trans-actuating subunit p65 yet others variations additionally happen. In nonstimulated cells, NFκB is sequestered in the cytoplasm in a latent non-DNA-restricting structure related with the IκBs, including IκBα, IκBβ, IκBγ, IκBε, Bcl-3, and antecedents p100 and p105 [10, 38]. On cell incitement with different NFκB inducers, the IKK complex quickly phosphorylates IκB on two serine buildups, focusing on the inhibitor proteins for ubiquitination and consequent debasement by the ubiquitin proteasome pathway. The IKK contains two catalytic subunits, IKKα and IKKβ, and the regulatory subunit NFκB essential modifier (NEMO or IKKγ).

The discharged NFκB dimer would then be able to translocate into the nucleus and initiates the statement of different genes. The actuated translation of NFκB is kept up through constant degradation of IκB, supported by an extracellular jolt, recommending that the gathering and debasement of IκB is a mechanism permitting the direction of NFκB. An assortment of other signaling events, including the phosphorylation of NFκB, the hyperphosphorylation of IKK, and handling of NFκB precursors, give extra components adjusting the level and term of NFκB movement. Polyphenols can apply their anti-inflammatory by tweaking NFκB actuation and acting at numerous steps of the enactment processes (Fig. **2**). Specifically, the impact of EGCG on the NFκB pathway has been broadly contemplated showing its inhibitory consequences for NFκB acquired by balancing the enactment of IKK and the degradation of IκBα. A fascinating *in vivo* study in rats demonstrated that EGCG particularly attenuated the myocardial damage after ischemia and reperfusion [39, 40]. This cardioprotection was related with diminished IL-6, lessened actuation of IKK, decreased debasement of IκB-α and diminish in initiated NFκB levels, with ensuing restraint of the inflammatory procedure at the early occasion of the interpretation intervened by the NFκB pathway. Also, EGCG, by restraining IκBα debasement and by blocking DNA-binding of NFκB, abrogated IL-12p40 production and iNOS articulation in LPS-enacted murine macrophages. EGCG hindered the phosphorylation of IκBα by TNFα-actuated IKK in fetal rat intestinal epithelial cell line. This may happen as an immediate impact on IKK or by meddling with the communication of IKK with IκBα [41, 42]. Eminently, the gallate assemble was practically fundamental for restraint of IKK movement, and the nearness of the catechin structure drastically upgraded this impact. In reality, IKK has all the earmarks of being a key control point for NFκB actuation and might be viewed as a reasonable focus for tweaking NFκB-intervened cell reactions. In initiated RAW 264.7 macrophages, the surge of iNOS mRNA and protein was insistently curbed by a mix of polyphenols got from grape seeds, likely through the decline of nuclear NFκB (p65) and of IκBα mRNA age. Furthermore, pretreatment of PMA-incited T cells with epicatechin and catechin reduced NFκB activity. This effect was likely procured by thwarting the phosphorylation of IKKβ, the subsequent defilement of IκBα, and the ensuing authoritative of NFκB to its DNA ascension progression. As such, the adjustment of the NFκB sanctioning course by flavonoids can occur at in front of timetable and late stages [43].

Exceptionally, the outcomes gained in RAW 264.7 macrophages treated with IFNγ and gliadin to prompt the provocative system. In these telephones, quercetin, tyrosol, and lycopene curbed the outpouring of iNOS, COX-2, and ace fiery qualities by keeping the atomic translocation of p50 and p65 subunits of NFκB, and the incitation of flag transduction and activator of interpretation (STAT) 1α and interferon regulative factor (IRF1) .Albeit moreover examinations are required evaluate the probability of envisioning or killing gliadin cytotoxicity through dietary confirmation, these results suggest that lycopene, quercetin, and tyrosol speak to potential nontoxic administrators for the control of intestinal aggravation in celiac sickness by keeping the inception of basic flag transduction pathways. Furthermore, the invaluable calming impacts connected by quercetin, both *in vitro* and *in vivo*, have all the earmarks of being a direct result of the limitation of IκBα protein phosphorylation, which by discouraging the institution of the NFκB pathway, neutralize the statement of cytokines and inducible NOS. Likewise, in impelled human pole cell line, quercetin diminished the outflow of star incendiary cytokines TNFα, IL-1β, IL-6, and IL-8 by upsetting the debasement of IκBα and the atomic translocation of p65, as such blocking NFκB order. Also, a progressing ex vivo consider showed that quercetin upset TNFα-prompted verbalization of ace incendiary cytokines interferon-inducible protein (IP) 10 and macrophage provocative protein (MIP) 2 in fundamental murine little intestinal epithelial cells. Quercetin applied this affect by preventing the enrollment of the NFκB cofactor CREB-limiting protein (CBP)/p300 (histone acetyl transferase) to the IP-10 and MIP-2 quality advertisers, recommending that quercetin may especially impact chromatin updating at local quality advertisers. In LPS-and IFNγ-treated BV-2 microglia, quercetin smothered NO age and iNOS quality interpretation by diminishing the authorization of IKK, NFκB, starting protein-1 (AP-1), STAT-1, and IRF-1. Also, quercetin prevented DNA-limiting activity of NFκB in a measurements subordinate way. These results prescribe that quercetin should give remedial focal points to covering of fiery related neuronal harm in neurodegenerative sicknesses. In the human hepatocyte-surmised Chang liver cells agonized with a cytokine blend, the limitation of mRNA verbalization of iNOS, COX-2, and CRP, started by quercetin and kaempferol, was connected with a decreased assembly of phosphorylated IκBα and IKKα and the obstacle of NFκB authorization. The calming activity of hydroxytyrosol in LPS-impelled murine macrophages was controlled by forestalling NFκB, STAT - 1α, and IRF-1 incitation, dependably limiting iNOS and COX-2 quality verbalization. By decreasing NFκB incitation, tyrosol propelled tantamount ramifications for NO discharge and COX-2 verbalization in PMA-started RAW 264.7 macrophages [44, 45]. Additionally, in LPS-invigorated human umbilical vein endothelial cells, hydroxytyrosol, oleuropein, and resveratrol, through hindrance of NFκB enactment, stifled the statement of VCAM-1 mRNA and protein, in a fixation subordinate mold. Additionally, reporter genes tests, performed utilizing deletional VCAM1 promoter builds, showed that extra translation factors, for example, AP-1 and GATA, could take an interest to the transcriptional direction of VCAM. In rundown, previously mentioned discoveries emphatically recommend that restraint of the NFκB pathways, along one or a few stages in their enactment course, could be an imperative piece of the systems in charge of the potential advantage of these dietary natural agents [45, 46].

Utilization of nourishments rich in phenolic mixes, at as high as 1 g for every day, is viewed as sheltered and advantageous for constant infection counteractive action. Phenolic mixes are the biggest gathering of characteristic cancer prevention agents of human dieting and have direct and indirect antioxidant and anti-inflammatory activities helping mitigate the oxidative stress at the cellular level. Flow explore shows that phytochemicals, including polyphenols, are solid anti-oxidant agents and radical scavenger for ROS *in vitro*; in any case, these mixes can go about as prooxidants at high doses. Besides, such direct radical-rummaging movement or diminishing energy of polyphenols is watched just at fixations fundamentally higher than the physiological levels found *in vivo*. Collecting proof is demonstrating that the *in vivo* antioxidant and anti-inflammatory impacts of polyphenols and their metabolites emerge from their capacity of tweaking cell signaling transductions. Ongoing examinations have built up that these mixes have a critical modulatory impact on cell biomarkers identified with oxidative stress and inflammation, prompting diminished danger of numerous chronic illnesses. Later *in vitro* and *in vivo* studies have uncovered that low groupings of phenolics enhance antioxidant enzyme activities, inhibit pro-inflammatory cytokines, and straightforwardly constrict NFκB-interceded or oxidative stress prompted inflammatory signaling pathways. By investigating the science and natural chemistry of dietary polyphenols and conceivable parts and systems in oxidative stress and inflammation-related biomarkers, future endeavors in polyphenols inquire about must spotlight on expanding the bio-openness and bioavailability from handling and plan of phenolics-rich functional foods, to at last create functional foods or nutraceuticals that lessen wellbeing danger of chronic diseases through the modulatory impacts of polyphenols.

Polyphenols in Cancer

Copious epidemiological confirmation underpins that an eating regimen rich in foods grown from the ground could bring down the danger of specific malignancies. The impact has been credited partially to regular polyphenols. Moreover, various investigations have exhibited that common polyphenols could be utilized for malignancy aversion and treatment. The potential instruments incorporate antioxidant, anti-inflammation, and balance of numerous atomic occasions associated with carcinogenesis. This substance condenses the anticancer viability of major polyphenol classes, in particular flavonoids, phenolic acids, lignans, and stilbenes, and examines the potential components of activity, in view of epidemiological, *in vitro*, *in vivo*, and clinical examinations.

Anticancer Properties and Mechanisms

An ongoing report of the US National Cancer Institute assessed that the malignancy costs surpassed US$124 billion in the United States in 2010; this number will increment in the coming years as a result of populace development and maturing. In any case, more current treatments expand quiet lives by just a couple of days or months and the subsequent personal satisfaction stays indeterminate. Subsequently, the advancement of treatments that can accomplish genuine (even discrete) measures of adequacy are critically required. Therefore, regular polyphenols (as talked about underneath) may offer some expectation. Plenteous data is currently accessible on cell components by which common polyphenols may meddle with carcinogenesis and tumor development and spread. Polyphenols have been appeared to follow up on various focuses in pathways identified with cell proliferation and passing, inflammation, angiogenesis, or medication and radiation opposition. By utilizing the data in late itemized audits (Fig. 3), we offer a concise outline on the components and targets possibly more applicable considering the sub-atomic bases for disease treatment approaches. By and by, the announced impacts guaranteed for polyphenols must be deliberately assessed as one discovers contrasts (even extensive and questionable) contingent upon disease cell write, trial conditions (*in vitro* or *in vivo*), fixations, galenic plans, and nanoparticle affiliations utilized.

Natural polyphenols may enhance the viability of biotherapy. In this unique situation, polyphenols may reestablish or actuate tumor cell affectability to TRAIL-incited cell passing with no clear harmfulness toward typical cells. A fundamental paper demonstrated in 2003 by Deeb *et al.* demonstrated that curcumin upgrades TRAIL-actuated apoptosis in LNCaP cells, which are just marginally susceptible to TRAIL [47]. Also, it was accounted for that the mix of TRAIL/Apo2L and genistein was powerful in restraining pancreatic disease growth. Furthermore, in resveratrol-treated tumor cells, TNF, anti-CD95 antibodies, and TRAIL initiate a caspase-subordinate passing pathway that escapes Bcl-2-interceded restraint. Resveratrol couldn't enhance the amount of death receptors at the surface of tumor cells however prompted their redistribution into lipid pontoons and encouraged the caspase cascade actuation in light of death receptor incitement [48]. Besides, thinks about have demonstrated that resveratrol

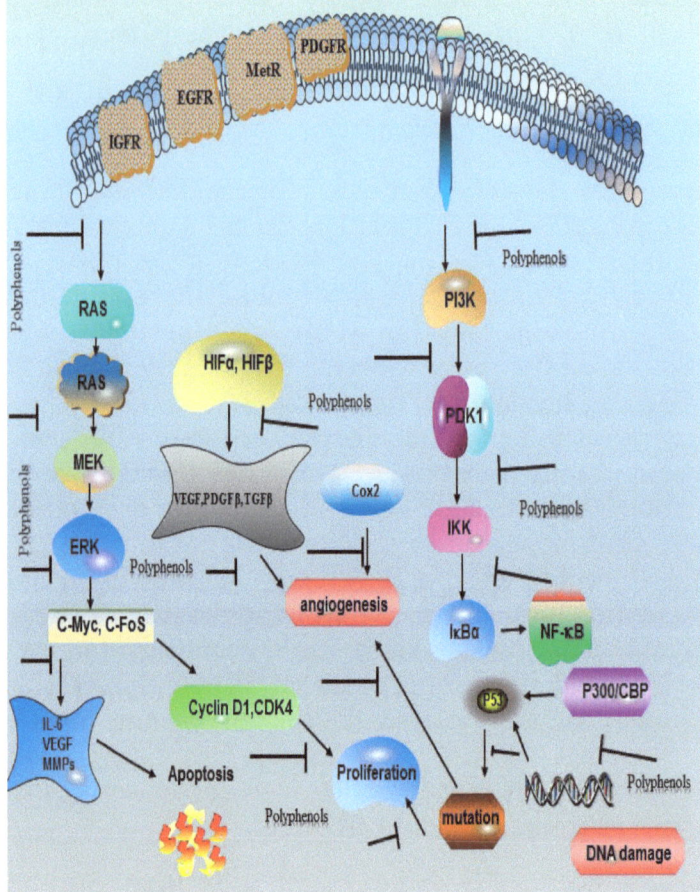

Fig. (3). Effect of polyphenols on different signaling cascades involved in cancer progression and dissemination. Polyphenols may interfere in pathways regulating tumor proliferation, apoptosis, adhesion, migration, invasion, angiogenesis, and metastasis.

is a strong sensitizer of tumor cells for TRAIL-initiated apoptosis through p53-autonomous acceptance of p21 and p21-interceded cell-cycle capture related to surviving consumption. In any case, overexpression of Bcl-2 or FADD-DN did not meddle with resveratrol-interceded cell-cycle capture or survivin exhaustion, yet obstructed the arrival of cytochrome c and Smac from mitochondria into the cytosol and upgraded caspase initiation and apoptosis on consolidated treatment with resveratrol and TRAIL, showing that overexpression of Bcl-2 or FADD-DN decoupled the impact of resveratrol on the cell cycle and apoptosis [48]. In this way, the mix of TRAIL and resveratrol might be incapable in tumors with improved Bcl-2 articulation or damaged passing receptor signaling. All things considered, quercetin was found to improve TRAIL-intervened apoptosis in colon cancer cells by prompting the aggregation of death receptors in lipid rafts [49]. In addition, in androgen heartless prostate cancer cells, resveratrol downregulated the outflow of Bcl-2, Bcl-X(L) and survivin and upregulated that of Bax, Bak, PUMA, Noxa, Bim, and the passing receptors TRAIL-R1/DR4 and TRAIL-R2/DR5, steady with a part of polyphenols in upregulation of death receptors. The treatment of prostate cancer cells with resveratrol brought about the age of ROS, translocation of Bax to mitochondria and diminish in mitochondrial film potential, the arrival of mitochondrial proteins (cytochrome c, Smac/DIABLO, and AIF) to the cytosol, enactment of effector caspase-3 and caspase-9, and acceptance of apoptosis [50].

Additionally tries demonstrated that curcumin restrained growth of LNCaP xenografts in naked mice by prompting apoptosis and hindering expansion, and sharpened these tumors to experience apoptosis by TRAIL [51]. In xenograft tumors, curcumin upregulated the declaration of TRAIL-R1/DR4, TRAIL-R2/DR5, Bax, Bak, p21/WAF1, and p27/KIP1 and restrained the actuation of NF-κB and its genes items, for example, cyclin D1, VEGF, uPA, MMP-2, MMP-9, Bcl-2, and Bcl-XL169. In this manner, the direction of death receptors and Bcl-2 relatives and inactivation of NF-κB may sharpen TRAIL-safe LNCaP xenografts. Moreover, curcumin repressed angiogenesis in tumors and coursing endothelial growth factor receptor 2-positive endothelial cells in mice. Besides, EGCG sharpened LNCaP cells to TRAIL-intervened apoptosis and synergistically repressed biomarkers related with angiogenesis and metastasis. Extra trials uncovered that curcumin repressed the phosphorylation of PI3K, AKT and mTOR in LNCaP cells; the hindrance of PI3K/AKT pathway prompted FOXO transcriptional action, bringing about the enlistment of Bim, TRAIL, p27/KIP1, DR4, and DR5 and restraint of cyclin D1 [51].

Based on the capacity of resveratrol to restrain tumor growth, metastasis, and angiogenesis and improve the remedial capability of TRAIL, resveratrol alone or in blend with TRAIL could be utilized for the administration of prostate cancer. Taken together, a developing assortment of trial prove recommends that polyphenols may sharpen TRAIL-safe cancer cells and expand TRAIL-actuated apoptosis in cancer cells with no evident poisonous toward typical cells. Nonetheless, these impacts may rely upon the cell type, the polyphenolic exacerbate, the treatment conditions, as well as the tumor microenvironment conditions [52].

1.3.2. Anticancer Effect of Polyphenol Structure and Activity

The connections amongst structure and anticancer action of certain polyphenols have been recorded. A superior comprehension of the structure-action relationship not just aides in settling the method of activities of the naturally occurring polyphenols yet in addition gives the premise of the sane outline of new and proficient polyphenols, which might be utilized as potential helpful operators. Larsen and partners utilized atomic docking to research how tea catechins may connect with the hepatocyte development factor receptor (otherwise called Met), which is regularly deregulated in different kinds of growth and is related with poor guess. The outcomes demonstrated that the gallate-containing catechins, including epicatechin gallate (ECG), EGCG, and gallocatechin gallate (GCG), fit positively into the Met-restricting site with hydrogen bonding set up between the aromatic hydroxyl gatherings of the gallate moiety and the spine NH of two Met kinase dynamic locales, to be specific Met1160 and Pro1158. By differentiate, tea catechins without the gallate gather did not communicate with Met1160 but rather display proclivity for the spine NH of Asp1222. This finding proposes that the gallate amass is a key auxiliary component for authoritative of tea catechins to the Met kinase domain33 [53, 54]. In a very recent study on the molecular structure–activity relationship of dietary polyphenols, Cerezo *et al.* known the structure options of a range of polyphenols that contributed to the variations within the IC50 values for the inhibition of VEGF-induced VEGFR-2 phosphorylation, as well as enclosed the (i) C2=C3 bond (in quercetin, luteolin, and orobol), (ii) 4-oxo cluster (in quercetin, luteolin, eriodictyol and taxifolin), (iii) electric charge (in cyanidin), and (iv) B-ring position within the C ring. for instance, the authors found that quercetin exhibited a 250-fold lower IC50 price compared with (+)-catechin, whose structure doesn't contain either the C2=C3 bond or 4-oxo cluster, suggesting that the presence of the C2=C3 bond or 4-oxo cluster powerfully contributes to the inhibition of VEGF-induced VEGFR-2 activation [55]. Shin and associates played out the quantitative structure-activity relationship concentrate to decide the auxiliary properties of 27 blended polyphenols with 8 scaffolds, which caused cell-cycle capture at the G1 stage to a fluctuating degree in the human colorectal cancer cell line HCT116 [56]. Based on the aftereffects of near molecular field examination and relative molecular similitude file investigation, a few moieties that were fundamental for the G1 cell-cycle capture were distinguished. In addition, the organic model of activity ponders uncovered that one of the combined polyphenols incited interpretation factor p53-interceded upregulation of the cell-cycle inhibitor P21, while quieting p53 brought about a diminishing in cell-cycle capture, recommending that the antitumor action of polyphenols is related with p53-intervened hindrance of cell-cycle movement at the G1 stage. By using a similar approach, Shin and coworkers also established that polyphenols manner cinnamaldehyde scaffold showed marked inhibitory effects on the clonogenicity of cisplatin-resistant A2780/Cis ovarian cancer cells [55].

Preclinical Studies on Anti-Metastatic Activities

On a fundamental level, genes articulation profiles and cellular heterogeneity of an essential tumor are saved in its far off metastasis; consequently, numerous sub-atomic pathways advancing tumorigenesis additionally advance metastasis. Notwithstanding, ongoing exploration has uncovered that the utilization of a similar remedial operator created divergent consequences for essential tumor development and metastatic cancer, recommending minor yet vital contrasts between essential tumors and metastases. For instance, treatment with 100 mg/kg RPI-1, a c-Met inhibitor, did not smother the improvement of subcutaneous H460 lung malignant growth xenografts, yet diminished metastases by 57%. In the course of recent decades, the potential cancer chemopreventive and anticancer exercises of different polyphenols have been broadly described in an assortment of preclinical models of human cancer. Despite the fact that most of the examinations have concentrated on the capacity of polyphenols to moderate tumor development and additionally the components included, various investigations utilizing refined cells and creature models have uncovered the inhibitory impact of polyphenols on tumor cell invasion and migration, proposing the capability of polyphenols against cancer metastases [57].

An ongoing report has demonstrated that piceatannol, a stillbenoid show in grapes and wine, stifled the invasion of AH109A hepatoma cells crosswise over culture rodent mesothelial cell monolayer in a focus subordinate way finished a scope of fixations from 12.5 to 200 mol/L. In another *in vitro* study, Lee and partners demonstrated the inhibitory effect of phyllanthus evacuates on the attack and relocation of both A549 human lung adenocarcinoma cells and MCF-7 human chest carcinoma cells by using storm cellar layer remove covered transwell intrusion measure, scratch wound-recovering test, and transwell movement analyze. An *in vivo* contemplate coordinated using a B16-F10 melanoma lung metastasis show exhibited that oligonol, a polyphenol containing 15.7% polyphenol monomer and 13.3% polyphenol dimer, basically hindered the advancement of B16-F10 lung metastases and extended the survival of metastatic tumor - bearing C57BL/6 mice. Hitherto, various examinations have investigated the components hidden the counter metastatic action of polyphenols, demonstrating that distinctive polyphenols cannot just hinder growth metastasis by meddling with a similar signaling pathway driving the multistep procedure of the metastatic course yet in addition inactivate diverse prometastatic factors [58].

Polyphenols on Epithelial–Mesenchymal Transition

Expanded epithelial– mesenchymal transition (EMT) and cell relocation and intrusion capacities of cancer cells assume critical roles in the metastatic procedure of malignancy. Several tests have analyzed polyphenols capacity to target assorted pathways related with carcinogenesis and malignant growth movement.

In the first place noted amid embryogenesis, EMT is a cell reinventing process changing nonmobile epithelial-like cells into portable mesenchymal-like cells. Over the previous decade, an energy on the part of EMT in disease movement and metastasis has advanced quickly. Numerous examinations utilizing as a part of vitro and *in vivo* models have unmistakably shown that a transient EMT process is one of the main thrusts of invasion and metastases of carcinomas (*i.e.*, epithelial tumors), which speak to roughly 90% of every single human tumor. At the cell level, a couple of key cell events are considered signs of the EMT system, including a change from the cuboidal morphology to the hub shaped morphology and the loss of epithelial cell-cell adhesion and apical-basal furthest point going to with the acquiring of increasingly motile and meddling behavior and front– raise limit [59]. At the molecular level, the start and culmination of EMT is managed by a few exceedingly planned molecular occasions including (i) changes in the statement of cell-surface proteins, for instance, the sorted out downregulation of the bond cell-surface protein E-cadherin and upregulation of proteins characterizing the mesenchymal phenotype, including vimentin, N-cadherin and α-smooth muscle actin; (ii) actuation of EMT-inciting translation factors, for example, the zinc finger proteins from the Snail superfamily, zinc finger and E-box-restricting proteins from the ZEB family (and the Twist bHLH proteins; and (iii) revamping of the actin cytoskeleton [60]. A few examinations have exhibited the impact of different natural polyphenols on EMT in light of the perceptions of diminished articulation of mesenchymal markers and the expanded articulation of epithelial markers.

The Hsieh lab detailed that the dark tea separate (BTE), containing numerous bioactive phenolic mixes including gallic corrosive, gallocatechin, and EGCG, hindered the invasion of invasion of SCC-4 human tongue squamous epithelial cells. This inhibitory effect was proposed to be connected with BTE started upregulation of epithelial markers, for instance, E-cadherin, and downregulation of mesenchymal markers, for example, SNAI1 and vimentin. Also, when SCC-9 cells were treated with EGCG alone, the verbalization dimensions of phosphorylated FAK, phosphorylated steroid receptor coactivator (Src), and vimentin were downregulated in a focus subordinate way [61]. FAK, a nonreceptor tyrosine kinase is a noteworthy restricting accomplice of Src. Enactment of the FAK– Src complex starts a course of phosphorylation occasions and in this way triggers a few signaling pathways, which in the end prompt diverse cellular reactions, including EMT [62].

A Sonenshein lab examine showed that EGCG propelled a less obtrusive profile of value explanation in Her-2/neu-overexpressing NF639 mouse mammary tumor cells, as displayed by upregulated epithelial genes, including E-cadherin, c - catenin, estrogen receptor an (ERa), and MTA3, and downregulated pro-invasive master regulators Snail1 and Snail3. EGCG additionally prompted the outflow of FOXO3a, which was appeared to instigate E-cadherin articulation through ERa signaling and avert TGFβ1-initiated EMT in NMuMG untransformed, deified mouse mammary epithelial cells. In addition, green tea in drinking water protected E-cadherin articulation in 7,12-dimethylbenz (a)anthracene (DMBA)- actuated rodent mammary ductal carcinoma *in situ in vivo*. In addition, EGCG downregulated the statement of co-expressed tumor-promoting genes, c-Rel and CK2; hindered articulation of the EMT controller Slug and its inducer fragrant hydrocarbon receptor [63, 64], and turned around the intrusive phenotype actuated by either DMBA or the mix of c-Rel and CK2 [65]. Another examination to researched on the effects of EGCG on tumourigenicity, migration, and intrusion of TW01 and TW06 nasopharyngeal carcinoma cells demonstrated that EGCG limited circle course of action and debilitated prominent like phenotypes described by EMT in cells created in without serum non adherent societies. EGCG were appeared to restrain the outflow of vimentin and Snail, however upregulate the statement of E-cadherin, proposing that EGCG hinders the EMT-included starting metastasis signaling [66]. Phenolic secoiridoids in additional virgin olive oil proficiently curbed the capacity of TGFβ to reconstruct MCF-7 chest cancer cells at the transcriptional level to express characteristics encoding EMT drivers, for instance, SNAI2, TCF4, VIM and FN, however fail to complete the EMT reversal program. S100A4, a cytoplasmic protein having a place with the S100 calcium-restricting protein family, is a known EMT middle person. Trial contemplates have connected the S100A4 gene product to the metastatic phenotype of tumor cells, anyway clinical insistence has demonstrated an association between' s up regulated S100A4 articulation and poor guess in a couple of growth forms. Studies have demonstrated that the counter interruption and unfriendly to metastatic exercises of two or three polyphenols are associated with their inhibitory impact on S100A4 explanation [67]. A past *in vivo* think about utilizing transgenic adenocarcinoma of the mouse prostate (TRAMP) demonstrate demonstrated that oral utilization of green tea downregulated S100A4 articulation and reestablished E-cadherin articulation in the prostate of the TRAMP display, bringing about a noteworthy abatement in the proportion of S100A4-to-E-cadherin articulation in mouse prostate tissues. The prenylated flavonoid xanthohumol has been appeared to weaken tumor cell-interceded rupturing of lymph endothelial boundary and avoid tumor cell intravasation and metastasis by repressing the statement of ICAM-1, paxillin, S100A4, and selectin E and decreasing the action of MLC2, NF-κB, and CYP1A1 [59].

Polyphenols in Clinical Trials

Albeit clinical trials researching the natural polyphenols for cancer treatment are fundamentally required, the aftereffects of clinical investigations with polyphenolic mixes have not been empowering. As per the indexed lists on ClinicalTrials.gov utilizing catchphrases "polyphenols" and "cancer," various clinical trials on the assessment of chemopreventive and chemotherapeutic impacts of different natural polyphenols are in progress or have been finished as of late. A considerable lot of these investigations have investigated the impacts of polyphenols in patients with beginning period cancers, though a couple have surveyed in patients with cutting edge cancer. For example, a randomized pilot arrange I preliminary is coordinated to survey whether quercetin overhauls the take-up of green tea polyphenols (GTPs) in the prostate tissue of men taking green tea extricate (GTE) and encountering radical prostatectomy. Given that quercetin was found to update the anticancer effects of green tea in preclinical examinations, this preliminary is expected to pass on the preclinical results forward in a transient human intervention consider. The most recent examination, a twofold visually impaired, fake treatment controlled randomized stage II preliminary, was directed to evaluate the effect of a polyphenol-rich whole sustenance supplement on the prostate specific antigen positive prostate cancer progression in 199 men. The intervention consisted of consumption of a tablet, containing 100 mg of broccoli powder, 100 mg of pomegranate whole fruit powder, and 20 mg of green tea 5:1 extract, three times a day [68].

The outcomes showed a huge here and now, great impact on the rate increment in PSA levels in men with prostate cancer, made do with dynamic observation or cautious reconnaissance for a PSA backslide after radical medicines, following ingestion of this all around endured, particular mix of concentrated sustenance. By differentiate, the outcomes from other clinical trials on green tea in the treatment of prostate cancer were poor. In a stage II trial of green tea for the treatment of patients with androgen-free metastatic prostate carcinoma, ingestion of non-standardized green tea powder neglected to instigate target tumor reaction characterized as a $\geq 50\%$ decrease in the gauge PSA levels. Just 1 of 42 demonstrated a short lived half reduction in the standard PSA level, which was not maintained past 2 months. Likewise, in a solitary establishment, planned, single-arm clinical trial announced by Choan *et al.*, the impact of an institutionalized GTE (250 mg/day) on PSA level or quantifiable pointers of ailment movement was assessed in patients with hormone unmanageable prostate cancer [69]. Of the 15 patients who finished in any event periods of treatment, 9 included dynamic ailment inside 2 months of beginning treatment, though 6 created dynamic sickness after extra 1– 4 months of treatment. Generally speaking, discoveries from those clinical examinations recommend that a bigger example estimate is expected to demonstrate a measurably critical contrast in fundamental biomarkers. What's more, polyphenols other than green tea ought to be investigated for the treatment of patients with prostate carcinoma [69].

Metastasis introduces the most impressive test to the effective treatment of malignancy. Numerous investigations have exhibited the capacities of natural polyphenols to smother tumor cell invasion and migration and metastasis arrangement in preclinical models. An expanding research exertion has been committed to recognizing potential systems hidden the counter metastatic activity of natural polyphenols. When all is said in done, those molecular and cellular instruments incorporate downregulation of MMP articulation, tweak of EMT controllers, impedance with Met signaling, hindrance of NF-κB interceded interpretation, and other conceivable components. Given the requirement for elective and less poisonous therapeutics for metastatic tumor, natural polyphenols' insignificant fundamental lethality and wide achieving systems of activity may make them appropriate as adjuvants and additionally corresponding drugs for metastatic malignancy administration. Regardless of epidemiological confirmation showing the potential advantages of polyphenols against malignancy improvement and movement, the quantity of excellent clinical trials investigating the impacts of polyphenols on dynamic tumors is constrained. So far, few randomized controlled trials have assess the impacts of polyphenols on disease metastasis endpoints. Since polyphenols are probably not going to be utilized as independent anticancer specialists, the future examinations must investigate the capability of consolidating natural polyphenols with other anticancer medications as a restorative technique to block movement of metastatic cancers impervious to the standard-of-mind treatment. Before dietary suggestions of natural polyphenols or clinical trials as anti-metastatic therapeutics, a better understanding of the molecular basis of the anti-metastatic effects mediated by polyphenols is necessary to develop surrogate endpoint biomarkers that can be correlated well with the efficacy of polyphenol-involved anti-metastatic treatment [59].

Risks and Safety of Polyphenol Utilization

Most investigations of polyphenols planned to decide the defensive impacts of polyphenols against illnesses or lethal medications, and generally couple of agents have analyzed their conceivable harmfulness. No intense lethality was seen after oral organization of a grape seed proanthocyanidin separate at a dosage of 0.5 or 2 g/kg body weight to rats or mice or after organization of punicalagin (an ellagitannin display in pomegranate juice) at a measurement of 60 g/kg eating regimen to rats [70]. Be that as it may, unending nephropathy was seen in rats when high dosages of quercetin (2% or 4%) were added to their eating regimen [71]. No impact on survival times was seen in that review, while expansion of quercetin (0.1%) to the eating regimen of mice fundamentally lessened their future [72]. Some polyphenols may have cancer-causing or genotoxic impacts at high measurements or fixations [73, 74]. Caffeic corrosive, for instance, when show at a 2% level in the eating regimen, incited forestomach and kidney tumors in rats and mice [75].

Direct extrapolation of these information demonstrates obvious hazard at ordinary dietary levels. Besides, catecholestrogens are hypothesized to intervene enlistment of renal tumors by estradiol. Quercetin represses O-methylation of catecholestrogens and builds kidney convergences of 2-and 4-hydroxyestrodiol by 60-80%. This may bring about improved redox cycling of catecholestrogens and estradiol-initiated tumorigenesis [75].

The danger of devouring high measurements of polyphenols from normally polyphenol rich sustenance is low, however we should consider the negative impacts of different fixings in these nourishments, for example, cholesterol expanding fats in espresso, liquor in wine, and fat in chocolate. Sustenance can be strengthened with polyphenols, however we should make sure that they are devoured by the objective populaces for which they are outlined and not by populaces that are possibly in danger, for example, kids and pregnant ladies [75]. Dietary supplements that contain high (*i.e.* pharmacologic) measurements of polyphenols can be created. The admission of polyphenols may then effortlessly achieve abnormal states; in such cases, toxicologic testing might be required to guarantee safe levels of admission. In this regard, a current provide details regarding the evaluation of the wellbeing of botanicals and natural arrangements for use in nourishment and sustenance supplements might just apply to the field of polyphenols [76].

The sort of wellbeing assessment would rely upon the idea of the polyphenol-containing item (a nourishment, a sustenance separate, or a pure compound) and on the proposed utilize possibly prompting a huge increment in the presentation. Before human mediation trials are intended to assess the impacts of polyphenols on constant sicknesses, with the utilization of invigorated nourishments or supplements (with either nutritious or pharmacologic measurements of polyphenols), a wellbeing evaluation of the connected dosage ought to be performed, to keep deceptive examinations from being directed. Before researchers, achieve that stage, in any case, and have to collect generous information from *in vitro*, animal, and observational epidemiologic examinations with just significant structures and dosages, to attribute a potential valuable impact to aggregate or particular polyphenol consumption. There is a proverb in

Tamil even elixir turns poisonous when taken in excess. A dosage that delivers a helpful impact in cell cultures might be noxious when connected in a human setting. On the other hand, a dosage utilized as a part of a trial study may never happen in a human setting, since utilization never achieves a similar level, on the grounds that the bioavailability is low, or in light of the fact that the proper measurement never achieves the objective site. The type of the phenolic compound is additionally critical, on the grounds that phenolic mixes happen in sustenance for the most part as conjugated mixes and the substances happening in plasma and tissues are for the most part mammalian conjugates, with the exception of certain isoflavones and flavonols. These viewpoints must be considered in the outline of future trial ponders in the field of polyphenols; there is a need to endeavor to show the human circumstance all the more firmly, regardless of whether examines are gone for assessing useful or antagonistic impacts.

Epigenetics Mechanism of Polyphenols

Since James Watson and Francis Crick initially found and clarified the sub-atomic structure of the DNA twofold helix in the 1950s, the possibility that DNA encodes the genetic data that decides inherited attributes has turned out to be generally acknowledged. This thought advanced the exploration of genetics, which advanced quickly in the decades following Watson and Crick's disclosure. To date, far reaching affiliation examines have distinguished roughly 25,000 human genes as a feature of the Human Genome Project. The greater part of these genes are associated with critical biological action and vitality homeostasis, and many genes with changes and varieties are related with different human maladies. Regardless of verification that DNA is the hereditary material, the genetic foundations and variable articulation levels watched can't totally clarify the subsequent complex phenotypes. For example, monozygous twins have the same chromosomal DNA sequence, however are frequently conflicting for some characteristics or complex ailments. The idea of acquired epigenetic changes may clarify these varieties in phenotypes and marvels [77]. In 1942, the term "epigenetics" was first presented by Conrad Hal Waddington, who characterized it as the part of science that reviews the causal connections among genes and their items, which are in charge of the phenotype of an organism. Epigenetics did not initially receive much attention following the discovery of DNA. However, after lying in the shadows for several decades, the topic of epigenetics became respectable when studies of chromatin structure developed in the 1980s. Later, in 1987, Robin Holliday re-imagined epigenetic as nuclear legacy that did not depend on contrasts in DNA grouping. Epigenetics is important for integrating genetics with developmental embryology; it offers acceptable explanations for certain features and phenomena in development, including cellular differentiation and parental imprinting in mammals. Moreover, epigenetic modifications play crucial roles in developmental patterning, biological processes, and pathological progression [77].

Epigenetic Modification in Mammals

Epigenetics is the investigation of heritable changes in the direction of genes articulation without an adjustment in DNA sequence, and these progressions can happen all through the genome. Not at all like hereditary changes, epigenetic adjustments are reversible. Epigenetic legacy is presently perceived as a basic and basic system in gene direction associated with the biological procedure and cellular memory of advancement. Over the previous decades, considers have set up the atomic components of epigenetic alterations, including DNA methylation, histone changes, and microRNA (Fig. **4**). The coordinated action of these modifications with genetic changes systematically modulates gene transcription and silencing progression [77].

DNA Methylation

DNA methylation epigenetics is characterized as the investigation of heritable however reversible changes in genes articulation happening without modifications in the succession of hidden DNA. Epigenetic adjustments frequently modify genes articulation, especially articulation of tumor silencers, promoters furthermore, oncogenes crucial for cell multiplication, separation, and survival in the midst of carcinogenesis (Table **2**). Among epigenetic changes, DNA methylation is the best-mulled over modification of DNA. S-adenosyl methionine (SAM) fills in as a comprehensive methyl total promoter in the methyl trade reactions catalyzed by DNA methyltransferases (DNMTs) in the eukaryotic center. Two sorts of DNMTs are accessible in eukaryotes including the upkeep methyltransferase DNMT1 and again methyltransferases DNMT3A and DNMT3B. The support methyltransferase keep up the pre-set up examples of DNA methylation, while the all over again methyltransferases build up new examples of methylation in the completely un-methylated DNA. DNA hyper-methylation of tumor silencer genes is a fairly visit occasion in a large portion of the cancers both amid the start or the movement occasions. Gene hyper-methylation may likewise start enlistment of the methylation-subordinate DNA-restricting proteins (MBDs) to the hyper-methylated DNA destinations. The MBDs additionally help in quieting of methylated genes by enrolling repressor edifices to these areas. These proteins are usually discovered possessing the hyper-methylated gene promoters in numerous cancers. Notwithstanding the

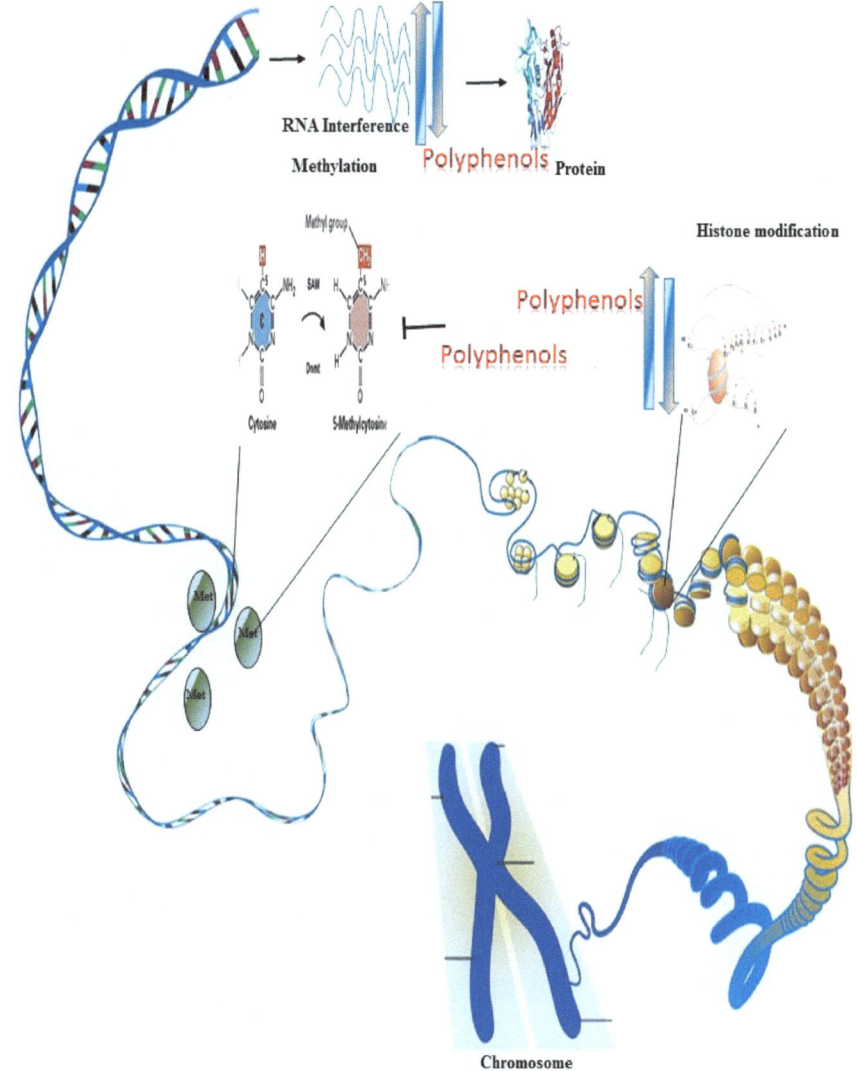

Fig. (4). Overview of epigenetic mechanisms regulating gene expression. Dietary phytochemicals impart anticancer properties through alteration in DNA methylation patterns, histone modification, and changes in non-coding RNAs levels. Up and down, arrows and inhibition.

MBDs, a transcriptional zone in DNMT1 starts histone deacetylase (HDACs) and other chromatin redesigning proteins to the target regions that can change acetylation and methylation status of histones, along these lines impeding transcriptional access to the chromatin. An instance of such surprising methylation-mediated genes quieting was shown ultra violet B (UVB) radiation-provoked skin tumors in the SKH-1 mouse appear. This examination clearly demonstrated the positive association between transcriptional limitation of the tumor silencer genes p16INK4a and RASSF1A and the UVB-intervened hyper-methylation and coming about enlistment of MeCP2 and MBDs at genes managerial territories in skin malignant growth exhibit *in vivo*. MeCP2 is the setting up individual from the MBD gathering of transcriptional repressors, which makes an abusive area at the target DNA site through enlistment of HDAC-containing transcriptional repressor structures to the methylated DNA. What's more, MeCP2 is additionally connected with higher H3K9 methylation, a vital heterochromatin stamp. Consequently, DNMTs inhibitors are imperative in cancer treatment and some FDA-endorsed inhibitors of DNMTs, for example, 5-azacytidine and 5-aza-2'-deoxycytidine, are being utilized as helpful medications against different cancer writes. Be that as it may, numerous engineered inhibitors have been appeared to cause unfavorable poisonous impacts, with a tight specificity [78]. Subsequently, phytochemicals which are broadly accessible with few reactions or unimportant toxicities are being tried for their part in immediate or roundabout hindrance of DNMT movement amid cancer aversion and treatment. DNMT-interceded differential consequences for promoter methylation and histone acetylation on gene control by bioactive phytochemicals are portrayed in Fig. (**4**).

Table 2. Polyphenols altering DNA methylation.

S.No.	Polyphenols	Molecular Mechanism	Pre-Clinical Model	Target Gene	Diseases Type
1	Curcumin	DNMT inhibitor	Leukemia, Esophageal	NA	Cancer
2	Apigenin	DNMT inhibitor	Skin cancer, Esophageal cells	Decreases CpG hypermethylation in Nrf2 promoter	Cancer
3	Epicatechin, Epicatechin-gallate, Epigalocatechin-3-gallate	DNMT inhibitor	Lung, Colon cancer cells, Esophageal, Oral,, Breast cancers	RAR˘, MGMT, MLH1, CDKN2A, RECK, TERT, RXR˛, CDX2, GSTP1, W1F1	Cancer
4	Genistein	DNMT inhibitor	Esophageal, Prostate Tumors	RAR˘, MGMT, CDKN2A, GSTP1, HMGNS, BTG3 RXR˛, CDX2, GSTP1, W1F1	Cancer
5	Quercetin	DNMT inhibitor	Breast, Colon, Esophageal cancers	CDKN2A	Cancer
6	Resveratrol	DNMT inhibitor	Breast, Lungs cancers	NA	Cancer

(Table 2) cont.....

S.No.	Polyphenols	Molecular Mechanism	Pre-Clinical Model	Target Gene	Diseases Type
7	Sulforaphane	DNMT inhibitor	Esophageal, Colon	NA	Cancer
8	Lycopene	DNMT inhibitor	Prostate, Breast cancers	GSTP1, RAR˘, HIN-1, Activation of GSTP1 promoter	Cancer

Histone Modifications and Chromatin Remodeling

Eukaryotic DNA is sorted out in a mind boggling structure known as chromatin, including DNA, histones and a few other DNA-binding proteins. Notwithstanding advancing a smaller structure, chromatin association likewise helps in the direction of genes articulation by confining the entrance of various DNA-restricting proteins or protein buildings to the genetic material. The procedures of "opening up" of chromatin and its compaction are related with various ATP-subordinate multienzyme edifices, known as chromatin renovating buildings. The chromatin upgrading is initiated by various histone tail modifications, which choose the state of activity of chromatin. The best-considered histone change lysine acetylation prompts opening up of the chromatin by virtue of the negative charge displayed by the acetyl moieties, in this manner reducing the histone–DNA affiliations. The lysine acetylation reactions are catalyzed by histone acetyltransferases (HATs), which trade the acetyl clusters from acetyl coenzyme A to the lysine moieties in the nucleosomes. Tops, requested into three families GCN5 N-acetyltransferase, MOZ/YBF2/SAS2/TIP60, and p300/CBP, accept basic parts in controlling the presentation of cell-cycle managerial proteins and can attach explicitly to the cell-cycle administrative mechanical assembly [79].

Histone deacetylases (HDACs) remove the acetyl packs from lysine developments to diminish the negative charge, thusly inciting chromatin compaction. Four unquestionable classes of HDACs in individuals have been recognized dependent on their assistant likeness to yeast proteins and also their impediment and acetylation works out. Class I, II, and IV HDACs are zinc-subordinate histone deacetylases, while class III HDACs are NAD+-subordinate HDACs. Distinctive HDACs work unmistakably with changed downstream targets, in this manner prompting their assorted tumor silencer and oncogenic exercises. Overexpression and modified HDAC exercises are for the most part connected with the hushing of tumor silencer genes and concealment of EMT and metastasis. HDAC1 overexpression brings about the downregulation of p53 and von Hippel–Lindau tumor silencer genes articulation and fortifies angiogenesis of human endothelial cells, while HDAC10 stifles metastasis of cervical malignancy through hindrance of MMP2 and MMP9 articulation. When all is said in done, histone acetylation is

Table 3. Polyphenols and histone modification.

S.No	Polyphenols	Molecular Mechanism	Pharmacological effects	Pre-Clinical Model	Target genes	Disease Type
1	Curcumin	HAT & HDAC inhibitor	anti-inflammatory anticancer, antioxidant, antiproliferative,	Leukemia, Prostate,Cervix, HIV, Hepatoma	GATA4, EOMES, GZMB, PRF1,H3/H4 deacetylation	Herpes,Malaria, Cancer
2	Apigenin	HDAC inhibitor	anticancer, antiproliferative, antidiabetic, antioxidant,	Skin cancer, Xenograft	P21	Prostate cancer
3	Epicatechin, Epicatechin-gallate, Epigalocatechin-3-gallate	HAT inhibitor	antioxidant, anticancer, anti–inflammatory	Lymphocytes, colon, keratinocytes	NF-kB, IL-6, BMI-1, EZH2, SUZ12,H3K27 trimethylation,H3/H4 acetylation	Cancer
4	Genistein	HAT inhibitor	anti–inflammatory anticancer, antiproliferative, antidiabetic, antioxidant, anti-migration,	Esophageal, Prostate, Breast, Renal	H2A/H2B/H3/H4, Acetylation	Cancer
5	Quercetin	SIRTI activator HAT inhibitor	anti-migration, anticancer, antiproliferative, antidiabetic, antioxidant,	Cervix, Drosophila Small intestine,Cancer Mouse Bowel inflammation	IP-10, MIP-2	Inflammatory diseases
6	Resveratrol	SIRTi activator	anti-migration, anticancer, antiproliferative, antidiabetic, antioxidant,	Embryonic kidney, Macrophages, Lungs, Liver, Cardiomyocytes,Yeast, Drosophila Mouse Rats	TNF-, IL-8, RBP	Colon cancer Lung cancer
7	Sulforaphane	HDAC inhibitor	anti-migration, anticancer, antiproliferative, antidiabetic, antioxidant,	Mouse, prostate cancer xenografts	H3/H4 acetylation RAR_, HBD-2, p21, Bax	Cancer
8	Indole-3 carbinol Diindolylmethane	HDAC inhibitor	anti-migration, anticancer, antiproliferative, antidiabetic, antioxidant,	Prostate cancer,Sprague-Dawley rats	IFN-_, TNF-_, IL-6, IL-2, NF-kB, COX-2, iNOS, IL-1_, IL-12	Cancer
9	Lycopene	reactivation of GSTP1 mRNA expression, associated with reduced promoter methylation	antioxidant, antiproliferation, anticancer, anti-invasive and antimetastatic	Breast cancer	glutathione S-transferase P1	Cancer

related with genes initiation and is inexhaustible in the euchromatin; by differentiate, deacetylation is connected to genes suppression and happens in the heterochromatin.

All things considered, genes suppression or initiation isn't totally reliant on histone acetylation or methylation, anyway is liable to the site and dimension of methylation or acetylation on histone tails. A segment of the dynamic chromatin markers related with genes verbalization are histone methylation on histone H3 at lysine 4 (H3K4), on histone H3 at lysine 36 (H3K36), on histone H3 at lysine 79 (H3K79), and on histone H4 at lysine 20 (H4K20); by separate, the inactivation markers related with genes concealment are methylation on histone H3 at lysine 9 (H3K9) and on histone H3 at lysine 27 (H3K27). HDACs are promising concentrations for threat balancing activity and treatment. A part of the simple much thought about HDAC inhibitors are trapoxin, trichostatin A, and suberoylanilide hydroxamic destructive (SAHA). Of these, SAHA (vorinostat) and romidepsin (Istodax) are modernly open FDA-attested HDAC inhibitors for treatment of cutaneous T-cell lymphoma. Some other HDAC inhibitors, for instance, panobinostat, valproic destructive, and belinostat, are in different times of clinical preliminaries [80] (Table **3**).

Sulforaphane

Sulforaphane (SFN), an isothiocyanate normally rich in generally expended cruciferous vegetables, for example, broccoli, broccoli sprouts, cabbage, and kale, has been appeared to diminish the danger of numerous basic cancers. SFN intervenes chemoprevention through a few systems, including cell-cycle arrest and enlistment of apoptosis and phase-2 detoxification enzymes. In any case, there has been developing enthusiasm for epigenetic control by SFN in chemoprevention in view of its HDAC restraint movement. The HDAC restraint movement of SFN has been appeared to prompt an expansion in the worldwide and nearby histone acetylation status of numerus genes. SFN-interceded epigenetic modifications are accepted to be unequivocally associated with the procedure of cancer chemoprevention by modifying the statement of different genes, incorporating tumor silencer genes in different cancers [81]. SFN was found to hinder DNMTs in MCF-7 and MDA-MB-231 breast cancer cells and in addition CaCo-2 colon cancer cells. Meeran *et al.* displayed that SFN treatment estimation and time-restrictively stifled human telomerase pivot transcriptase (hTERT), the reactant authoritative subunit of telomerase, in both MCF-7 and MDA-MB-231 cells and influenced typical control cells [79]. Besides, the levels of DNMTs, especially DNMT1 and DNMT3a, were likewise diminished in the SFN-treated breast cancer cells. Strikingly, downregulation of DNMTs actuated site-particular CpG demethylation happening principally in the primary exon of hTERT, in this manner encouraging CTCF restricting related with hTERT restraint, trailed by apoptosis in breast cancer cells [78]. SFN has moreover been found to have HDAC inhibitory development in various other disease *in vitro* and *in vivo* malignant growth models. SFN dose restrictively extended the development of a β-catenin-responsive columnist (TOPflash) and diminished HDAC activity in human embryonic kidney. In HCT116 cells, SFN repressed HDAC action, along these lines expanding histone acetylation at the p21WAF1/CIP1 promoter to upgrade its demeanor. Human prostate cancer cells BPH-1, LNCaP, and PC-3 likewise demonstrated noteworthy restraint of HDAC action after SFN treatment. Besides, SFN-initiated histone acetylation expanded the outflow of p21WAF1/CIP1, in this manner restraining cell-cycle capture and inciting cell apoptosis in these prostate cancer cell lines. SFN also has HDAC inhibitory effects *in vivo* as showed up in creature and human models. Myzak *et al.* demonstrated that mice treated with a lone oral estimations of 10 μM SFN had basic HDAC inhibitory development in colonic mucosa with extended acetylated histones H3 and H4. Besides, the expanded acetylation upgraded the statement of the p21WAF1/CIP1 and Bax genes, consequently smothering tumorigenesis in Apc/+ mice. Another examination showed that the organization of 7.5 μM SFN per animal for 21 days fundamentally killed prostate cancer PC-3 tumor xenografts by repressing HDAC action *in vivo* [82]. Outstandingly, in human subjects, a solitary dosage of 68 g of broccoli grows fundamentally repressed HDAC action in fringe blood mononuclear cells at 3 and 6 h following utilization. All in all, SFN is a powerful HDAC inhibitor both *in vitro* and *in vivo* models [82].

Genistein

Genistein, an isoflavone having a place with the flavonoids gathering of mixes, is found in various plants, including fava bean, soybean, lupin, kudzu, and psoralea. Genistein and different isoflavones have anticancer and antiangiogenic properties against different cancers. A few examinations have discovered direct measurements of genistein to affect the cancers of the prostate, cervix, mind, breast, and colon. It is winding up progressively evident that genistein applies numerous consequences for cancer cell development. The few systems basic the counter proliferative and anticancer properties of genistein incorporate avoidance of DNA change, lessening in cancer cell expansion, hindrance of angiogenesis, and acceptance of cell apoptosis. A potential system that has as of late gotten impressive consideration is that genistein is associated with control of genes translation or hushing action by regulating epigenetic occasions, for example, DNA methylation and additionally chromatin adjustments. A few reports have discovered that genistein exhibits DNMT inhibitory and histone alteration exercises in cancer cells. In prostate cancer cells, genistein actuated the statement of the tumor silencer genes p21WAF1/CIP1 and p16INK4a by modifying promoter methylation and histone alteration [79]. Moreover, genistein expanded acetylated histones H3 and H4 and H3K4 at the p21WAF1/CIP1 and p16INK4a translation begin destinations, intervened by HAT enlistment. Genistein-interceded advertiser hypomethylation and hyperacetylation reactivate verbalization of tumor silencer genes in human prostate malignant growth cells and are trailed by cell-cycle catch and cell apoptosis affected by cyclin and caspase pathways, separately [63]. This dietary bioactive compound likewise reactivates BTG3, a tumor silencer genes, in the renal carcinoma cell lines A498, ACHN, and HEK-293. Genistein actuates the epigenetic re-articulation of BTG3 by modifying promoter DNA methylation by hindering DNMT and methyl-Cp--restricting area 2 in these cells, however expands histone acetylation by improving HAT action, trailed by advancement of acetylated histones H3 and H4, dimethyl H3K4, and trimethyl H3K4 close to the translation begin site at the BTG3 promoter. This is reliable with different reports that genistein upregulated mRNA articulation of the BRCA1, p16INK4a, RARb, MGMT, and p21WAF1/CIP1 genes [83]. Studies have additionally demonstrated that genistein in blend with different DNMTs or HDAC inhibitors upgraded the reactivation of methylation-silenced genes [63, 84].

Genistein not just reactivates tumor silencer genes through epigenetic changes yet in addition hinders the declaration of tumor promoter genes, for example, hTERT. Genistein hinders DNMT1, DNMT3a, and DNMT3b and advances inactivating histone trimethyl H3K9, trailed by transcriptional restraint of hTERT articulation in human breast cancer cells [85]. In another investigation with human breast cancer cells MDA-MB-468, low convergences of genistein mostly demethylated tumor silencer GSTP1 promoter and reactivated its expression [86]. Notwithstanding *in vitro* epigenetic adjustment, genistein treated neonatal CD-1 mice indicated oddly hypomethylated nucleosomal restricting protein-1 promoter than hypermethylated control (nongenistein) mice. As opposed to genistein-instigated DNA hypomethylation intervened through DNMT restraint, considers have demonstrated that genistein prompted hypermethylation in some animal models. Furthermore, genistein expanded hypermethylation in human examinations randomized with particular cancer-related genes. Thirty-four sound premenopausal ladies were randomized to take 40 or 140 mg isoflavones day by day through one menstrual cycle, and the methylation status of p16INK4a, RASSF1A, RARβ2, ER, and CCND2 were surveyed in intraductal examples. The outcomes demonstrated that RARβ2 and CCND2 were hypermethylated after genistein organization, and these outcomes connected well with serum genistein levels [87].

Curcumin

Curcumin, a yellow color displays in the flavor turmeric (*Curcuma longa*), has been connected with different accommodating activities including anti-inflammatory, antiangiogenic, wound-healing, antioxidant, and anticancer properties. Curcumin has showed up in various creature models and human examinations to be to an awesome degree secured, even at high dosages; in any case, its dissolvability and bioavailability is an obstacle for medicinal solution headway. Curcumin-intervened chemoprevention is prevalently empowered through cell-cycle catch and cell apoptosis acknowledgment in various malignancy cells. Curcumin-prompted apoptosis is locked in with intrinsic and outward apoptosis pathways, the NF-κB-intervened pathway, and the PI3K/Akt hailing pathway. Late verification has exhibited that curcumin in like manner limits DNMT activities and histone change, for instance, HDAC limitation in tumorigenesis [88]. Molecular docking of the curcumin– DNMT1 cooperation recommended that curcumin covalently obstructs the synergist thiolate of C1226 of DNMT1 to apply its inhibitory impact. This hindrance is by all accounts relatively lower than other bioactive dietary parts, for example, EGCG and genistein. Besides, curcumin treatment with extricated genomic DNA from a leukemia cell line incited worldwide hypo-methylation [89]. These outcomes give solid confirmation that curcumin is an intense DNA hypo-methylating specialist, essential for its wide range inhibitory movement in irritation, cancer, and numerous different illnesses. Curcumin likewise has solid inhibitory movement against HDACs and HATs in a few *in vitro* cancer models. Curcumin indicated solid multiplication restraint strength on Burkitt's lymphoma cells *in vitro*, with the IC50 esteem for 24 h of 25 µM. Critical lessening was identified in the p300, HDAC1, HDAC3, and HDAC8 levels after treatment with curcumin, trailed by avoidance of IκBα debasement and restraint of atomic translocation of the NFκB/p65 subunit. Meja *et al*. shown that even low centralizations of curcumin (*i.e.*, 30 and 200 nM) reestablished corticosteroid work in human monocytes presented to oxidants. This happened as a result of HDAC2 movement kept up by counteracting oxidant-actuated debasement of HDAC2 by downregulating gene articulation related with protein degradation [90].

Curcumin has been distinguished as a solid inhibitor of HATs in both *in vitro* and *in vivo* growth models. An early epigenetic contemplate demonstrated that curcumin is a particular inhibitor of p300/CBP HAT action, however not of p300/CBP-related factor, *in vitro* and *in vivo*. Curcumin-interceded p300/CBP hindrance was related with the constraint of histones H3 and H4 and nonhistone protein, for example, p53 and HIV-TAT proteins. Another structural investigation think about by Marcu *et al*. uncovered that α-and β-unsaturated carbonyl gatherings in the curcumin sidechain work as Michael response locales, which is required for its HAT inhibitory movement. Moreover, the creators exhibited that curcumin specifically advances proteasome-subordinate debasement of p300 and the firmly related CBP protein, without influencing the HATs, for example, PCAF or GCN5, in prostate PC3-M and peripheral blood lymphocytes [91]. Remarkably, curcumin could successfully square histone hyperacetylation in both PC3-M prostate cancer cells and fringe blood lymphocytes initiated by the HDAC inhibitor MS-275. Kang *et al.* demonstrated a solid hindrance of curcumin-intervened HAT inhibitory action related with a reduction in histone H3 and H4 acetylation in brain cancer cells. Further, curcumin-initiated histone alteration related with caspase-interceded cellular apoptosis in mind cancer cells and upgraded neurogenesis, synaptogenesis, and migration of neural ancestor cells in brain-derived adult neural stem cells *in vitro* [92]. Another investigation showed that curcumin reestablished bright radiation-instigated hyperacetylation in the promoter district of ATF3, COX2, and MKP1, which are inflammatory-related genes in human keratinocytes. Moreover, thinks about have additionally demonstrated that curcumin-intervened hypoacetylation of the promoters of specific genes was firmly associated with genes quieting. An exceptionally late examination demonstrated that curcumin represses high glucose-instigated pro-inflammatory cytokines by epigenetic change in human monocytic cells THP-1. Curcumin treatment altogether diminished HAT action, p300 and acetylated CBP/p300 genes articulation, and instigated HDAC2 articulation in THP-1 cells, along these lines restraining high glucose-prompted pro-inflammatory cytokines, an imperative atomic focus in decreasing diabetic inconveniences. In a rat models, curcumin was observed to be protective against cardiovascular disappointment, aggravation, and fibrosis through the downregulation of NFκB, GATA4, and TGFβ motioning and additionally hindrance of HAT movement. Curcumin was additionally observed to be extremely powerful against streptozotocin-actuated diabetes in male Sprague Dawley rats through the restraint of H3 hyperacetylation, NFκB binding, and p300 and H3S10 phosphorylation [79].

Resveratrol

Resveratrol, a dietary polyphenol got from grapes, berries, peanuts, and other plant sources, was found to have solid anticancer properties by modifying signal transduction pathways that control cell division and improvement, apoptosis, irritation, angiogenesis, and metastasis. The anticancer property of resveratrol has been reinforced by its ability to prevent expansion of a wide combination of human tumor cells, for instance, those in skin, bosom, prostate, lung, and colon. These *in vitro* comes about have prompted various preclinical creature concentrates to assess the capability of this medication for cancer chemoprevention and chemotherapy. Different biochemical and molecular activities appear to add to resveratrol's belongings against precancerous or cancer cells.

Resveratrol has been appeared to have weaker DNMT inhibitory movement than other dietary bioactive parts, for example, EGCG. Resveratrol avoids epigenetic quieting of BRCA-1 incited by AHR in human bosom cancer cells MCF-7. AHR-intervened improvement of monomethylated-H3K9, DNMT1, and methyl-restricting space protein-2 at the BRCA1 promoter was reestablished, at any rate somewhat by resveratrol treatment, which was related with BRCA1 reactivation in MCF-7 cells. By differentiate, resveratrol did not altogether incite retinoic corrosive receptor beta (RARβ) 2 articulation by hindering RARβ2 promoter methylation in MCF-7 cells contrasted and other adenosine analogs. Resveratrol is likewise connected with the enactment of the sort III HDAC inhibitors, sirtuin (SIRT) 1, and p300, in various *in vitro* and *in vivo* models. Enacted SIRT1 contrarily controls survivin articulation through its deacetylase action. Wang *et al.* (2008) found that human BRCA1-related breast cancers have bring down levels of SIRT1 articulation. Nonetheless, bioactive dietary parts related with SIRT1 initiation intervened an expanded articulation of human BRCA1 by adjusting H3 acetylation, which is an imperative procedure for focused treatment for BRCA1-related bosom cancer. Likewise, SIRT1-related BRCA1 signaling is critical for hindering tumorigenesis by initiating oncoproteins in human bosom cancer cells. In APC/+ mice, SIRT1-encoded proteins were appeared to be required for resveratrol-interceded chemoprevention. SIRT1 additionally assumes imperative parts in the maturing processes in light of the fact that SIRT1-invalid mice couldn't endure caloric confinement and did not broaden their life expectancy contrasted and control mice [93].

EGCG

EGCG, the major polyphenol in green tea, has been broadly examined as a potential demethylating administrator. EGCG is methylated by catechol-O-methyltransferase, the compound trustworthy of the inactivation of catechol atoms, for instance, dietary polyphenols. This synthetic familiarizes a methyl pack with the catecholamine gathering, which is given by SAM. Demethylation of SAM achieves the improvement of S-adenosyl-l-homocysteine (SAH), a groundbreaking inhibitor of DNMT. Generation of SAH has been conjectured as one of the components for the demethylating properties of this compound. By differentiate, EGCG can shape hydrogen bonds with various deposits in the synergist pocket of DNMT, in this way going about as an immediate inhibitor of DNMT1. The restraint of DNMT may keep the methylation of the recently integrated DNA strand, bringing about the inversion of the hyper-methylation and re-articulation of the hushed genes. At long last, EGCG has been appeared to be a productive inhibitor of human dihydrofolate reductase. Like other antifolate mixes, EGCG acts through communication with folic corrosive digestion in cells, causing the restraint of DNA and RNA union and modifying DNA methylation [94].

In an original paper in 2003, Fang *et al.* shown that treatment of human esophageal malignancy cells with EGCG caused an obsession and time-subordinate reversal of hyper-methylation of a couple of known tumor silencer genes, for instance, the p16, RAR, MGMT, and MLH1 genes. In a comparable work, reactivation of some methylation-calmed genes by EGCG was similarly appeared human colon and prostate malignancy cells. From that point forward, a few gatherings discovered comparative *in vitro* result [95]. Incomplete demethylation of hyper-methylated RARβ by EGCG was shown in MCF-7 and MDA-MB-231 cells. Kato *et al.* demonstrated that treatment of oral cancer cells with EGCG in part turned around the hyper-methylation status of RECK and essentially upgraded the articulation level of RECK mRNA [96]. Pandey *et al.* displayed that introduction of human prostate malignant growth LNCaP cells to GTPs caused a concentration and time-subordinate re-articulation of a known herald to the beginning of prostate disease, and methylation examination revealed expansive demethylation in the GSTP1 advertiser region [97]. Berletch *et al.* demonstrated that treatment of MCF-7 cells with EGCG brought about a period subordinate decline in hTERT advertiser methylation [98].

By differentiate, a few authors did not report this noteworthy demethylation and actuation of a few genes by EGCG. Chuang *et al.* analyzed an aggregate of six genes or dull components, to be specific p16, RARβ, MAGE-A1, MAGE-B2, and Alu, in three separate cell lines, to be specific T24, HT29, and PC3, for their DNA methylation levels and their mRNA articulation levels utilizing a few demethylating operators. Treatment with EGCG incited neither DNA demethylation nor re-articulation of the broke down genes. What's more, Stresemann *et al.* likewise played out a similar investigation of mixes already answered to restrain DNMT movement in cancer cell lines, including EGCG. These creators decided the cytosine methylation level and methylation status of TIMP3 in various cell lines and found that EGCG did not restrain DNA methylation. The numerous potential purposes behind the inconsistencies among contemplates incorporate contrasts in investigation techniques, conceivable genes or cell line-specificity of EGCG, or ineffectual treatment strategy. In light of their outcomes, Stresemann *et al.* contended that cell impacts initiated by EGCG could probably be ascribed to the oxidative pressure actuated by this compound [99].

Notwithstanding whether EGCG can switch DNA hyper-methylation and reactivate methylation-quieted genes *in vivo* remains to be settled. Mittal *et al.*

exhibited that topical treatment of EGCG using a hydrophilic cream prevents UVB-instigated overall DNA hypo-methylation plan in continually UVB-uncovered mice. Immunohistochemical area of DNA methylation configuration was performed using against 5-methylcytosine monoclonal neutralizer. Since overall DNA hypo-methylation is a wonder typically associated with hyper-methylation and inactivation of specific genes in the midst of carcinogenesis, the makers guessed that their observation was solid with the possibility that EGCG can maintain a strategic distance from or pivot the hyper-methylation of specific genes [100].

Kinney *et al.* recently tested whether oral consumption of GTPs could affect normal or cancer-specific DNA methylation *in vivo* by using a mice model [101]. Wild-sort and TRAMP mice were given 0.3% GTPs in drinking water starting at multi month of age. To screen DNA methylation, the producers assessed 5-methyl-deoxycytidine levels, methylation of the B1 dull part, and methylation of the Mage-a8 qualities. GTP treatment did not smother tumor movement in TRAMP mice and no estimations subordinate changes in DNA methylation status were observed. Yuasa *et al.* played out a review examination looking at the methylation status of a few genes in essential gastric carcinomas in connection to past way of life of the patients, including dietary propensities [102]. Methylation of CDX2 and BMP-2, estimated through methylation-specific PCR, connected with the diminished admission of green tea and cruciferous vegetables. At long last, Tsao *et al.* as of late distributed a stage II, randomized, fake treatment controlled trial of GTE in patients with high-chance oral premalignant injuries (OPL). The OPL clinical reaction rate was higher in all GTE arms at various measurements (n = 28; half) contrasted and the fake treatment arm (n = 11; 18.2%), however it didn't achieve factual noteworthiness (P = 0.09). Just two patients in the GTE arm had pattern p16 promoter methylation that could be assessed following treatment, which did not invert methylation status in either patient [103]. Albeit most confirmation on the epigenetic properties of tea common mixes has concentrated on EGCG, different catechins, for example, catechin, epicatechin, ECG, and apigallocatechin, have been found to have comparative highlights, however with much lower DNMT inhibitory movement contrasted and that of EGCG [94].

Lycopene

Lycopene, a bright red carotene pigment belonging to tetraterpenoids, is a phytochemical naturally occurring in tomatoes, carrot, watermelon, papaya, cherries, and other plants. It is an intense cell reinforcement and has been appeared to adjust different genes associated with DNA repair, cell-cycle control, and apoptosis in bosom cancer cells. Concentrates by Chalabi *et al.* detailed the impacts of lycopene on GSTP1 in bosom cancer cells. Lycopene (2 µM /week) was appeared to instigate GSTP1 articulation and demethylate the GSTP1 promoter in MDA-MB-468 cells, however not in MCF-7 cells. The declaration of different genes, for example, RARβ2 and HIN1, stayed unaltered by lycopene treatment in both MCF-7 and MDA-MB-468 cells. In spite of the fact that this investigation demonstrated that lycopene might be DNA methylating operator, extra examinations are expected to unravel the lycopene-interceded consequences for the epigenetic systems [104]. The protective impact of lycopene on the prostate is distinctive between androgen-responsive and androgen-headstrong inferred prostate cancer cells. Fu *et al.* exhibited that lycopene treatment altogether diminished methylation levels of the GSTP1 promoter and expanded the mRNA and protein levels of GSTP1 in an androgen-obstinate PC-3 cells. It likewise diminished in DNMT3A articulation in PC-3 cells; nonetheless, no such change was seen in LNCaP cells [105].

CONCLUSION AND FUTURE DIRECTIONS

The developing field of wholesome genomics targets supplement related hereditary and epigenetic changes for counteractive action and treatment of different ailments, including cancer. As indicated by the investigations depicted in this, since they change different epigenetic adjustments, bioactive dietary parts have an extraordinary potential in the avoidance and treatment of a wide assortment of cancers. Cancer is a multistep processes and uses numerous survival pathways to beat typical cells. Hence, bioactive segments, for example, EGCG, that have various atomic targets and stifle numerous cell pathways may have solid potential for cancer avoidance and treatment. Albeit individual bioactive dietary segments have indicated extraordinary potential in avoidance and treatment of different cancers, the consolidated utilization of these segments ought to be more proficient in focusing on the numerous cell processes engaged with tumorigenesis. Extra clinical examinations are required to investigate the wellbeing profile of dosages, organization courses, organ specificity, and bioavailability of these bioactive parts in people. Antiquated restorative uses and current logical proof unequivocally support the utilization of these bioactive dietary parts for medicate disclosure and advancement against cancer anticipation and treatment.

ABBREVIATIONS

ALS	Amyotrophic Lateral Sclerosis
AP-1	Activating Protein–1
AA	Arachidonic Acid
CURC	Curcumin

Cy3G	Cyanidin-3-Glucoside
COX	Ciclooxygenase
EGCG	Eigallocatechin-3-Gallate
ERK	Extracellular Signal-Related Kinases
EVOO	Extra Virgin Olive Oil
HMC-1	Human Mast-Cell Line
HPLC	High Performance Liquid Chromatography
HPLC-DAD	High-Performance Liquid Chromatography–Diode Array Detection
ICAM-1	Intercellular Adhesion Molecule 1
IKB	Inhibitor kB, Ub, Ubiquitin
IKK	IkB-Kinase
IL-8	Interleukin-8
IFNγ	Interferon-γ
IL-1β	Interleukin-1β
IARC	International Agency for Research on Cancer
IP	Intraperitoneal
IV	Intravenous
IL-6	Interleukin-6
INOS	Inducible Nitric Oxide Synthase
IRF-1	Interferon Regulatory Factor-1
LC-MS/MS	liquid Chromatography Tandem Mass Spectrometry
LOX	Lipoxygenase
MCP-1	Monocyte Chemoattractant Protein-1
MDR	Multidrug Resistance
MRP	Multidrug Resistance Protein
MAPKKK	MAPK Kinase Kinase
MIP-2	Macrophage Inflammatory Protein-2
MMPs	Matrix Metalloproteinases
NCI	National Cancer Institute
NMR	Nuclear Magnetic Resonance; NO, Nitric Oxide
NOAEL	No-Observed-Adverse-Effect-Level
NOS	Nitric Oxide Synthase
NSCLC	Non-Small-Cell Lung Carcinoma
OAT	Organic Anion Transporters
PLA2	Phospholipase A2. ADI, Acceptable Daily Intake

Quer	Quercetin
JNK	C-Jun Amino-Terminal Kinases; p38 (or p38-MAPK), p38-Mitogen-Activated Protein Kinase MEK (or MKK), MAPK-Kinase
LPS	Lipopolysaccharides
Resv	Resveratrol
SCLC	Small-Cell Lung Carcinoma
TRAIL	TNF-Related Apoptosis-Inducing Ligand
TGFβ	Tissue Growth Factor-β
TNF-α	Tumour Necrosis Factor-α
UGT	UDP-Glucuronosyltransferases
UV	Ultraviolet
UVB	Ultraviolet B Radiation
VCAM	Vascular Cell Adhesion Molecule

CONSENT FOR PUBLICATION

Not applicable.

CONFLICT OF INTEREST

The authors declare no conflict of interest, financial or otherwise.

ACKNOWLEDGEMENTS

This work was supported in part by grants R01DA040537, R01DA037838, and R01DA034547 from the National Institutes of Health.

REFERENCES

[1] Zhou Y, Zheng J, Li Y, *et al.* Natural polyphenols for prevention and treatment of cancer. Nutrients 2016; 8(8): 515.
[http://dx.doi.org/10.3390/nu8080515] [PMID: 27556486]

[2] Li F, Li S, Li H-B, *et al.* Antiproliferative activity of peels, pulps and seeds of 61 fruits. J Funct Foods 2013; 5(3): 1298-309.
[http://dx.doi.org/10.1016/j.jff.2013.04.016]

[3] Laura A, Alvarez-Parrilla E, Gonzalez-Aguilar GA. Fruit and vegetable phytochemicals: Chemistry, nutritional value and stability. John Wiley & Sons 2009.

[4] Han X, Shen T, Lou H. Dietary polyphenols and their biological significance. Int J Mol Sci 2007; 8(9): 950-88.
[http://dx.doi.org/10.3390/i8090950]

[5] Scalbert A, Williamson G. Dietary intake and bioavailability of polyphenols. J Nutr 2000; 130(8S) (Suppl.): 2073S-85S.
[http://dx.doi.org/10.1093/jn/130.8.2073S] [PMID: 10917926]

[6]   Bohn T. Dietary factors affecting polyphenol bioavailability. Nutr Rev 2014; 72(7): 429-52.
      [http://dx.doi.org/10.1111/nure.12114] [PMID: 24828476]

[7]   Santhakumar AB, Battino M, Alvarez-Suarez JM. Dietary polyphenols: Structures, bioavailability and protective effects against atherosclerosis. Food Chem Toxicol 2018; 113: 49-65.
      [http://dx.doi.org/10.1016/j.fct.2018.01.022] [PMID: 29360556]

[8]   Rajendran P, Chen YF, Chen YF, *et al.* The multifaceted link between inflammation and human diseases. J Cell Physiol 2018; 233(9): 6458-71.
      [http://dx.doi.org/10.1002/jcp.26479] [PMID: 29323719]

[9]   Pandey KB, Rizvi SI. Plant polyphenols as dietary antioxidants in human health and disease. Oxid Med Cell Longev 2009; 2(5): 270-8.
      [http://dx.doi.org/10.4161/oxim.2.5.9498] [PMID: 20716914]

[10] Santangelo C, Varì R, Scazzocchio B, Di Benedetto R, Filesi C, Masella R. Polyphenols, intracellular signalling and inflammation. Ann Ist Super Sanita 2007; 43(4): 394-405.
      [PMID: 18209273]

[11] Dinarello CA. Proinflammatory cytokines. Chest 2000; 118(2): 503-8.
      [http://dx.doi.org/10.1378/chest.118.2.503] [PMID: 10936147]

[12] Calixto JB, Campos MM, Otuki MF, Santos AR. Anti-inflammatory compounds of plant origin. Part II. modulation of pro-inflammatory cytokines, chemokines and adhesion molecules. Planta Med 2004; 70(2): 93-103.
      [http://dx.doi.org/10.1055/s-2004-815483] [PMID: 14994184]

[13] García-Lafuente A, Guillamón E, Villares A, Rostagno MA, Martínez JA. Flavonoids as anti-inflammatory agents: implications in cancer and cardiovascular disease. Inflamm Res 2009; 58(9): 537-52.
      [http://dx.doi.org/10.1007/s00011-009-0037-3] [PMID: 19381780]

[14] González-Gallego J, García-Mediavilla MV, Sánchez-Campos S, Tuñón MJ. Anti-inflammatory and immunomodulatory properties of dietary flavonoids In: Watson RR, Preedy VR and Zibadi S, Eds. Polyphenols in Human Health and Disease. Amsterdam: Elsevier 2014; pp. 435-52.
      [http://dx.doi.org/10.1016/B978-0-12-398456-2.00032-3]

[15] Leyva-López N, Gutierrez-Grijalva EP, Ambriz-Perez DL, Heredia JB. Flavonoids as cytokine modulators: a possible therapy for inflammation-related diseases. Int J Mol Sci 2016; 17(6): 921.
      [http://dx.doi.org/10.3390/ijms17060921] [PMID: 27294919]

[16] Miles EA, Zoubouli P, Calder PC. Differential anti-inflammatory effects of phenolic compounds from extra virgin olive oil identified in human whole blood cultures. Nutrition 2005; 21(3): 389-94.
      [http://dx.doi.org/10.1016/j.nut.2004.06.031] [PMID: 15797683]

[17] Santangelo C, Varì R, Scazzocchio B, Di Benedetto R, Filesi C, Masella R. Polyphenols, intracellular signalling and inflammation. Ann Ist Super Sanita 2007; 43(4): 394-405.
      [PMID: 18209273]

[18] Bitler CM, Viale TM, Damaj B, Crea R. Hydrolyzed olive vegetation water in mice has anti-inflammatory activity. J Nutr 2005; 135(6): 1475-9.
      [http://dx.doi.org/10.1093/jn/135.6.1475] [PMID: 15930455]

[19] Lyu SY, Park WB. Production of cytokine and NO by RAW 264.7 macrophages and PBMC *in vitro* incubation with flavonoids. Arch Pharm Res 2005; 28(5): 573-81.
      [http://dx.doi.org/10.1007/BF02977761] [PMID: 15974445]

[20] Batra P, Sharma A. Sharma, Anti-cancer potential of flavonoids: recent trends and future perspectives 3 Biotech 2013; 3(6): 439-59. Back to cited text (13)

[21] Lorenz M, Wessler S, Follmann E, *et al.* A constituent of green tea, epigallocatechin-3-gallate, activates endothelial nitric oxide synthase by a phosphatidylinositol-3-OH-kinase-, cAMP-dependent

[22] Sutherland BA, Shaw OM, Clarkson AN, Jackson DN, Sammut IA, Appleton I. Neuroprotective effects of (-)-epigallocatechin gallate following hypoxia-ischemia-induced brain damage: novel mechanisms of action. FASEB J 2005; 19(2): 258-60.
[http://dx.doi.org/10.1096/fj.04-2806fje] [PMID: 15569775]

protein kinase-, and Akt-dependent pathway and leads to endothelial-dependent vasorelaxation. J Biol Chem 2004; 279(7): 6190-5.
[http://dx.doi.org/10.1074/jbc.M309114200] [PMID: 14645258]

[23] Xu Z, Chen S, Li X, Luo G, Li L, Le W. Neuroprotective effects of (-)-epigallocatechin-3-gallate in a transgenic mouse model of amyotrophic lateral sclerosis. Neurochem Res 2006; 31(10): 1263-9.
[http://dx.doi.org/10.1007/s11064-006-9166-z] [PMID: 17021948]

[24] Kawser Hossain M, Abdal Dayem A, Han J, et al. Molecular mechanisms of the anti-obesity and anti-diabetic properties of flavonoids. Int J Mol Sci 2016; 17(4): 569.
[http://dx.doi.org/10.3390/ijms17040569] [PMID: 27092490]

[25] Terra X, Valls J, Vitrac X, et al. Grape-seed procyanidins act as antiinflammatory agents in endotoxin-stimulated RAW 264.7 macrophages by inhibiting NFkB signaling pathway. J Agric Food Chem 2007; 55(11): 4357-65.
[http://dx.doi.org/10.1021/jf0633185] [PMID: 17461594]

[26] Dai J, Mumper RJ. Plant phenolics: extraction, analysis and their antioxidant and anticancer properties. Molecules 2010; 15(10): 7313-52.
[http://dx.doi.org/10.3390/molecules15107313] [PMID: 20966876]

[27] García-Martínez O, De Luna-Bertos E, Ramos-Torrecillas J, et al. Phenolic compounds in extra virgin olive oil stimulate human osteoblastic cell proliferation. PLoS One 2016; 11(3): e0150045.
[http://dx.doi.org/10.1371/journal.pone.0150045] [PMID: 26930190]

[28] Bonni A, Brunet A, West AE, Datta SR, Takasu MA, Greenberg ME. Cell survival promoted by the Ras-MAPK signaling pathway by transcription-dependent and -independent mechanisms. Science 1999; 286(5443): 1358-62.
[http://dx.doi.org/10.1126/science.286.5443.1358] [PMID: 10558990]

[29] Zhang W, Liu HT. MAPK signal pathways in the regulation of cell proliferation in mammalian cells. Cell Res 2002; 12(1): 9-18.
[http://dx.doi.org/10.1038/sj.cr.7290105] [PMID: 11942415]

[30] Dunn KL, Espino PS, Drobic B, He S, Davie JR. The Ras-MAPK signal transduction pathway, cancer and chromatin remodeling. Biochem Cell Biol 2005; 83(1): 1-14.
[http://dx.doi.org/10.1139/o04-121] [PMID: 15746962]

[31] Zhou HY, Shin EM, Guo LY, et al. Anti-inflammatory activity of 4-methoxyhonokiol is a function of the inhibition of iNOS and COX-2 expression in RAW 264.7 macrophages via NF-kappaB, JNK and p38 MAPK inactivation. Eur J Pharmacol 2008; 586(1-3): 340-9.
[http://dx.doi.org/10.1016/j.ejphar.2008.02.044] [PMID: 18378223]

[32] González-Gallego J, García-Mediavilla MV, Sánchez-Campos S, Tuñón MJ. Fruit polyphenols, immunity and inflammation. Br J Nutr 2010; 104(S3) (Suppl. 3): S15-27.
[http://dx.doi.org/10.1017/S0007114510003910] [PMID: 20955647]

[33] Cazarolli LH, Zanatta L, Alberton EH, et al. Flavonoids: prospective drug candidates. Mini Rev Med Chem 2008; 8(13): 1429-40.
[http://dx.doi.org/10.2174/138955708786369564] [PMID: 18991758]

[34] Watson RR, Preedy VR, Zibadi S. Polyphenols in human health and disease. Academic press 2013.

[35] Li W, Mei X, Tu YY. Effects of tea polyphenols and their polymers on MAPK signaling pathways in cancer research. Mini Rev Med Chem 2012; 12(2): 120-6.
[http://dx.doi.org/10.2174/138955712798995011] [PMID: 22372602]

[36] Wang T, Zhang X, Li JJ. The role of NF-kappaB in the regulation of cell stress responses. Int

Immunopharmacol 2002; 2(11): 1509-20.
[http://dx.doi.org/10.1016/S1567-5769(02)00058-9] [PMID: 12433052]

[37] Tak PP, Firestein GS. NF-kappaB: a key role in inflammatory diseases. J Clin Invest 2001; 107(1): 7-11.
[http://dx.doi.org/10.1172/JCI11830] [PMID: 11134171]

[38] Wajant H. TRAIL and NFκB signaling-a complex relationship, Vitamins & Hormones. Elsevier 2004; pp. 101-32.

[39] Nam N-H. Naturally occurring NF-Kappa B inhibitors. Mini Rev Med Chem 2006; 6(8): 945-51.
[http://dx.doi.org/10.2174/138955706777934937] [PMID: 16918500]

[40] Syed DN, Afaq F, Kweon MH, et al. Green tea polyphenol EGCG suppresses cigarette smoke condensate-induced NF-kappaB activation in normal human bronchial epithelial cells. Oncogene 2007; 26(5): 673-82.
[http://dx.doi.org/10.1038/sj.onc.1209829] [PMID: 16862172]

[41] Park J-W, Choi YJ, Suh S-I, Kwon TK. Involvement of ERK and protein tyrosine phosphatase signaling pathways in EGCG-induced cyclooxygenase-2 expression in Raw 264.7 cells. Biochem Biophys Res Commun 2001; 286(4): 721-5.
[http://dx.doi.org/10.1006/bbrc.2001.5415] [PMID: 11520057]

[42] Wheeler DS, Catravas JD, Odoms K, Denenberg A, Malhotra V, Wong HR. Epigallocatechin--gallate, a green tea-derived polyphenol, inhibits IL-1 β-dependent proinflammatory signal transduction in cultured respiratory epithelial cells. J Nutr 2004; 134(5): 1039-44.
[http://dx.doi.org/10.1093/jn/134.5.1039] [PMID: 15113942]

[43] Mackenzie GG, Carrasquedo F, Delfino JM, Keen CL, Fraga CG, Oteiza PI. Epicatechin, catechin, and dimeric procyanidins inhibit PMA-induced NF-kappaB activation at multiple steps in Jurkat T cells. FASEB J 2004; 18(1): 167-9.
[http://dx.doi.org/10.1096/fj.03-0402fje] [PMID: 14630700]

[44] Hussain T, Tan B, Yin Y, Blachier F, Tossou MC, Rahu N. Oxidative stress and inflammation: what polyphenols can do for us? Oxid Med Cell Longev 2016; 2016: 7432797.
[http://dx.doi.org/10.1155/2016/7432797] [PMID: 27738491]

[45] Rahman I, Biswas SK, Kirkham PA. Regulation of inflammation and redox signaling by dietary polyphenols. Biochem Pharmacol 2006; 72(11): 1439-52.
[http://dx.doi.org/10.1016/j.bcp.2006.07.004] [PMID: 16920072]

[46] Stalińska K, Guzdek A, Rokicki M, Koj A. Transcription factors as targets of the anti-inflammatory treatment. A cell culture study with extracts from some Mediterranean diet plants. J Physiol Pharmacol 2005; 56(1) (Suppl. 1): 157-69.
[PMID: 15800392]

[47] Deeb D, Xu YX, Jiang H, et al. Curcumin (diferuloyl-methane) enhances tumor necrosis factor-related apoptosis-inducing ligand-induced apoptosis in LNCaP prostate cancer cells. Mol Cancer Ther 2003; 2(1): 95-103.
[PMID: 12533677]

[48] Delmas D, Rébé C, Lacour S, et al. Resveratrol-induced apoptosis is associated with Fas redistribution in the rafts and the formation of a death-inducing signaling complex in colon cancer cells. J Biol Chem 2003; 278(42): 41482-90.
[http://dx.doi.org/10.1074/jbc.M304896200] [PMID: 12902349]

[49] Psahoulia FH, Drosopoulos KG, Doubravska L, Andera L, Pintzas A. Quercetin enhances TRAIL-mediated apoptosis in colon cancer cells by inducing the accumulation of death receptors in lipid rafts. Mol Cancer Ther 2007; 6(9): 2591-9.
[http://dx.doi.org/10.1158/1535-7163.MCT-07-0001] [PMID: 17876056]

[50] Wen S, Zhu D, Huang P. Targeting cancer cell mitochondria as a therapeutic approach. Future Med

Chem 2013; 5(1): 53-67.
[http://dx.doi.org/10.4155/fmc.12.190] [PMID: 23256813]

[51] Shankar S, Ganapathy S, Chen Q, Srivastava RK. Curcumin sensitizes TRAIL-resistant xenografts: molecular mechanisms of apoptosis, metastasis and angiogenesis. Mol Cancer 2008; 7(1): 16.
[http://dx.doi.org/10.1186/1476-4598-7-16] [PMID: 18226269]

[52] Asensi M, Ortega A, Mena S, Feddi F, Estrela JM. Natural polyphenols in cancer therapy. Crit Rev Clin Lab Sci 2011; 48(5-6): 197-216.
[http://dx.doi.org/10.3109/10408363.2011.631268] [PMID: 22141580]

[53] Larsen CA, Bisson WH, Dashwood RH. Tea catechins inhibit hepatocyte growth factor receptor (MET kinase) activity in human colon cancer cells: kinetic and molecular docking studies. J Med Chem 2009; 52(21): 6543-5.
[http://dx.doi.org/10.1021/jm901330e] [PMID: 19839593]

[54] Larsen CA. Suppression of Met signaling by the green tea polyphenol (-) epigallocatechin-3-gallate (EGCG). Oregon State University 2010.

[55] Cerezo AB, Winterbone MS, Moyle CW, Needs PW, Kroon PA. Molecular structure-function relationship of dietary polyphenols for inhibiting VEGF-induced VEGFR-2 activity. Mol Nutr Food Res 2015; 59(11): 2119-31.
[http://dx.doi.org/10.1002/mnfr.201500407] [PMID: 26250940]

[56] Shin SY, Yoon H, Ahn S, et al. Structural properties of polyphenols causing cell cycle arrest at G1 phase in HCT116 human colorectal cancer cell lines. Int J Mol Sci 2013; 14(8): 16970-85.
[http://dx.doi.org/10.3390/ijms140816970] [PMID: 23965967]

[57] Kidd PM. Bioavailability and activity of phytosome complexes from botanical polyphenols: the silymarin, curcumin, green tea, and grape seed extracts. Altern Med Rev 2009; 14(3): 226-46.
[PMID: 19803548]

[58] Gangehei L, Ali M, Zhang W, Chen Z, Wakame K, Haidari M. Oligonol a low molecular weight polyphenol of lychee fruit extract inhibits proliferation of influenza virus by blocking reactive oxygen species-dependent ERK phosphorylation. Phytomedicine 2010; 17(13): 1047-56.
[http://dx.doi.org/10.1016/j.phymed.2010.03.016] [PMID: 20554190]

[59] Zhou Q, Bennett LL, Zhou S. Multifaceted ability of naturally occurring polyphenols against metastatic cancer. Clin Exp Pharmacol Physiol 2016; 43(4): 394-409.
[http://dx.doi.org/10.1111/1440-1681.12546] [PMID: 26773801]

[60] Foubert E, De Craene B, Berx G. Key signalling nodes in mammary gland development and cancer. The Snail1-Twist1 conspiracy in malignant breast cancer progression. Breast Cancer Res 2010; 12(3): 206.
[http://dx.doi.org/10.1186/bcr2585] [PMID: 20594364]

[61] Chang YC, Chen PN, Chu SC, Lin CY, Kuo WH, Hsieh YS. Black tea polyphenols reverse epithelial-to-mesenchymal transition and suppress cancer invasion and proteases in human oral cancer cells. J Agric Food Chem 2012; 60(34): 8395-403.
[http://dx.doi.org/10.1021/jf302223g] [PMID: 22827697]

[62] Bolós V, Gasent JM, López-Tarruella S, Grande E. The dual kinase complex FAK-Src as a promising therapeutic target in cancer. OncoTargets Ther 2010; 3: 83-97.
[http://dx.doi.org/10.2147/OTT.S6909] [PMID: 20616959]

[63] Majid S, Dar AA, Ahmad AE, et al. BTG3 tumor suppressor gene promoter demethylation, histone modification and cell cycle arrest by genistein in renal cancer. Carcinogenesis 2009; 30(4): 662-70.
[http://dx.doi.org/10.1093/carcin/bgp042] [PMID: 19221000]

[64] Belguise K, Guo S, Sonenshein GE. Activation of FOXO3a by the green tea polyphenol epigallocatechin-3-gallate induces estrogen receptor α expression reversing invasive phenotype of breast cancer cells. Cancer Res 2007; 67(12): 5763-70.

[http://dx.doi.org/10.1158/0008-5472.CAN-06-4327] [PMID: 17575143]

[65] Belguise K, Guo S, Yang S, *et al.* Green tea polyphenols reverse cooperation between c-Rel and CK2 that induces the aryl hydrocarbon receptor, slug, and an invasive phenotype. Cancer Res 2007; 67(24): 11742-50.
[http://dx.doi.org/10.1158/0008-5472.CAN-07-2730] [PMID: 18089804]

[66] Lin CH, Shen YA, Hung PH, Yu YB, Chen YJ. Epigallocathechin gallate, polyphenol present in green tea, inhibits stem-like characteristics and epithelial-mesenchymal transition in nasopharyngeal cancer cell lines. BMC Complement Altern Med 2012; 12(1): 201.
[http://dx.doi.org/10.1186/1472-6882-12-201] [PMID: 23110507]

[67] Fei F, Qu J, Zhang M, Li Y, Zhang S. S100A4 in cancer progression and metastasis: A systematic review. Oncotarget 2017; 8(42): 73219-39.
[http://dx.doi.org/10.18632/oncotarget.18016] [PMID: 29069865]

[68] Thomas R, Williams M, Sharma H, Chaudry A, Bellamy P. A double-blind, placebo-controlled randomised trial evaluating the effect of a polyphenol-rich whole food supplement on PSA progression in men with prostate cancer--the U.K. NCRN Pomi-T study. Prostate Cancer Prostatic Dis 2014; 17(2): 180-6.
[http://dx.doi.org/10.1038/pcan.2014.6] [PMID: 24614693]

[69] Choan E, Segal R, Jonker D, *et al.* A prospective clinical trial of green tea for hormone refractory prostate cancer: an evaluation of the complementary/alternative therapy approach, Urologic Oncology: Seminars and Original Investigations. Elsevier 2005; pp. 108-13.

[70] Cerdá B, Cerón JJ, Tomás-Barberán FA, Espín JC. Repeated oral administration of high doses of the pomegranate ellagitannin punicalagin to rats for 37 days is not toxic. J Agric Food Chem 2003; 51(11): 3493-501.
[http://dx.doi.org/10.1021/jf020842c] [PMID: 12744688]

[71] Dunnick JK, Hailey JR. Toxicity and carcinogenicity studies of quercetin, a natural component of foods. Fundam Appl Toxicol 1992; 19(3): 423-31.
[http://dx.doi.org/10.1016/0272-0590(92)90181-G] [PMID: 1459373]

[72] Jones E, Hughes RE. Quercetin, flavonoids and the life-span of mice. Exp Gerontol 1982; 17(3): 213-7.
[http://dx.doi.org/10.1016/0531-5565(82)90027-4] [PMID: 7140862]

[73] Hirose M, Takesada Y, Tanaka H, Tamano S, Kato T, Shirai T. Carcinogenicity of antioxidants BHA, caffeic acid, sesamol, 4-methoxyphenol and catechol at low doses, either alone or in combination, and modulation of their effects in a rat medium-term multi-organ carcinogenesis model. Carcinogenesis 1998; 19(1): 207-12.
[http://dx.doi.org/10.1093/carcin/19.1.207] [PMID: 9472713]

[74] Snyder RD, Gillies PJ. Evaluation of the clastogenic, DNA intercalative, and topoisomerase II-interactive properties of bioflavonoids in Chinese hamster V79 cells. Environ Mol Mutagen 2002; 40(4): 266-76.
[http://dx.doi.org/10.1002/em.10121] [PMID: 12489117]

[75] Mennen LI, Walker R, Bennetau-Pelissero C, Scalbert A. Risks and safety of polyphenol consumption. Am J Clin Nutr 2005; 81(1) (Suppl.): 326S-9S.
[http://dx.doi.org/10.1093/ajcn/81.1.326S] [PMID: 15640498]

[76] Schilter B, Andersson C, Anton R, *et al.* Guidance for the safety assessment of botanicals and botanical preparations for use in food and food supplements. Food Chem Toxicol 2003; 41(12): 1625-49.
[http://dx.doi.org/10.1016/S0278-6915(03)00221-7] [PMID: 14563389]

[77] Pan MH, Lai CS, Wu JC, Ho CT. Epigenetic and disease targets by polyphenols. Curr Pharm Des 2013; 19(34): 6156-85.
[http://dx.doi.org/10.2174/1381612811319340010] [PMID: 23448446]

[78]   Shukla S, Meeran SM, Katiyar SK. Epigenetic regulation by selected dietary phytochemicals in cancer chemoprevention. Cancer Lett 2014; 355(1): 9-17.
[http://dx.doi.org/10.1016/j.canlet.2014.09.017] [PMID: 25236912]

[79]   Meeran SM, Ahmed A, Tollefsbol TO. Epigenetic targets of bioactive dietary components for cancer prevention and therapy. Clin Epigenetics 2010; 1(3-4): 101-16.
[http://dx.doi.org/10.1007/s13148-010-0011-5] [PMID: 21258631]

[80]   Shankar E, Kanwal R, Candamo M, Gupta S. Dietary phytochemicals as epigenetic modifiers in cancer: Promise and challenges, Seminars in cancer biology. Elsevier 2016; pp. 82-99.

[81]   Herman-Antosiewicz A, Xiao H, Lew KL, Singh SV. Induction of p21 protein protects against sulforaphane-induced mitotic arrest in LNCaP human prostate cancer cell line. Mol Cancer Ther 2007; 6(5): 1673-81.
[http://dx.doi.org/10.1158/1535-7163.MCT-06-0807] [PMID: 17513615]

[82]   Myzak MC, Tong P, Dashwood W-M, Dashwood RH, Ho E. Sulforaphane retards the growth of human PC-3 xenografts and inhibits HDAC activity in human subjects. Exp Biol Med (Maywood) 2007; 232(2): 227-34.
[PMID: 17259330]

[83]   Majid S, Kikuno N, Nelles J, et al. Genistein induces the p21WAF1/CIP1 and p16INK4a tumor suppressor genes in prostate cancer cells by epigenetic mechanisms involving active chromatin modification. Cancer Res 2008; 68(8): 2736-44.
[http://dx.doi.org/10.1158/0008-5472.CAN-07-2290] [PMID: 18413741]

[84]   Li Y, Meeran SM, Patel SN, Chen H, Hardy TM, Tollefsbol TO. Epigenetic reactivation of estrogen receptor-α (ERα) by genistein enhances hormonal therapy sensitivity in ERα-negative breast cancer. Mol Cancer 2013; 12(1): 9.
[http://dx.doi.org/10.1186/1476-4598-12-9] [PMID: 24063558]

[85]   Li Y, Liu L, Andrews LG, Tollefsbol TO. Genistein depletes telomerase activity through cross-talk between genetic and epigenetic mechanisms. Int J Cancer 2009; 125(2): 286-96.
[http://dx.doi.org/10.1002/ijc.24398] [PMID: 19358274]

[86]   Mense SM, Hei TK, Ganju RK, Bhat HK. Phytoestrogens and breast cancer prevention: possible mechanisms of action. Environ Health Perspect 2008; 116(4): 426-33.
[http://dx.doi.org/10.1289/ehp.10538] [PMID: 18414622]

[87]   Qin W, Zhu W, Shi H, et al. Soy isoflavones have an antiestrogenic effect and alter mammary promoter hypermethylation in healthy premenopausal women. Nutr Cancer 2009; 61(2): 238-44.
[http://dx.doi.org/10.1080/01635580802404196] [PMID: 19235040]

[88]   Reuter S, Gupta SC, Park B, Goel A, Aggarwal BB. Epigenetic changes induced by curcumin and other natural compounds. Genes Nutr 2011; 6(2): 93-108.
[http://dx.doi.org/10.1007/s12263-011-0222-1] [PMID: 21516481]

[89]   Henning SM, Wang P, Carpenter CL, Heber D. Epigenetic effects of green tea polyphenols in cancer. Epigenomics 2013; 5(6): 729-41.
[http://dx.doi.org/10.2217/epi.13.57] [PMID: 24283885]

[90]   Meja KK, Rajendrasozhan S, Adenuga D, et al. Curcumin restores corticosteroid function in monocytes exposed to oxidants by maintaining HDAC2. Am J Respir Cell Mol Biol 2008; 39(3): 312-23.
[http://dx.doi.org/10.1165/rcmb.2008-0012OC] [PMID: 18421014]

[91]   Marcu MG, Jung Y-J, Lee S, et al. Curcumin is an inhibitor of p300 histone acetylatransferase. Med Chem 2006; 2(2): 169-74.
[http://dx.doi.org/10.2174/157340606776056133] [PMID: 16787365]

[92]   Kang S-K, Cha S-H, Jeon H-G. Curcumin-induced histone hypoacetylation enhances caspase---dependent glioma cell death and neurogenesis of neural progenitor cells. Stem Cells Dev 2006; 15(2):

165-74.
[http://dx.doi.org/10.1089/scd.2006.15.165] [PMID: 16646663]

[93] Wang R-H, Zheng Y, Kim H-S, *et al.* Interplay among BRCA1, SIRT1, and Survivin during BRCA1-associated tumorigenesis. Mol Cell 2008; 32(1): 11-20.
[http://dx.doi.org/10.1016/j.molcel.2008.09.011] [PMID: 18851829]

[94] Link A, Balaguer F, Goel A. Cancer chemoprevention by dietary polyphenols: promising role for epigenetics. Biochem Pharmacol 2010; 80(12): 1771-92.
[http://dx.doi.org/10.1016/j.bcp.2010.06.036] [PMID: 20599773]

[95] Fang M, Chen D, Yang CS. Dietary polyphenols may affect DNA methylation. J Nutr 2007; 137(1)(Suppl.): 223S-8S.
[http://dx.doi.org/10.1093/jn/137.1.223S] [PMID: 17182830]

[96] Kato K, Long NK, Makita H, *et al.* Effects of green tea polyphenol on methylation status of RECK gene and cancer cell invasion in oral squamous cell carcinoma cells. Br J Cancer 2008; 99(4): 647-54.
[http://dx.doi.org/10.1038/sj.bjc.6604521] [PMID: 18665171]

[97] Pandey M, Shukla S, Gupta S. Promoter demethylation and chromatin remodeling by green tea polyphenols leads to re-expression of GSTP1 in human prostate cancer cells. Int J Cancer 2010; 126(11): 2520-33.
[PMID: 19856314]

[98] Berletch JB, Liu C, Love WK, Andrews LG, Katiyar SK, Tollefsbol TO. Epigenetic and genetic mechanisms contribute to telomerase inhibition by EGCG. J Cell Biochem 2008; 103(2): 509-19.
[http://dx.doi.org/10.1002/jcb.21417] [PMID: 17570133]

[99] Stresemann C, Brueckner B, Musch T, Stopper H, Lyko F. Functional diversity of DNA methyltransferase inhibitors in human cancer cell lines. Cancer Res 2006; 66(5): 2794-800.
[http://dx.doi.org/10.1158/0008-5472.CAN-05-2821] [PMID: 16510601]

[100] Mittal A, Piyathilake C, Hara Y, Katiyar SK. Exceptionally high protection of photocarcinogenesis by topical application of (--)-epigallocatechin-3-gallate in hydrophilic cream in SKH-1 hairless mouse model: relationship to inhibition of UVB-induced global DNA hypomethylation. Neoplasia 2003; 5(6): 555-65.
[http://dx.doi.org/10.1016/S1476-5586(03)80039-8] [PMID: 14965448]

[101] Morey Kinney SR, Zhang W, Pascual M, *et al.* Lack of evidence for green tea polyphenols as DNA methylation inhibitors in murine prostate. Cancer Prev Res (Phila) 2009; 2(12): 1065-75.
[http://dx.doi.org/10.1158/1940-6207.CAPR-09-0010] [PMID: 19934341]

[102] Yuasa Y, Nagasaki H, Akiyama Y, *et al.* Relationship between CDX2 gene methylation and dietary factors in gastric cancer patients. Carcinogenesis 2005; 26(1): 193-200.
[http://dx.doi.org/10.1093/carcin/bgh304] [PMID: 15498792]

[103] Tsao AS, Liu D, Martin J, *et al.* Phase II randomized, placebo-controlled trial of green tea extract in patients with high-risk oral premalignant lesions. Cancer Prev Res (Phila) 2009; 2(11): 931-41.
[http://dx.doi.org/10.1158/1940-6207.CAPR-09-0121] [PMID: 19892663]

[104] Chalabi N, Delort L, Le Corre L, Satih S, Bignon Y-J, Bernard-Gallon D. Gene signature of breast cancer cell lines treated with lycopene 2006.
[http://dx.doi.org/10.2217/14622416.7.5.663]

[105] Sun Y, Jiang X, Chen S, Price BD. Inhibition of histone acetyltransferase activity by anacardic acid sensitizes tumor cells to ionizing radiation. FEBS Lett 2006; 580(18): 4353-6.
[http://dx.doi.org/10.1016/j.febslet.2006.06.092] [PMID: 16844118]

CHAPTER 5

Glioblastoma Multiforme; Drug Resistance & Combination Therapy

Megha Gautam[1], Saumya Singh[1], Mehak Aggarwal[1], Manish K Sharma[2], Shweta Dang[1] and Reema Gabrani[1,*]

[1] *Jaypee Institute of Information Technology, A-10, Sector 62, Noida, Uttar Pardesh, India*
[2] *Pioneer Center of Biosciences, Mohan Nagar, Ghaziabad, Uttar Pardesh, India*

Abstract: Brain tumors are most aggressive lethal types of cancer and have been reported to have poor prognosis. Patients diagnosed with glioblastoma multiforme (GBM) have an aggressive, tough and resistant brain tumor with average survival 12 to 16 months. The most common age for diagnosis of GBM is reported to be in between 45 and 70 years. GBM arises from glial cells which are glue like supportive cells of the brain that help to maintain and protect the neurons of central and peripheral nervous system from any damage.

GBM is usually treated with surgery and radiation followed by chemotherapy where temozolomide (TMZ) is a part of therapy. TMZ is an alkaline agent that destroys the glioblastoma cells by forming O_6-methylgunine in DNA. TMZ is an anticancer drug popularly used sometimes along with ionizing radiation. However, one of the downsides of chemotherapy is the development of resistance against the drug which results in the failure of the treatment and hence poor prognosis. The alternate treatment strategies are being explored to prolong the survival of GBM. The treatment of GBM by using HDACi (histone deacetylase inhibitors), MGMT (O6-methylguanine DNA methyltransferase) inhibitors, beta blockers, statins, antimetabolites, and some phyto-therapeutics in synergistic combinations may be beneficial for outcome. A number of drugs are being investigated in synergistic combination and will offer a substantial survival advantage in GBM patients. The present chapter discusses the synergistic combinations of mainly TMZ with various other anti-cancer or FDA approved drugs for other indications that can enhance different molecular mechanisms, increase cell death, reduce drug resistance or decrease the drug toxicity in glioblastomas.

Keywords: Bcl-2, Cancer Stem Cells, Chemotherapeutics, Combination, GBM, Hypoxia, MGMT, Resistance, Temozolomide, Therapy.

---

[*] **Corresponding author Reema Gabrani:** Jaypee Institute of Information Technology, A-10, Sector 62, Noida, Uttar Pardesh, India; Tel: +91-120-2594211; Fax: 0120-2400986; Email: reema.gabrani@jiit.ac.in

Atta-ur-Rahman and M. Iqbal Choudhary (Eds.)
All rights reserved-© 2019 Bentham Science Publishers

INTRODUCTION

The abnormal growth of cells which originate in the brain is categorised as primary brain tumor. It could also reach the brain due to metastatic spread from other parts of the body termed as secondary tumor. The tumor rate of growth along with its location determines its effect on the function of the nervous system [1]. The cranial bones are fixed and there is no space for tumor mass to grow. Consequently, the symptoms occur due to increase in intracranial pressure which causes headaches, memory loss, seizures and behaviour changes. It may also include loss of sensation or movement of a body part, speech irregularities and issues with recognition skills. Symptoms usually rest on the location of tumor occurrence and their respective mass. This can result in severe brain damage which could be life-threatening [1].

Glioblastoma (GBM) classified as grade IV is the most common and lethal type of brain tumor with poor prognosis [2]. GBM is generally reported between 45 to 70 years of age [3]. GBM treatment involves chemotherapy accompanied with surgery and radiotherapy [2]. The most common chemotherapeutic drug used for the treatment of GBM is temozolomide (TMZ). Regardless of the present treatment, prognosis of GBM is poor and the average survival is around one year [3]. However, the problem with current treatment is the occurrence of TMZ resistance. Still, there is no other alternative treatment approach that can extend the overall survival in GBM patients. Some factors which are involved in the drug resistance mechanism are Bcl-2 family of proteins, O6- methylguanine- DNA-methyltransferase (MGMT), cancer stem cells (CSCs), epidermal growth factor receptor mutations and hypoxia [4 - 7].

The alkylating agent TMZ causes DNA methylation and leads to cell death. GBM cells show TMZ resistance which is mediated by MGMT that can result in demethylation [4]. The TMZ resistance is a major hurdle to cure GBM and many drugs have been developed to target the demethylation mediated by MGMT. Epidermal growth factor receptor (EGFR) amplification as well as overexpression has been seen in GBM. Truncated and deleted version of EGFR has been identified and EGFRvIII mutation is very common which changes the protein sequences resulting in altered antigenicity [8]. Hedgehog aberrant signaling has also been linked to GBM. Hedgehog pathway is crucial during embryogenesis and supports CNS development. This signaling pathway can also contribute towards GBM resistance and be a potential target for its therapy [9].

GBM undergoes extensive changes in its epigenome which can alter the expression of gene. These alterations are also the suitable target to restrict the growth of cancer. Histone deacetylase inhibitors (HDACi) are characterized as anticancer drugs that can alter the epigenome and lead to cell cycle arrest or cell death [10].

The development of novel therapeutics is still in need that can increase the survival rate in GBM patients. The identification of more drugs in synergistic combination with TMZ might be promising and significantly improve the overall survival in GBM patients. The chapter focuses on drug resistance in GBM and the various therapeutic combinations targeting several disrupted cellular pathways.

CLASSIFICATION OF ASTROCYTIC TUMORS

Astrocytoma is malignant brain tumor, arising from the astrocytes, star shape like cells of the brain. Astrocyte is a type of glial cell which is glue like in connective tissue that provides support to the nerve cell. The entire tumor arising from the glial cells is known as glioma, the most common primary brain tumor. WHO classified the astrocytomas on the basis of cellular proliferation and necrotic tissue found in between the tumor mass which shows the tumor as a high grade type. According to the 2016 WHO classification, astrocytomas are further classified on the basis of their molecular parameters [11]. Now according to the WHO 2016 classification, brain tumor is categorized on the basis of isocitrate dehydrogenase (IDH)-mutant or IDH-wildtype markers status.

Diffusive Astrocytomas and Anaplastic Astrocytomas

Diffuse gliomas include the WHO grade II and grade III astrocytic tumors, grade II and grade III oligodendroglioma, grade IV glioblastoma (GBM), diffusive gliomas of childhood and some other types of astrocytomas. The WHO grade II diffuse astrocytomas and WHO grade III anaplastic astrocytomas are classified according to their IDH mutant status, and NOS (Not other specified) categories. Tumor is designated as NOS when there is no facility for molecular tests. Most of the grade II and grade III tumors are classified as *IDH* mutant category. *IDH* mutation could be at genes located at its codon 132 or/and 172 and they have been mainly identified as single amino acid missense mutation. *IDH* wild type does not contain any of these mutations [12].

There are two types of glioblastomas (grade IV tumor)-

1. Glioblastoma, IDH-wildtype: This brain tumor is primary GBM (arising *de novo*) which is aggressive in nature and the most common type affecting more than 90% of the cases [13].

2. Glioblastoma, IDH mutant: Secondary GBM (arising from a lower-grade tumor): These tumors originate as lower grade and can be slow growing and

may take longer to become higher grade tumor. They are generally found in younger age group and can represent around 10% cases [11].

DRUG RESISTANCE

Glioblastoma (GBM) is the most common primary malignant brain tumor and also one of the deadliest tumors in humans. Standard of care for this disease includes maximal surgical resection, radiation, and chemotherapy with alkylating agent temozolomide (TMZ). Despite aggressive treatment the majority of tumors eventually recur and intrinsic molecular signaling as well as tumor cellular heterogeneity are among the most challenging factors leading to recurrence. These mechanisms quickly adapt GBM cells to cytotoxic therapeutics and drive adaptive evolution of tumor cells through interaction with the complex tumor microenvironment. The key players in these mechanisms are cancer stem cells (CSC), which actively utilize a wide variety of complex progenitor-like behaviors and signaling pathways to expand tumor cell population.

Despite the aggressive treatment, occurrence of resistance in tumor is becoming a common problem. The intrinsic molecular signaling and GBM heterogeneity are main factors leading to recurrence [6]. The intrinsic mechanisms cause TMZ resistance to tumor cells where complex tumor microenvironment is also involved. The GBM stem like cells (GSC) play a role in heterogeneity as well as in drug resistance mechanisms, which are associated with the molecular pathways that promote the growth of tumor cell population and metastasis [5].

GSCs have the ability for self-renewal and are also involved in tumorigenic initiation and resistance mechanisms [14]. The radiotherapy and chemotherapy can enhance the GSC side population, categorized by the expression of stem cell markers, thus, making the GBM cells more resistant to treatment. GSCs subpopulations have been recently characterized by Lan *et al.* [14]. According to the study, the group A clones have neutral growth dynamics and TMZ was effective in restricting the growth of these cells. A minority population group B GSC showed different growth pattern and were resistant to TMZ. The population of slow cycling GSC can evolve to stem cells having rapid self-maintenance ability that gives rise to non-dividing cells. Moreover, the rare 'outlier' group B clones could result in the expansion of GSC population resistant to chemotherapy [14].

Recent studies have shown that there is over-expression of nucleolin, a protein that plays a role in ribosome biogenesis and in RNA maturation, in GBM. Nucleolin lessens the GSCs enrichment and may lower the risk of drug resistance [15]. It has been observed recently that nucleolin decreased the levels of stem cell markers like Sox2 and Oct4 and made GBM cells more sensitive to TMZ [15]. Hence it was reported that nucleolin has inverse relationship with GSC [15].

Ahmed *et al.* have linked hypoxia to upregulation of GSC population which makes the GBM cells more resistant to treatment. The study showed that hypoxia inducible factors (HIF) HIF-1α and HIF-2α enhanced the expression of stem cell marker CD133. The knock down of HIF-1α and HIF-2α by siRNA decreased CD133 expression and sensitized the cells to chemotherapy. It was observed that HIF-1α and HIF-2α were associated with resistance mediated by TMZ and cisplatin, respectively [16].

Some of the drugs owe their biological response on cancer due to their ability to cause DNA damage. The DNA repair mechanism can counter the DNA damage caused by drugs and can also play a role in drug resistance. TMZ causes cell death as DNA methylation agent where O^6-methylguanine DNA methyltransferase (MGMT) can cause demethylation hence counter the effect of the drug. Thus the population of GBM cells in the presence of MGMT becomes ineffective and resistant to TMZ. Dysregulation in other molecular mechanisms such as nucleotide excision repair (NER), homologous recombination (HR) and also mismatch repair (MMR) can reverse the DNA damage caused by TMZ and hence can also contribute to resistance. There has been an effort to predict TMZ resistance based on the analysis of these DNA repair markers [17].

COMBINATION THERAPY AGAINST GLIOBLASTOMA

The standard therapies used against GBM are not sufficient since their cytotoxic effects lead to lifelong morbidity in a number of patients. Novel therapeutic strategies are required to overcome the issue of increasing drug resistance. The recent approach is the use of synergistic compounds or drugs that can work on different targets such that their combined effects will reduce the tumor growth. The *in vitro* screening of FDA approval drugs which are not previously identified as GBM therapeutics [18] or novel compounds could be useful for GBM treatment in combinations with approved drugs (Table **1**).

Table 1. Selected drug combinations and their mechanism of action against glioblastoma.

S.No	Combinatorial Therapy	Class of Drug	Mechanism of Action in GBM Cells	Reference
1	Thalidomide (THD) + TMZ	Immunomodulatory drug	Tumor necrosis factor (TNF-α) which induces angiogenesis, THD inhibits the expression of TNF-α	[19]
2	Lomeguatrib + TMZ	Anti-cancer	Inactivates MGMT, decreased MGMT expression, increased p53 expression, and did not change MGMT methylation	[20]

(Table 1) cont.....

S.No	Combinatorial Therapy	Class of Drug	Mechanism of Action in GBM Cells	Reference
3	TMZ + Cisplatin	Anti-cancer	Downregulates the expression of MGMT	[21]
4	Bevacizumab + Irinotecan	monoclonal antibody + anti-cancer	Reduce the expression of angiogenic factors and shows anti-neoplastic activity	[22]
5	Pitavastatin + Irinotecan	Statins	Anti- tumor activity by targeting MDR-1	[23]
6	LEV + TMZ	Antiepileptic + anti-cancer	Inhibition of MGMT	[24]
7	2DG (2-deoxyglucose) + metformin	Anti-metabolite + anti-hyperglycemic	Effectively reduced the stemness and invasive properties by downregulating the expression of nestin, Sox-2, and Notch2, CD133 in GBM cell line	[25]
8	Cisplatin + TMZ	Anti-cancer	Significantly enhanced apoptosis, activated caspase-3 and PARP levels	[26]
9	2-DG + Cisplatin	Antimetabolite + anticancer	Reduction of the levels of intracellular ATP	[27]
10	Hydroxychloroquine + TMZ	Antimalarial + anti-cancer	Regulates GBM chemoresistance	[28]
11	Valproate + TMZ	Anti-epileptic + anti-cancer	Regulates TMZ sensitivity *via* downregulation of MGMT	[29]
12	Ciprofloxacin + TMZ	Antibiotic + anti-cancer	Sensitized MDR to chemotherapy or increased the efficacy of chemotherapeutic agents	[30]
13	Paclitaxel+ TMZ	Anti-cancer	Inhibition of glucose metabolism	[31]
14	Fluoxetine + TMZ	SSRIs + anti-cancer	Activates the endoplasmic reticulum (ER) stress-related apoptotic	[32]
15	Bortezomib + TMZ	Proteasome inhibitor + anti-cancer	Overcomes MGMT-mediated GBM resistance to temozolomide	[33]
16	Olaparib + TMZ	Anti-cancer + anti-cancer	Enhanced radio-sensitisation responses to PARP inhibitors	[34]
17	Vorinostat + TMZ	HDACi + anti-cancer	Vorinostat being histone deacetylase (HDAC) inhibitor has shown radiosensitizing properties in clinical trial in combination with TMZ	[35]

(Table 1) cont.....

S.No	Combinatorial Therapy	Class of Drug	Mechanism of Action in GBM Cells	Reference
18	Sulfasalazine + Valproic Acid	Rheumatoid arthritis + anti- epilepsy	Causes cell death via dysregulation in the intracellular oxidative response	[36]
19	Copanlisib + Gemcitabine	PI3-Kinase inhibitor + anti-cancer	Preclinical studies have shown that copanlisib with gemcitabine in combination have anti-tumor activity *in vivo*	[37]
20	ABT263 + Crizotinib	Bcl-2 family protein inhibitor + anti-cancer	Inhibits Bcl-2 and Bcl-xL	[38]
21	GDC-0941 + ABT263	PI3K inhibitor + Bcl-2 family protein inhibitor	Overcomes endogenous resistance to apoptosis by Mcl-1 mediated cell death	[39]
22	sFRP4 (secreted Frizzled-Related Protein 4) +TMZ	Wnt antagonist + anti-cancer	Inhibits glioma stem- like cells by modulating EMT via Wnt/β-catenin pathway	[40]

Based on target mechanism, various combinations of drugs being studied for their efficacy against GBM are discussed below.

MGMT Inhibitors

GBM cells appear resistant to TMZ which is mediated by DNA repair protein, MGMT, that removes the TMZ-generated DNA adduct [41].

Resistance to TMZ is a major obstacle for the successful treatment of GBM. It has been reported that GBM patients with a methylated MGMT promoter have an increased overall survival and better response to combinatorial TMZ and radiation therapy compared with radiation itself [42]. Lack of MGMT expression at protein level is considered good prognostic factor in TMZ-treated GBM patients [43].

It is well known that genetic and epigenetic silencing of MGMT as well as DNA repair genes is associated with number of glioblastoma cases. Many drugs have been developed to target this methylation site. As GBM develops resistance to TMZ, it has been combined with other drugs such as cisplatin, lomeguatrib. Clinical studies of cisplatin in combination with TMZ showed promising results [21].

Bobustuc *et al.* [44] found significant reduction of cell proliferation when treated with Levetiracetam plus TMZ in several GBM cell lines. Levetiracetam has also been reported to have an inhibitory effect on MGMT protein expression in GBM cell lines but not in normal human astrocyte cells. Another alkylating agent lomustine has shown efficacy in association with TMZ in GBM resistant cells.

The effect was more pronounced in MMR deficient GBM cells [45]. Other inhibitors like poly ADP ribose polymerase (PARP) inhibitor (olaparib) can also be combined with TMZ for treatment against GBM [34].

Anti-angiogenic Compounds

Angiogenesis is the process where new blood vessels are made from the already existing vessels to provide nutrients to growing mass of tumor and further facilitate metastasis. Hypoxia in GBM is associated with expression of HIF and can induce pro-angiogenic factors like vascular endothelial growth factor (VEGF), platelet derived growth factor (PDGF), fibroblast growth factor (FGF). Various drugs are being explored to target angiogenesis to reduce metastasis. Earlier studies were conducted upon combining temozolomide with thalidomide, an anti-angiogenic agent [20]. Despite the initial promise, the drug did not exhibit any efficacy in the presence of TMZ and radiation therapy. Studies have been conducted on GBM using the drug bevacizumab, a monoclonal antibody, that inhibits VEGF. Bevacizumab is the first anti-angiogenic therapy approved for use in patients with cancer. This is FDA approved drug for treating recurrent GBM. It is reported to show positive effects when combined with radiation therapy and temozolomide against grade 3 and grade 4 gliomas by sensitizing the GBM cells to drugs and radiotherapy. However, many of the clinical trials with other anti-angiogenic drugs like enzastaurin, dasatinib did not show any significant improvement in progression free survival [46].

Apart from VEGF, other molecules which promote angiogenesis have also been targeted to restrict GBM. These molecules include matrix metalloproteinases (MMPs), integrins, key mediators of Delta-Notch and Wnt pathways [47]. Wnt signaling *via* β-catenin pathway increased glycolytic pathway resulting in accumulation of lactate which promotes lactate transporter and thus angiogenesis [47]. There is ongoing clinical trial against selected solid malignancies using LGK974, Wnt inhibitor [48], which covers head and neck and cervical squamous cell cancer. LGK974 in GBM cell lines could reduce tumor growth and deplete GSC population [49]. So far, only bevacizumab has shown success in restricting GBM and is being combined with various other agents like antigens as vaccine candidates [50 - 53] to boost the immune system.

Bcl-2 Family Inhibitors

Programmed cell death or apoptosis is the natural and very important response of the cell towards damage. Cancer cells evade apoptosis either by increasing expression of anti-apoptotic factors like Bcl2 or reducing levels of pro-apoptotic factors Bax, Bad. These mediators of the apoptosis along with their regulators like IAPs (inhibitors of apoptosis proteins) are one of the prime targets for anticancer therapy. It has been observed that phosphatidyl inositol 3 kinase (PI3K) inhibitor (GDC-0941) and Bcl2 inhibitor (ABT-263) reduced resistance to apoptosis and mediated cell death [39]. The anti-cancerous effects were evident by alteration in membrane potential and increased activity of both initiator and effector caspases [48, 52]. Another study indicated that anti-BH3 domain molecule, ABT263 and cMET pathway inhibitor called crizotinib, exhibited synergistic activity in GBM tumor reduction by decreasing the levels of Bcl2 and Bcl-xL [46, 50]. Another study indicated IAP inhibitor, GDC-0152, showed tumor reduction in mice model for GBM [54].

Histone Deacetylase Inhibitors

HDACs are over-expressed in many cancer types including GBM. They have been linked to silencing of genes which are involved in regulation of cell cycle, DNA damage, cellular repair and apoptotic pathways. HDACi can trigger hyper-acetylation of histones or non-histone proteins, promoting growth arrest and apoptosis [55, 56]. Some studies have shown a potential benefit of HDACi such as vorinostat, valproic acid in the treatment of GBM [57, 58]. These inhibitors can radio sensitize GBM cells to standard drug and also enhance the effect of chemotherapy drugs. HDACi can also be combined with other agents like lysine-specific histone demethylase 1 (LSD1) which can be more effective against GBM cells [57].

Overall the clinical studies have shown very little success towards the efficacy of these drugs. New isoforms of HDACi (PCI-34051, ACY-1215) are currently being explored. Further research in finding effective combinations of HDACi is warranted [57]. Vorinostat along with TMZ and pembrolizumab (approved for cervical cancer) clinical trials are ongoing for GBM treatment [59].

Epidermal Growth Factor Receptor Inhibitor

EGFR dysregulation in terms of its mutation or over-expression has been observed in numerous cases in GBM. EGFR aberrant mutations in colorectal carcinoma, squamous cell carcinoma and head and neck cancer are very well documented and FDA approved small molecule based inhibitors are used as line of therapy. However, the clinical data using some of the approved tyrosine kinase inhibitors (erlotinib, gefitinib, lapatinib) for the treatment of GBM was ineffective. The failure in clinical trials was attributed to EGFRvIII mutant expression and also to loss of phosphatase and tensin homolog (PTEN). Continuous EGFR signaling leads to proliferation of cells by mitogen activated protein kinase (MAPK) pathway and PI3K pathway. PTEN is tyrosine phosphatase which specifically inactivates phosphatidylinositol 3,4,5 triphosphate. PTEN mutation keeps the PI3K in the active form for much longer duration and promotes proliferation of cells [60].

Development of resistance in GBM due to expression of mutated EGFR has been linked to increased expression of Bcl-xL protein [61].

New devised immunotherapy, chimeric antigen receptor (CAR)-T cells, helps T cells to recognize antigen, without being presented along with MHC. Specific CAR-T cells were designed by fusing single-chain antibody variable fragment (scFv) (specific to mutant EGFvIII) to T cell receptor and are being tested in clinical trials [62].

Erlotinib (EGFR inhibitor) in combination with arsenic trioxide (multifunctional inhibitor) synergistically induced cell death, promoted reactive oxygen species response, decreased survival and migration of GBM cells [63]. *In silico* analysis of various drugs in combination and their effect on various mitogenic pathways in terms of cell death revealed that EGFR amplification or PTEN loss did not correlate with combinatorial drugs suggesting that other approaches are required to address the GBM resistance [64].

Targeting Hedgehog Pathway

Hedgehog signaling is an important embryogenic pathway. When hedgehog ligand binds to the patched receptor, it relieves the smoothened receptor from inhibitory effect of patched receptor. As a result, Gli signaling protein enters nucleus, acts as transcription factor and promotes the transcription of target genes. A recent study linked MGMT positive GBM tissues with increased expression of Gli. Many different small molecular based inhibitors like GDC0449, LDE225 and natural products (curcumin, resveratrol) have shown promising results towards inhibition of hedgehog pathway by inducing apoptosis and inhibiting PI3K pathway [65]. Cyclopamine administration along with TMZ displayed synergistic effect on GBM tumor inhibition [9]. GSCs inhibition has also been shown to increase multiple folds in the presence of Gli inhibitor and TMZ and reduced the size of neurospheres [66].

Other Target Mechanisms

Other than the common targets such as angiogenesis and MGMT gene silencing, researchers have focused and tried to examine the role of other potential targets in glioblastomas. These include the potassium channels Kv1.3 expressed in the inner mitochondrial membrane of many cancer cells. Kv1.3 channels are known to modulate cell proliferation in endothelial cells, T lymphocytes, macrophages and cancer cells. By inhibiting Kv1.3 channels, a drug can induce apoptosis in several tumor cells at doses that will not be lethal for normal cells. Studies have been conducted upon various Kv1.3 inhibitors including mitochondria-targeted derivatives (PAPTP or PCARBTP) obtained from 5-(4-phenoxybutoxy) psoralen (PAP-1) as well as clofazimine [67]. *In vitro* studies of these drugs have shown a positive result, however these drugs still need to be optimized to translate the results *in vivo* with similar efficacy. Another potential target is MDR1 (multi drug resistance) protein which aids glioblastoma to acquire resistance to many drugs like TMZ. MDR1 is part of ABC transporter which is responsible for efflux of drugs and toxins and hence, confers resistance [68].

Statins are prescribed to treat hypercholesterolemia. Statins were indicated as possible adjunctive treatments in several cancers, due to inhibitory effects on cell signaling pathways which are involved in proliferation, migration, invasion and induction of apoptosis [69, 70]. Several recent *in vitro* studies have found statins to have proapoptotic and cytotoxic effects on glioma and other cancer cells [23, 71]. Many of the FDA approved statins (HMG-Co A reductase inhibitors) have also been combined with anti-neoplastic agents such as irinotecan and their effect has been studied to overcome the resistance [23]. Among different statins, pitavastatin when combined with irinotecan reported the best results. Pitavastatin is highly efficient in reducing tumor growth. It acts as a substrate for MDR1 protein which is highly expressed in glioblastoma cells upon drug treatment and increases resistance to chemotherapy. Irinotecan, topoisomerase inhibitor, also has shown a synergistic effect by lowering IC_{50} in combination with pitavastatin by inhibiting the MDR1 activity by suppressing its glycosylation [23].

Psychotropic Drugs

The psychotropic drugs are used to stimulate neurotransmission and several studies have reported their anti-proliferative activity [72, 73]. Some subclasses of psychotropic drugs including tricyclic antidepressants (TCAs), selective serotonin reuptake inhibitors (SSRIs), antiepileptic drugs (AEDs) are being investigated as possible adjuvants for treatment of cancer [72, 74 - 76]. These drugs might reduce the proliferation of cells by promoting autophagic cell death by inhibiting PI3K pathway. Some antipsychotics like pimozide are selective serotonin receptor 7 inhibitor and they can be combined with other drugs.

Recently studies have been reported that antidepressants (amitriptyline, imipramine) and SSRIs (paroxetine, fluoxetine and sertraline) increased the caspase-3 activity and reduced tumor cell proliferation in cell lines, including rat C6 glioma, human neuroblastoma and human astrocytoma cell lines [73, 77].

Beta-Blockers

Beta blockers, also known as beta-adrenergic blocking agents are commonly prescribed in the treatment of hypertension and in prevention of cardiovascular diseases [78, 79]. Some studies have proposed that these agents may inhibit angiogenesis, invasion and cellular proliferation and also increase apoptosis in several cancer cell lines [80, 81].

Several studies have shown the efficacy of beta-blocker propranolol as an adjunctive treatment of cancer. Propranolol is a nonselective beta-blocker that competes with adrenaline and noradrenaline binding at beta-1- and -2 adreno-receptor sites [25, 82]. Pasquier *et al.* [80] investigated the use of propranolol in several cell lines, including human breast cancer, neuroblastoma and U87 GBM cell lines. Higher dose of propranolol was required to decrease the proliferation in all cell lines. However, propranolol in combination with paclitaxel and 5-fluorouracil decreased angiogenesis and was most effective against breast cancer cell lines. Results were not reported for antiangiogenic effects of propranolol in the U87 GBM cell line. Propranolol and butoxamine were shown to induce apoptosis by increasing caspase activity [81]. Wolter *et al.* have also shown that propranolol could activate tumor suppressor protein p53 and thus inhibit proliferation of cells [83].

Anti-Metabolites

2-Deoxyglucose (2DG) is known as a glycolytic inhibitor. In a recent study, GBM cell viability was significantly decreased by the combination of 2-deoxyglucose (2DG) and metformin [25]. The combination was effective in reducing cellular metabolism, invasion ability and also reduced stemness ability of the GBM cells. Pistollato *et al.* [84] have also shown that 2-DG increased succinate dehydrogenase activity which resulted in decreased succinate and hence HIF-1α which forced the GBM cells towards differentiation [84]. 2-Deoxyglucose (2DG) has also been shown to inhibit cancer cell proliferation in pancreatic cancer [82] and also in breast cancer [85]. It has also been reported that metformin, a well-known biguanide (anti-diabetic), inhibits cancer cell migration and proliferation [86].

CONCLUSION

The difficulty in treating glioblastoma disease lies in its inherent complexity and numerous mechanisms of drug resistance. Comprehending the molecular relationship between GBM cells and their environment is critical since these abnormalities can indicate tumor formation and progression, a process that can be reversible *via* therapeutic targeting for restoration of sensitivity to drugs. Thus, the identification of the cellular and molecular mechanisms that confer drug resistance is an important goal for the treatment of glioblastomas.

Resistance in GBM cells can develop due to various factors like hypoxia, GBM stem cells, and modulation of various proteins involved in cell cycle regulation and apoptosis. Other factors like aberrations in developmental pathways like Wnt, hedgehog have also been linked to resistance in GBM. Alterations in genetic as well as epigenetic pathways like EGFR-MAPK, PI3K can contribute towards GBM resistance. The most reported case of resistance for GBM is towards TMZ. The main players like MGMT and other DNA repair enzymes can reverse the methylation caused by TMZ and aid in development of resistance.

Various factors involved in GBM development are the potential sites for targeted therapy. Crossing the blood brain barrier poses a major hurdle to the efficient drug targeting to restrict the uncontrolled tumor. Some of the drugs like erlotinib which is FDA approved for restricting squamous cell carcinoma of the lung, was not effective against GBM in clinical trials. There are other instances like inefficacy of HDACi against GBM also corroborates that GBM is very tough to cure. Novel and combinatorial approach is being explored to find an effective cure for GBM. Various combinations like TMZ with HDACi, PI3K inhibitor or hedgehog inhibitor have shown encouraging data for restricting GBM.

Several researches have shown that the number of drugs currently in market like anti-depressants, anti-epileptic, statins, beta-blockers and other antihypertensive agents, exhibit promising antineoplastic effects *in vitro*. The ability to use currently marketed drugs in the treatment of GBM provides a financially practical approach to encourage the development of new therapeutic treatments to improve outcome survival in patients with GBM. Despite lot of data, success rate in clinical trials has not been very encouraging. The reason could be many times *in vitro* analysis and animal model cannot predict the actual biological response in humans. So far, the data related to Bevacizumab, anti-VEGF antibody, has been encouraging. Its various combinations with antigens as vaccine candidates and immune boosters are in various stages of clinical trials. Many individually approved drugs separately for GBM or other cancer indication has been combined like Vorinostat, TMZ and pembrolizumab and is in clinical trials.

Glioblastoma remains a challenging disease and alternative strategies are required to develop well-organized and appropriate therapeutic options against GBM.

CONSENT FOR PUBLICATION

Not applicable.

CONFLICT OF INTEREST

The authors declare no conflict of interest, financial or otherwise.

ACKNOWLEDGEMENTS

We thank Department of Biotechnology, Jaypee Institute of Information Technology, Noida, UP, India, for providing the infrastructural facility to support the work.

REFERENCES

[1] Hanif F, Muzaffar K, Perveen K, Malhi SM, Simjee ShU. Glioblastoma multiforme: A review of its epidemiology and pathogenesis through clinical presentation and treatment. Asian Pac J Cancer Prev 2017; 18(1): 3-9.
[http://dx.doi.org/10.22034/APJCP.2017.18.1.3] [PMID: 28239999]

[2] Tamimi AF, Juweid M. Epidemiology and Outcome of Glioblastoma. In: De Vleeschouwer S, Ed. Glioblastoma Brisbane, Australia: Codon Publications. 2017; pp. 143-53.
[http://dx.doi.org/10.15586/codon.glioblastoma.2017.ch8]

[3] Stupp R, Mason WP, van den Bent MJ, et al. Radiotherapy plus concomitant and adjuvant temozolomide for glioblastoma. N Engl J Med 2005; 352(10): 987-96.
[http://dx.doi.org/10.1056/NEJMoa043330] [PMID: 15758009]

[4] Lee SY. Temozolomide resistance in glioblastoma multiforme. Genes Dis 2016; 3(3): 198-210.
[http://dx.doi.org/10.1016/j.gendis.2016.04.007] [PMID: 30258889]

[5] Safari M, Khoshnevisan A. Cancer stem cells and chemoresistance in glioblastoma multiform: A review article. J Stem Cells 2015; 10(4): 271-85.
[http://dx.doi.org/jsc.2015.10.4.271]

[6] Kouri FM, Jensen SA, Stegh AH. The role of Bcl-2 family proteins in therapy responses of malignant astrocytic gliomas: Bcl2L12 and beyond. Sci World J 2012; 2012: 838916.
[http://dx.doi.org/10.1100/2012/838916] [PMID: 22431925]

[7] Chou CW, Wang CC, Wu CP, et al. Tumor cycling hypoxia induces chemoresistance in glioblastoma multiforme by upregulating the expression and function of ABCB1. Neuro-oncol 2012; 14(10): 1227-38.
[http://dx.doi.org/10.1093/neuonc/nos195] [PMID: 22946104]

[8] Chistiakov DA, Chekhonin IV, Chekhonin VP. The EGFR variant III mutant as a target for immunotherapy of glioblastoma multiforme. Eur J Pharmacol 2017; 810: 70-82.
[http://dx.doi.org/10.1016/j.ejphar.2017.05.064] [PMID: 28583430]

[9] Wang K, Chen D, Qian Z, Cui D, Gao L, Lou M. Hedgehog/Gli1 signaling pathway regulates MGMT expression and chemoresistance to temozolomide in human glioblastoma. Cancer Cell Int 2017; 17: 117.
[http://dx.doi.org/10.1186/s12935-017-0491-x] [PMID: 29225516]

[10] Eckschlager T, Plch J, Stiborova M, Hrabeta J. Histone deacetylase inhibitors as anticancer drugs. Int J Mol Sci 2017; 18(7): E1414.
[http://dx.doi.org/10.3390/ijms18071414] [PMID: 28671573]

[11] Louis DN, Ohgaki H, Wiestler OD, Cavenee WK. World Health Organization Histological Classification of Tumours of the Central Nervous System. International Agency for Research on Cancer, France 2016; 26(25): 4189-99.

[12] Reuss DE, Mamatjan Y, Schrimpf D, et al. IDH mutant diffuse and anaplastic astrocytomas have similar age at presentation and little difference in survival: a grading problem for WHO. Acta Neuropathol 2015; 129(6): 867-73.
[http://dx.doi.org/10.1007/s00401-015-1438-8] [PMID: 25962792]

[13] Ohgaki H, Kleihues P. The definition of primary and secondary glioblastoma. Clin Cancer Res 2013;

19(4): 764-72.
[http://dx.doi.org/10.1158/1078-0432.CCR-12-3002] [PMID: 23209033]

[14] Lan X, Jörg DJ, Cavalli FMG, *et al.* Fate mapping of human glioblastoma reveals an invariant stem cell hierarchy. Nature 2017; 549(7671): 227-32.
[http://dx.doi.org/10.1038/nature23666] [PMID: 28854171]

[15] Ko CY, Lin CH, Chuang JY, Chang WC, Hsu TI. MDM2 degrades deacetylated nucleolin through ubiquitination to promote glioma stem-like cell enrichment for chemotherapeutic resistance. Mol Neurobiol 2018; 55(4): 3211-23.
[http://dx.doi.org/10.1007/s12035-017-0569-4] [PMID: 28478507]

[16] Ahmed EM, Bandopadhyay G, Coyle B, Grabowska A. A HIF-independent, CD133-mediated mechanism of cisplatin resistance in glioblastoma cells. Cell Oncol (Dordr) 2018; 41(3): 319-28.
[http://dx.doi.org/10.1007/s13402-018-0374-8] [PMID: 29492900]

[17] Nagel ZD, Kitange GJ, Gupta SK, *et al.* DNA repair capacity in multiple pathways predicts chemoresistance in glioblastoma multiforme. Cancer Res 2017; 77(1): 198-206.
[http://dx.doi.org/10.1158/0008-5472.CAN-16-1151] [PMID: 27793847]

[18] Kast RE, Boockvar JA, Brüning A, *et al.* A conceptually new treatment approach for relapsed glioblastoma: coordinated undermining of survival paths with nine repurposed drugs (CUSP9) by the International Initiative for Accelerated Improvement of Glioblastoma Care. Oncotarget 2013; 4(4): 502-30.
[http://dx.doi.org/10.18632/oncotarget.969] [PMID: 23594434]

[19] Son MJ, Kim JS, Kim MH, *et al.* Combination treatment with temozolomide and thalidomide inhibits tumor growth and angiogenesis in an orthotopic glioma model. Int J Oncol 2006; 28(1): 53-9.
[PMID: 16327979]

[20] Taspinar M, Ilgaz S, Ozdemir M, *et al.* Effect of lomeguatrib-temozolomide combination on MGMT promoter methylation and expression in primary glioblastoma tumor cells. Tumour Biol 2013; 34(3): 1935-47.
[http://dx.doi.org/10.1007/s13277-013-0738-7] [PMID: 23519841]

[21] Wang Y, Kong X, Guo Y, Wang R, Ma W. Continuous dose-intense temozolomide and cisplatin in recurrent glioblastoma patients. Medicine (Baltimore) 2017; 96(10): e6261.
[http://dx.doi.org/10.1097/MD.0000000000006261] [PMID: 28272232]

[22] Mesti T, Moltara ME, Boc M, Rebersek M, Ocvirk J. Bevacizumab and irinotecan in recurrent malignant glioma, a single institution experience. Radiol Oncol 2015; 49(1): 80-5.
[http://dx.doi.org/10.2478/raon-2014-0021] [PMID: 25810706]

[23] Jiang P, Mukthavaram R, Chao Y, *et al.* Novel anti-glioblastoma agents and therapeutic combinations identified from a collection of FDA approved drugs. J Transl Med 2014; 12: 13.
[http://dx.doi.org/10.1186/1479-5876-12-13] [PMID: 24433351]

[24] Kim YH, Kim T, Joo JD, *et al.* Survival benefit of levetiracetam in patients treated with concomitant chemoradiotherapy and adjuvant chemotherapy with temozolomide for glioblastoma multiforme. Cancer 2015; 121(17): 2926-32.
[http://dx.doi.org/10.1002/cncr.29439] [PMID: 25975354]

[25] Kim EH, Lee JH, Oh Y, *et al.* Inhibition of glioblastoma tumorspheres by combined treatment with 2-deoxyglucose and metformin. Neuro-oncol 2017; 19(2): 197-207.
[http://dx.doi.org/10.1093/neuonc/now174] [PMID: 27571886]

[26] Qi Q, Liu X, Li S, Joshi HC, Ye K. Synergistic suppression of noscapine and conventional chemotherapeutics on human glioblastoma cell growth. Acta Pharmacol Sin 2013; 34(7): 930-8.
[http://dx.doi.org/10.1038/aps.2013.40] [PMID: 23708557]

[27] Jalota A, Kumar M, Das BC, Yadav AK, Chosdol K, Sinha S. Synergistic increase in efficacy of a combination of 2-deoxy-D-glucose and cisplatin in normoxia and hypoxia: switch from autophagy to

apoptosis. Tumour Biol 2016; 37(9): 12347-58.
[http://dx.doi.org/10.1007/s13277-016-5089-8] [PMID: 27306214]

[28] Adamski V, Schmitt C, Ceynowa F, *et al.* Effects of sequentially applied single and combined temozolomide, hydroxychloroquine and AT101 treatment in a long-term stimulation glioblastoma *in vitro* model. J Cancer Res Clin Oncol 2018; 144(8): 1475-85.
[http://dx.doi.org/10.1007/s00432-018-2680-y] [PMID: 29858681]

[29] Ryu CH, Yoon WS, Park KY, *et al.* Valproic acid downregulates the expression of MGMT and sensitizes temozolomide-resistant glioma cells. J Biomed Biotechnol 2012; 2012: 987495.
[http://dx.doi.org/10.1155/2012/987495] [PMID: 22701311]

[30] Zandi A, Zanjani TM, Ziai SA, *et al.* Evaluation of the cytotoxic effects of ciprofloxacin on human glioblastoma. Middle East J Cancer 2017; 8(3): 119-26.

[31] Guan DG, Chen HM, Liao SF, Zhao TZ. Combination of temozolomide and Taxol exerts a synergistic inhibitory effect on Taxol-resistant glioma cells *via* inhibition of glucose metabolism. Mol Med Rep 2015; 12(5): 7705-11.
[http://dx.doi.org/10.3892/mmr.2015.4405] [PMID: 26459853]

[32] Ma J, Yang YR, Chen W, *et al.* Fluoxetine synergizes with temozolomide to induce the CHOP-dependent endoplasmic reticulum stress-related apoptosis pathway in glioma cells. Oncol Rep 2016; 36(2): 676-84.
[http://dx.doi.org/10.3892/or.2016.4860] [PMID: 27278525]

[33] Kong XT, Nguyen NT, Choi YJ, *et al.* Phase 2 study of bortezomib combined with temozolomide and regional radiation therapy for upfront treatment of patients with newly diagnosed glioblastoma multiforme: Safety and efficacy assessment. Int J Radiat Oncol Biol Phys 2018; 100(5): 1195-203.
[http://dx.doi.org/10.1016/j.ijrobp.2018.01.001] [PMID: 29722661]

[34] Fulton B, Short SC, James A, *et al.* PARADIGM-2: Two parallel phase I studies of olaparib and radiotherapy or olaparib and radiotherapy plus temozolomide in patients with newly diagnosed glioblastoma, with treatment stratified by MGMT status. Clin Transl Radiat Oncol 2017; 8: 12-6.
[http://dx.doi.org/10.1016/j.ctro.2017.11.003] [PMID: 29594237]

[35] Galanis E, Anderson SK, Miller CR, *et al.* Phase I/II trial of vorinostat combined with temozolomide and radiation therapy for newly diagnosed glioblastoma: results of Alliance N0874/ABTC 02. Neuro-oncol 2018; 20(4): 546-56.
[http://dx.doi.org/10.1093/neuonc/nox161] [PMID: 29016887]

[36] Garcia CG, Kahn SA, Geraldo LHM, *et al.* Combination therapy with sulfasalazine and valproic acid promotes human glioblastoma cell death through imbalance of the intracellular oxidative response. Mol Neurobiol 2018; 55(8): 6816-33.
[http://dx.doi.org/10.1007/s12035-018-0895-1] [PMID: 29349577]

[37] Kim RD, Alberts SR, Peña C, *et al.* Phase I dose-escalation study of copanlisib in combination with gemcitabine or cisplatin plus gemcitabine in patients with advanced cancer. Br J Cancer 2018; 118(4): 462-70.
[http://dx.doi.org/10.1038/bjc.2017.428] [PMID: 29348486]

[38] Zhang Y, Ishida CT, Shu C, *et al.* Inhibition of Bcl-2/Bcl-xL and c-MET causes synthetic lethality in model systems of glioblastoma. Sci Rep 2018; 8(1): 7373.
[http://dx.doi.org/10.1038/s41598-018-25802-0] [PMID: 29743557]

[39] Pareja F, Macleod D, Shu C, *et al.* PI3K and Bcl-2 inhibition primes glioblastoma cells to apoptosis through downregulation of Mcl-1 and Phospho-BAD. Mol Cancer Res 2014; 12(7): 987-1001.
[http://dx.doi.org/10.1158/1541-7786.MCR-13-0650] [PMID: 24757258]

[40] Bhuvanalakshmi G, Arfuso F, Millward M, Dharmarajan A, Warrier S. Secreted frizzled-related protein 4 inhibits glioma stem-like cells by reversing epithelial to mesenchymal transition, inducing apoptosis and decreasing cancer stem cell properties. PLoS One 2015; 10(6): e0127517.
[http://dx.doi.org/10.1371/journal.pone.0127517] [PMID: 26030909]

[41] Ochs K, Kaina B. Apoptosis induced by DNA damage O6-methylguanine is Bcl-2 and caspase-9/3 regulated and Fas/caspase-8 independent. Cancer Res 2000; 60(20): 5815-24.
[PMID: 11059778]

[42] Hegi ME, Diserens AC, Gorlia T, *et al.* MGMT gene silencing and benefit from temozolomide in glioblastoma. N Engl J Med 2005; 352(10): 997-1003.
[http://dx.doi.org/10.1056/NEJMoa043331] [PMID: 15758010]

[43] Hegi ME, Liu L, Herman JG, *et al.* Correlation of O6-methylguanine methyltransferase (MGMT) promoter methylation with clinical outcomes in glioblastoma and clinical strategies to modulate MGMT activity. J Clin Oncol 2008; 26(25): 4189-99.
[http://dx.doi.org/10.1200/JCO.2007.11.5964] [PMID: 18757334]

[44] Bobustuc GC, Baker CH, Limaye A, *et al.* Levetiracetam enhances p53-mediated MGMT inhibition and sensitizes glioblastoma cells to temozolomide. Neuro-oncol 2010; 12(9): 917-27.
[http://dx.doi.org/10.1093/neuonc/noq044] [PMID: 20525765]

[45] Stritzelberger J, Distel L, Buslei R, Fietkau R, Putz F. Acquired temozolomide resistance in human glioblastoma cell line U251 is caused by mismatch repair deficiency and can be overcome by lomustine. Clin Transl Oncol 2018; 20(4): 508-16.
[http://dx.doi.org/10.1007/s12094-017-1743-x] [PMID: 28825189]

[46] Lombardi G, Pambuku A, Bellu L, *et al.* Effectiveness of antiangiogenic drugs in glioblastoma patients: A systematic review and meta-analysis of randomized clinical trials. Crit Rev Oncol Hematol 2017; 111: 94-102.
[http://dx.doi.org/10.1016/j.critrevonc.2017.01.018] [PMID: 28259301]

[47] McCord M, Mukouyama YS, Gilbert MR, Jackson S. Targeting WNT signaling for multifaceted glioblastoma therapy. Front Cell Neurosci 2017; 11: 318.
[http://dx.doi.org/10.3389/fncel.2017.00318] [PMID: 29081735]

[48] A phase I, open-label, dose escalation study of oral LGK974 in patients with malignancies dependent on wnt ligands Clinicaltrialsgov, NIH 2018. https://clinicaltrials.gov/ct2/show/ NCT01351103

[49] Kahlert UD, Suwala AK, Koch K, *et al.* Pharmacologic Wnt inhibition reduces proliferation, survival, and clonogenicity of glioblastoma cells. J Neuropathol Exp Neurol 2015; 74(9): 889-900.
[http://dx.doi.org/10.1097/NEN.0000000000000227] [PMID: 26222502]

[50] Safety and efficacy study of SL-701, a glioma-associated antigen vaccine to treat recurrent glioblastoma multiforme. Clinicaltrialsgov, NIH 2018; 11(7) https://clinicaltrials.gov/ct2/show/ NCT02078648

[51] Vaccine Therapy With Bevacizumab Versus Bevacizumab Alone in Treating Patients With Recurrent Glioblastoma Multiforme That Can Be Removed by Surgery. ClinicalTrialsgov, NIH 2018; 11(7) https://clinicaltrials.gov/ct2/show/NCT01814813

[52] Pembrolizumab +/- bevacizumab for recurrent GBM. Clinicaltrialsgov, NIH 2018; 11(7) https://clinicaltrials.gov/ct2/show/NCT02337491

[53] Phase 2 study of MEDI4736 in patients with glioblastoma. Clinicaltrialsgov, NIH 2018; 11(7) https://clinicaltrials.gov/ct2/show/NCT02336165

[54] Tchoghandjian A, Soubéran A, Tabouret E, *et al.* Inhibitor of apoptosis protein expression in glioblastomas and their *in vitro* and in vivo targeting by SMAC mimetic GDC-0152. Cell Death & Disease 2016; 7(8): e2325-5.
[http://dx.doi.org/10.1038/cddis.2016.214]

[55] Aras Y, Erguven M, Aktas E, Yazihan N, Bilir A. Antagonist activity of the antipsychotic drug lithium chloride and the antileukemic drug imatinib mesylate during glioblastoma treatment *in vitro*. Neurol Res 2016; 38(9): 766-74.
[http://dx.doi.org/10.1080/01616412.2016.1203096] [PMID: 27367429]

[56] Weller M, Gorlia T, Cairncross JG, *et al.* Prolonged survival with valproic acid use in the EORTC/NCIC temozolomide trial for glioblastoma. Neurology 2011; 77(12): 1156-64.
[http://dx.doi.org/10.1212/WNL.0b013e31822f02e1] [PMID: 21880994]

[57] Lee DH, Ryu HW, Won HR, Kwon SH. Advances in epigenetic glioblastoma therapy. Oncotarget 2017; 8(11): 18577-89.
[http://dx.doi.org/10.18632/oncotarget.14612] [PMID: 28099914]

[58] Alvarez AA, Field M, Bushnev S, Longo MS, Sugaya K. The effects of histone deacetylase inhibitors on glioblastoma-derived stem cells. J Mol Neurosci 2015; 55(1): 7-20.
[http://dx.doi.org/10.1007/s12031-014-0329-0] [PMID: 24874578]

[59] A phase I trial of pembrolizumab and vorinostat combined with temozolomide and radiation therapy for newly diagnosed glioblastoma March 16, 2018. ClinicalTrialsgov, NIH 2018. https://clinicaltrials.gov/ct2/show/NCT03426891

[60] Xu H, Zong H, Ma C, *et al.* Epidermal growth factor receptor in glioblastoma. Oncol Lett 2017; 14(1): 512-6.
[http://dx.doi.org/10.3892/ol.2017.6221] [PMID: 28693199]

[61] Taylor TE, Furnari FB, Cavenee WK. Targeting EGFR for treatment of glioblastoma: molecular basis to overcome resistance. Curr Cancer Drug Targets 2012; 12(3): 197-209.
[http://dx.doi.org/10.2174/156800912799277557] [PMID: 22268382]

[62] Westphal M, Maire CL, Lamszus K. EGFR as a target for glioblastoma treatment: An unfulfilled promise. CNS Drugs 2017; 31(9): 723-35.
[http://dx.doi.org/10.1007/s40263-017-0456-6] [PMID: 28791656]

[63] Mesbahi Y, Zekri A, Ahmadian S, Alimoghaddam K, Ghavamzadeh A, Ghaffari SH. Targeting of EGFR increase anti-cancer effects of arsenic trioxide: Promising treatment for glioblastoma multiform. Eur J Pharmacol 2018; 820: 274-85.
[http://dx.doi.org/10.1016/j.ejphar.2017.12.041] [PMID: 29274334]

[64] Barrette AM, Bouhaddou M, Birtwistle MR. Integrating transcriptomic data with mechanistic systems pharmacology models for virtual drug combination trials. ACS Chem Neurosci 2018; 9(1): 118-29.
[http://dx.doi.org/10.1021/acschemneuro.7b00197] [PMID: 28950062]

[65] Liu Y, Liu X, Chen LC, *et al.* Targeting glioma stem cells *via* the Hedgehog signaling pathway. Neuroimmunol Neuroinflamm 2014; 1(2): 51-9.
[http://dx.doi.org/10.4103/2347-8659.139715]

[66] Melamed JR, Morgan JT, Ioele SA, Gleghorn JP, Sims-Mourtada J, Day ES. Investigating the role of Hedgehog/GLI1 signaling in glioblastoma cell response to temozolomide. Oncotarget 2018; 9(43): 27000-15.
[http://dx.doi.org/10.18632/oncotarget.25467] [PMID: 29930746]

[67] Venturini E, Leanza L, Azzolini M, *et al.* Targeting the potassium channel Kv1.3 kills glioblastoma cells. Neurosignals 2017; 25(1): 26-38.
[http://dx.doi.org/10.1159/000480643] [PMID: 28869943]

[68] Fujihara T, Mizobuchi Y, Nakajima K, *et al.* Down-regulation of MDR1 by Ad-DKK3 *via* Akt/NFκB pathways augments the anti-tumor effect of temozolomide in glioblastoma cells and a murine xenograft model. J Neurooncol 2018; 139(2): 323-32.
[http://dx.doi.org/10.1007/s11060-018-2894-5] [PMID: 29779087]

[69] Cemeus C, Zhao TT, Barrett GM, Lorimer IA, Dimitroulakos J. Lovastatin enhances gefitinib activity in glioblastoma cells irrespective of EGFRvIII and PTEN status. J Neurooncol 2008; 90(1): 9-17.
[http://dx.doi.org/10.1007/s11060-008-9627-0] [PMID: 18566746]

[70] Yongjun Y, Shuyun H, Lei C, Xiangrong C, Zhilin Y, Yiquan K. Atorvastatin suppresses glioma invasion and migration by reducing microglial MT1-MMP expression. J Neuroimmunol 2013; 260(1-2): 1-8.

[http://dx.doi.org/10.1016/j.jneuroim.2013.04.020] [PMID: 23707077]

[71] Gaist D, Hallas J, Friis S, Hansen S, Sørensen HT. Statin use and survival following glioblastoma multiforme. Cancer Epidemiol 2014; 38(6): 722-7.
[http://dx.doi.org/10.1016/j.canep.2014.09.010] [PMID: 25455652]

[72] Levkovitz Y, Gil-Ad I, Zeldich E, Dayag M, Weizman A. Differential induction of apoptosis by antidepressants in glioma and neuroblastoma cell lines: evidence for p-c-Jun, cytochrome c, and caspase-3 involvement. J Mol Neurosci 2005; 27(1): 29-42.
[http://dx.doi.org/10.1385/JMN:27:1:029] [PMID: 16055945]

[73] Sachlos E, Risueño RM, Laronde S, et al. Identification of drugs including a dopamine receptor antagonist that selectively target cancer stem cells. Cell 2012; 149(6): 1284-97.
[http://dx.doi.org/10.1016/j.cell.2012.03.049] [PMID: 22632761]

[74] Bielecka-Wajdman AM, Lesiak M, Ludyga T, Sieroń A, Obuchowicz E. Reversing glioma malignancy: a new look at the role of antidepressant drugs as adjuvant therapy for glioblastoma multiforme. Cancer Chemother Pharmacol 2017; 79(6): 1249-56.
[http://dx.doi.org/10.1007/s00280-017-3329-2] [PMID: 28500556]

[75] Barker CA, Bishop AJ, Chang M, Beal K, Chan TA. Valproic acid use during radiation therapy for glioblastoma associated with improved survival. Int J Radiat Oncol Biol Phys 2013; 86(3): 504-9.
[http://dx.doi.org/10.1016/j.ijrobp.2013.02.012] [PMID: 23523186]

[76] Walker AJ, Grainge M, Bates TE, Card TR. Survival of glioma and colorectal cancer patients using tricyclic antidepressants post-diagnosis. Cancer Causes Control 2012; 23(12): 1959-64.
[http://dx.doi.org/10.1007/s10552-012-0073-0] [PMID: 23065071]

[77] Erdemir F, Atilgan D, Firat F, Markoc F, Parlaktas BS, Sogut E. The effect of sertraline, paroxetine, fluoxetine and escitalopram on testicular tissue and oxidative stress parameters in rats. Int Braz J Urol 2014; 40(1): 100-8.
[http://dx.doi.org/10.1590/S1677-5538.IBJU.2014.01.15] [PMID: 24642156]

[78] Lamy S, Lachambre MP, Lord-Dufour S, Béliveau R. Propranolol suppresses angiogenesis *in vitro*: inhibition of proliferation, migration, and differentiation of endothelial cells. Vascul Pharmacol 2010; 53(5-6): 200-8.
[http://dx.doi.org/10.1016/j.vph.2010.08.002] [PMID: 20732454]

[79] Larochelle P, Tobe SW, Lacourcière Y. β-Blockers in hypertension: studies and meta-analyses over the years. Can J Cardiol 2014; 30(5) (Suppl.): S16-22.
[http://dx.doi.org/10.1016/j.cjca.2014.02.012] [PMID: 24750978]

[80] Pasquier E, Ciccolini J, Carre M, et al. Propranolol potentiates the anti-angiogenic effects and anti-tumor efficacy of chemotherapy agents: implication in breast cancer treatment. Oncotarget 2011; 2(10): 797-809.
[http://dx.doi.org/10.18632/oncotarget.343] [PMID: 22006582]

[81] Zhang D, Ma Q, Shen S, Hu H. Inhibition of pancreatic cancer cell proliferation by propranolol occurs through apoptosis induction: the study of beta-adrenoceptor antagonist's anticancer effect in pancreatic cancer cell. Pancreas 2009; 38(1): 94-100.
[http://dx.doi.org/10.1097/MPA.0b013e318184f50c] [PMID: 19106745]

[82] Cheng G, Zielonka J, McAllister D, Tsai S, Dwinell MB, Kalyanaraman B. Profiling and targeting of cellular bioenergetics: inhibition of pancreatic cancer cell proliferation. Br J Cancer 2014; 111(1): 85-93.
[http://dx.doi.org/10.1038/bjc.2014.272] [PMID: 24867695]

[83] Wolter JK, Wolter NE, Blanch A, et al. Anti-tumor activity of the beta-adrenergic receptor antagonist propranolol in neuroblastoma. Oncotarget 2014; 5(1): 161-72.
[http://dx.doi.org/10.18632/oncotarget.1083] [PMID: 24389287]

[84] Pistollato F, Abbadi S, Rampazzo E, et al. Hypoxia and succinate antagonize 2-deoxyglucose effects

on glioblastoma. Biochem Pharmacol 2010; 80(10): 1517-27.
[http://dx.doi.org/10.1016/j.bcp.2010.08.003] [PMID: 20705058]

[85] Ciavardelli D, Rossi C, Barcaroli D, *et al.* Breast cancer stem cells rely on fermentative glycolysis and are sensitive to 2-deoxyglucose treatment. Cell Death Dis 2014; 5(7): e1336.
[http://dx.doi.org/10.1038/cddis.2014.285] [PMID: 25032859]

[86] Bao B, Wang Z, Ali S, *et al.* Metformin inhibits cell proliferation, migration and invasion by attenuating CSC function mediated by deregulating miRNAs in pancreatic cancer cells. Cancer Prev Res (Phila) 2012; 5(3): 355-64.
[http://dx.doi.org/10.1158/1940-6207.CAPR-11-0299] [PMID: 22086681]

CHAPTER 6

Recent Advances in the Development of Mesoporous Anti-Cancer Drug Nanocarriers

Jessica Flood-Garibay, Lucila I. Castro-Pastrana[*] and Miguel A. Méndez-Rojas[*]

Department of Chemical & Biological Sciences and Laboratory of Nanotechnology and Molecular Biomedicine Research, School of Sciences, Universidad de las Américas Puebla, San Andrés Cholula, Puebla, México

Abstract: The application of nanomaterials in biomedicine is a very active field of research, as it has the potential for developing several innovations in health care, diagnosis, medical imaging and therapy. In particular, the use of nanostructured materials for drug formulations is drawing the attention of pharmaceutical companies and research groups around the world. The development of new systems for controlled drug transportation and delivery is a very complex multidisciplinary field since they must possess unique physical and chemical features to improve the stability of the active pharmaceutical ingredient, to enhance drug bioavailability and delivery efficiency, as well as to control the drug clearance rate. Nanomaterials present unique physical properties that offer several advantages over traditional carrier systems. There are several systems that can be selected for a specific formulation, depending on the administration route, such as carbon nanostructures (*e.g.*, graphene, graphene oxide and carbon nanotubes), nanoliposomes, micelles, dendrimers, polymeric and inorganic nanoparticles (*e.g.*, metallic, metal oxides and composites), among several others. All the aforementioned systems will require intensive research to thoroughly understand their safety and long-term effects in order for them to be included in health products in the future. This chapter reviews the most recent progress on the development of mesoporous nanocarriers for controlled transport and delivery of anti-cancer drugs. First, some fundamental ideas are discussed on the actual benefits and risks of using nanomaterials in pharmaceutical formulations, compared with current existing technologies. Some of the most representative mesoporous materials used to develop efficient nanocarriers are presented. Their physical and chemical properties are introduced to better understand their advantages in terms of the design of efficient systems for the controlled delivery and release of anti-cancer drugs. Moreover, the design of novel anti-cancer drug transport and delivery systems that harness the unique characteristics of mesoporous nanomaterials is addressed. Finally, some of the potential risks associated with the biomedical use of nanostructured materials, related to their diverse chemical compositions, physical properties and technological applications, are

---

[*] **Corresponding authors Lucila I. Castro-Pastrana and Miguel A. Méndez-Rojas**: Department of Chemical & Biological Sciences, Universidad de las Américas Puebla, Ex-Hda. de Sta. Catarina Mártir s/n, San Andrés Cholula, 72820, Puebla, México; Tel: +52 (222) 229 2607; Fax: +52 (222) 229 2416; Emails: lucila.castro@udlap.mx and miguela.mendez@udlap.mx.

Atta-ur-Rahman and M. Iqbal Choudhary (Eds.)
All rights reserved-© 2019 Bentham Science Publishers

examined along with proposed ways to minimize their potential health and environmental impact.

Keywords: *Anticancer Drugs, Bioavailability, Cancer, Controlled Release, Drug Delivery, Drug Release, Mesoporous, Metal Oxides, Nanomaterials, Nanocarriers, Nanocarbon, Nanotoxicity, Pharmaceutical Formulation, Targeted Delivery.*

INTRODUCTION

Tackling the Global Cancer Burden

According to the American Cancer Society, cancer mortality has now fallen by around 1.5% compared to the statistics of the last 10 years (2006-2015). However, it is estimated that in the United States (U.S.) alone, in 2018 1,735,350 new cases will be diagnosed and there will be 609,640 cases of death from some type of cancer [1]. It has been suggested that changes in patients' lifestyle as well as more timely diagnoses and treatments have contributed significantly to this positive scenario, at least for the U.S. Yet, according to the Global Cancer Observatory, over 14 million new cancer patients are detected every year and this number is expected to rise to 23.6 million by 2030. Globally, nearly 1 in 6 deaths is due to cancer and a third of those deaths are related to widely recognized risk factors such as obesity, lack of exercise, low fruit and vegetable intake, as well as tobacco and alcohol use [2]. Moreover, late-stage presentation and inaccessible diagnosis and treatment exacerbate the risk of death especially in low-income countries while cancer survival rates have increased only for countries and people with high incomes.

The recently published CONCORD-3 study presents the true face of this disparity in access to medicine. While in Australia and in the U.S. the five-year survival rate of breast cancer is 90%, in India it is only 66%; in Finland, more than 95% of children diagnosed with acute lymphoblastic leukemia are still alive after five years, in Ecuador, only 49.8% of them. A child with a brain tumor has a 5-year survival of 80% in Denmark, 66% in Spain, 36% in Mexico and 28.9% in Brazil [3]. This study also noted that in high-income countries, social classes and less-favored races are also lagging behind in survival. In the U.S., white patients achieve a 65% survival rate for colon cancer, compared to African Americans, who are 9% below the former. Given this scenario, the importance of reinforcing the development of new anti-cancer drugs that contribute to not only abate deaths and improve the quality of life of cancer survivors, but also to shorten the gap in access to cancer medication between developed economies and the so-called *'pharmerging'* markets is evident. It will also be necessary to find a rational and efficient balance between the development of brand new anticancer drugs and the optimization of existing formulations of antineoplastic agents with which there is already good clinical experience.

Present and Future of Cancer Medications

The development of novel oncology drugs and companion diagnostic tests has revolutionized in recent years the traditional sequence of stages and processes of preclinical and clinical studies, as well as the regulatory methods for clinical research and new medicines' approval. While always prioritizing safety over speed, innovative regulatory pathways have introduced modalities like 'fast track', 'expedited development', 'breakthrough therapy designation', 'priority review', 'limited approval', 'first cycle approval' and 'accelerated approval'. These approval statuses have been introduced mainly to favor the development of new anticancer agents along with the definition of new clinical endpoints to broaden the conceptualization of survival and quality of life in cancer. Still, close post-marketing activities must follow these flexible approaches to test the real-life performance of each drug in order to achieve formal full approval in a reasonable time and without negative surprises.

In 2017, cancer medications dominated the list of all new molecules approved by the FDA and conventional chemically synthesized drugs represented almost two-thirds of the new molecular entities approved over biotech drugs [4]. Over the period 2016-2020, about 225 new active substances are forecasted to come to market globally where cancer treatments represent the largest category of the expected new products. Of these 225 new substances, around 30% will be biologics. Over 90% of expected new cancer treatments will be targeted therapies, of which one-third will use a biomarker. Oncology, as the leading class of specialty medicines, will account for 11% of global medicine spending in 2020 [5]. According to the U.S. National Cancer Institute, there are currently more than 250 licensed cancer drugs and drug combinations [6]. The *WHO Collaborating Centre for Drug Statistics Methodology* classifies antineoplastic agents (Anatomical Therapeutic Chemical code, first and second level: L01) in 5 groups: alkylating agents (L01A), antimetabolites (L01B), plant alkaloids and other natural products (L01C), cytotoxic antibiotics and related substances (L01D), platinum compounds (L01XA), methylhydrazines (L01XB), monoclonal antibodies (L01XC), sensitizers used in photodynamic/radiation therapy (L01XD), protein kinase inhibitors (L01XE), and other antineoplastic agents (L01XX) [7].

Another category that currently has very active research is represented by immunotherapies, which are subclassified according to their antigen specificity.

The main groups are: tumor-targeting monoclonal antibodies; anti-CTLA-4 and anti-PD-1/PD-L1 immune checkpoint blockers; immunostimulatory cytokines; oncolytic viruses; vaccines (peptide-based, immune- or dendritic-cell–based and tumor-cell–based), adoptive T-cell, dendritic cell and chimeric antigen receptor (CAR-T) therapies [8, 9]. Immunotherapies belong to the so-called 'targeted therapies' along with hormone therapies, signal transduction inhibitors, gene expression modulators, apoptosis inducers, angiogenesis inhibitors, and toxin delivery molecules. Targeted therapies act on specific molecular targets that are associated with cancer; they are often cytostatic and may be restricted to patients whose tumor has a specific gene mutation that codes for the target. Sometimes, patients whose cancer did not respond to other therapies, has spread, or is inoperable, are those who are considered candidates to receive this type of therapies. Thus, targeted therapies are considered the cornerstone of precision medicine and are currently the focus of much anticancer drug development [10]. This therapeutic arsenal is very vast and hence the importance not only of optimizing its pharmacological and pharmaceutical properties but also its use by health professionals and patients.

Reaching Cancerous Tissues More Efficiently

Particularly for antineoplastic drugs, a large part of the current efforts in optimizing new dosage forms as well as the formulations already existing in the market focus on local delivery and controlled release, from any route of administration, so that the drug reaches the cancerous tissues with greater specificity, efficiency and safety. In fact, cancer medications have opened administration routes that were not common due to the need to deliver drugs in a more localized manner. For example, bleomycin sulfate reconstituted solution can be administered by intrapleural (intracavitary) injection through a thoracostomy tube; goserelin is available as 28-day and 12-week implants that are injected at a 30- to 45-degree angle into the anterior abdominal wall below the navel line; reconstituted mitomycin is administered into the pre-heated bladder using the so-called electromotive mitomycin therapy, and carmustine wafers are implanted and left in the cavity after surgical removal of a brain tumor [11, 12]. Unfortunately, these sophisticated forms of administration are costly and require patient hospitalization to administer the drug.

Modulation of drug release from the dosage forms should serve to maintain a prolonged exposure of tumors to drugs, which is of particular importance in the case of cell cycle specific agents that exert a cytostatic effect such as signal transduction inhibitors (*e.g.*, erlotinib, gefinitib, imatinib, trastuzumab and cetuximab) and angiogenesis inhibitors (*e.g.*, bevacizumab, everolimus, lenalidomide, regorafenib, sorafenib, sunitinib and thalidomide) [13]. The optimization of drug delivery forms also depends on the understanding of the characteristics of the tumor tissues as well as the physiological barriers that surround them and that could prevent drugs from reaching them. Hence, delivery systems should try to exploit differences in accessibility and in physiological and anatomical factors between cancer and normal cells in order to increase the concentration of drug to tumor cells and to decrease the amount of drug delivered to normal tissues. In addition, targeted drug delivery systems can act in a passive (*e.g.*, by means of antiphagocytic coating substances) or in an active way (*e.g.*, by means of antibodies or materials responsive to pH, temperature or magnetic fields) [14, 15].

In terms of the pathophysiological features of tumor tissues, the Enhanced Permeability and Retention effect (EPR) has been described, where tumor vasculature tends to be more permeable to larger molecules, which are then retained in the tumor bed due to reduced lymphatic drainage. Thus, modulating the tumor blood flow (*e.g.*, by vasoconstrictive agents or vasodilators like nitric oxide or botulinum neurotoxin) as well as its vasculature (*e.g.*, by sonoporation, hyperthermia, antiangiogenic agents) and stroma (*e.g.*, by collagenase or hyaluronidase), together with killing the cancer cells to reduce their barrier function (*e.g.*, by radiation or near infrared photoimmunotherapy), are promising methods to enhance the EPR effect and to improve cancer drug delivery [16]. They can even be combined with small size particles (*e.g.*, nanoparticles and liposomes) and the use of hydrophilic polymers (*e.g.*, polyethylene oxide/glycol) to coat the particles in order to overcome the mononuclear phagocytic system and be able to circulate longer and accumulate at tumor sites [14, 15]. Furthermore, pinocytosis rates and degradative enzymes (*e.g.*, cathepsins) could be increased in tumor cells, which may also present changes in pH of extracellular matrix, thereby presenting a very particular microenvironment that can be taken as an advantage by certain drug delivery systems.

Anticancer drugs usually have a narrow therapeutic index and a steep dose-response curve thus requiring complete and consistent absorption processes to avoid sub-therapeutic or toxic doses reaching the body. Some of them have very short elimination half-lives, possess unstable and reactive chromophores, or are susceptible to both *physical and chemical instability* such as the biotechnological products. These challenges may combine with *their non-selective mechanisms of action,* the need to cross-physiological barriers to get to the extracellular space of the tumor, and the development of multiple drug resistance by the tumor cells. Therefore, drug delivery systems with better targeting ability are needed either to protect the drug or to preserve some tissues from exposure to drug (*e.g.*, microcapsules, liposomes, microspheres, micro and nanoparticles, polymer drug conjugates) or to improve pharmacokinetic and pharmacodynamic drug properties like many nanocarriers used as controlled delivery vehicles (*e.g.*, dendrimers, protein and polymeric nanoparticles, iron oxide and mesoporous silica nanoparticles, carbon nanotubes), in addition to quantum dots, self-emulsifying drug delivery systems (SEDDS), nanocrystals, drug-antibody and lipid-drug conjugates, among many others [13, 15, 17]. Consequently, the main aim in the development of drug delivery systems is to successfully carry drugs to the desired sites of therapeutic action while reducing adverse side effects by controlling the rate, time and place of release.

A drug that has been used recurrently to develop and test the most recent advances and investigations related to anticancer drug delivery systems is doxorubicin (DOX). DOX is a high solubility-low permeability cytotoxic anthracycline antibiotic with a short half-life and limited clinical application due to its acute cardiotoxicity [18]. It is indicated in acute lymphoblastic and acute myeloblastic leukemia, Wilms' tumor, neuroblastoma, soft tissue and bone sarcomas, breast and ovarian carcinoma, transitional cell bladder carcinoma, thyroid carcinoma and gastric carcinoma, among others [11]. Photodegradation of DOX solutions is well documented and it has a pH-dependent stability in solution [19]. Several transporters have been shown to be involved in transporting DOX including ABCB1, ABCC1, ABCC2, ABCG2, RALBP1 (export) and SLC22A16 (import) which may affect considerably its distribution and metabolism pharmacokinetics [20]. Thus, DOX is a very good candidate to explore novel and promising targeted drug delivery vehicles. Table **1** shows some of these innovative methods investigated for DOX as an illustrative example of the race to successfully address most common and challenging delivery-related problems.

Table 1. Recent *in vitro* investigations using doxorubicin (DOX) as a drug model towards improving its efficient, safe and targeted delivery.

System	Findings/Advantages	Ref.
Nanocomposite hydrogel films obtained through incorporation of graphene quantum dot (GQD) as a nanoparticle into carboxymethyl cellulose (CMC) hydrogel	High DOX loading and prolonged release through pH-sensitive drug delivery.	[21]
Smart photosensitive nanoscopic vehicles made of dihydroindolizine (DHI) encapsulated in liposome.	Photoinduced isomerization from closed (hydrophobic) to open isomeric form (hydrophilic) of DHI leading to DOX delivery from liposome to cervical cancer cell line HeLa, enhanced cellular uptake of DOX and 40% reduction in cell *via*bility.	[22]

(Table 1) cont.....

System	Findings/Advantages	Ref.
Encapsulation system of self-assembled hyaluronic acid (HA)-testosterone conjugates obtained by functionalization of either natural sodium hyaluronate or hydrazide-modified HA derivatives with testosterone hemisuccinate.	Sustained release of DOX over 96 hours at pH 7.4 and comparable cytotoxicity against MCF-7 cancer cell line regarding cytotoxicity of free DOX.	[23]
Complexation system made of depolymerized polyanionic holothurian glycosaminoglycans (DHG).	DOX encapsulation efficiency over 60% plus combined release profile showing an initial fast release and subsequent slow and sustained release. Improved cell killing ability of DOX for HepG-2, MCF-7 and A549 tumor cells.	[24]
Chitosan-folate conjugated colloidal ZnO-Mn(+2) quantum dots bearing DOX.	Almost complete entrapment efficiency, sustained release pattern at the lysosomal pH (pH 5.0), enhanced cytotoxicity, cellular uptake and preferentially taken up by the cancerous cells *via* receptor-mediated endocytosis mechanism.	[25]
pH-sensitive micelles based on hydrazine-containing amphiphilic block copolymer of hydrophilic polyethylene glycol and hydrophobic polylactic-co-glycolic acid.	DOX release was significantly faster at pH 4.0 and pH 5.0 compared to pH 7.4, and assays on HepG-2 and MCF-7 cells revealed higher antitumor activity than pH-insensitive micelles.	[26]
Nanogel consisting of sodium alginate-modified graphene oxide and *N*-isopropylacrylamide	Thermo-responsive sustained delivery of DOX.	[27]
Mesoporous silica-based core–shell urease-powered nanomotors (nanobots).	Nanobots able to self-propel in ionic media showing a four-fold increase in DOX release with an enhanced anticancer efficiency toward HeLa cells due to a synergistic effect of the enhanced drug release and the ammonia produced at high concentrations of urea substrate.	[28]

Cancer medication formulations are also undergoing a switch trend from parenteral routes to oral delivery. In Europe, 67% of the commercially available oral oncolytics are physical mixture formulations while only 4% use solid dispersion technology even when the latter have demonstrated to better overcome dissolution-limited absorption, which is a common challenge of half of the currently licensed oral anticancer drugs [29]. Incomplete and highly variable oral absorption of anticancer agents is detrimental to maintaining an optimal drug concentration in plasma and in the vicinity of tumors and might result in treatment failure or toxicity. Therefore, to enhance oral absorption, a combination of pharmaceutical and pharmacological approaches have to come into play.

Among the biopharmaceutical aspects, much emphasis is placed on the solubility and permeability of a drug, although more recently the pharmacokinetic processes have been incorporated into the equation to be able to predict needs in terms of formulation and methods to enhance oral deliverability. In 1995, the Biopharmaceutics Classification System (BCS) was enacted by the FDA in order to provide an official drug classification based in four classes according to their solubility in aqueous medium and their intestinal permeability properties [30]. Later in 2005, the Biopharmaceutics Drug Disposition Classification System (BDDCS) was proposed in order to include drug disposition aspects such as first-pass metabolism, transporter-mediated drug uptake and efflux and biliary versus renal excretion, taking the extent of metabolism as a surrogate for permeability [31]. The relevance of considering drug transporters also lies in their crucial role in multidrug resistance of tumor cells. Table **2** shows examples of oral oncolytics registered in Europe belonging to the four classes of the combined BCS/BDDCS system.

Table 2. Examples of anticancer drugs of each BCS/BDDCS class [29].

		High Solubility	Low Solubility
		Class I	Class II
High Permeability Extensive Metabolism		**5-Amino levulinic acid hydrochloride (L01XD04)** **Capecitabine (L01BC06)** Cobimetinib hemifumarate (L01XE38) **Cyclophosphamide monohydrate (L01AA01)** **Fludarabine phosphate (L01BB05)** Hydroxycarbamide (L01XX05) **Idarubicin hydrochloride (L01DB06)** **Letrozole (L02BG04)** **Tegafur (L01BC03 and L01BC53)** **Toremifene citrate (L02BA02)**	**Bicalutamide (L02BB03)** **Busulfan (L01AB01)** **Enzalutamide (L02BB04)** **Erlotinib hydrochloride (L01XE03)** Exemestane (L02BG06) **Gefitinib (L01XE02)** **Imatinib mesilate (L01XE01)** **Mercaptopurine monohydrate (L01BB02)** **Methotrexate disodium (L01BA01 and L04AX03)** **Tamoxifen citrate (L02BA01)**
		Class III	Class IV
Low Permeability Poor Metabolism		**Anastrozole (L02BG03)** **Gimeracil (n.a.)** **Lenalidomide (L04AX04)** **Osimertinib mesylate (L01XE35)** **Oteracil monopotassium (n.a.)** **Tipiracil hydrochloride (n.a.)** **Topotecan hydrochloride (L01XX17)** Trifluridine (L01BC59)	Abiraterone acetate (L02BX03) Bosutinib monohydrate (L01XE14) Ceritinib (L01XE28) Etoposide (L01CB01) Everolimus (L01XE10 and L04AA18) **Methotrexate disodium (L01BA01 and L04AX03)** Olaparib (L01XX46) Vinorelbine ditartrate (L01CA04)

In brackets: Anatomical Therapeutic Chemical (ATC) code [7]. n.a. = not available.

Briefly, class I in the combined BCS / BDDCS classification has such favorable conditions that it does not require assistance from apical uptake transporters in the gastrointestinal tract, nor is its oral disposition affected by efflux transporters. As for class II drugs, they do not require the aid of absorptive enterocyte transporters to diffuse passively through them but they may be pumped back by efflux transporters in the gut and taken by influx transporters when they reach the hepatocytes, undergoing first pass metabolism and thus affecting their bioavailability. Both class III and IV require the assistance of absorptive transporters due to their low permeability, which is why they do not saturate enterocyte efflux transporters having the potential to be influenced by them [32]. In addition, the BDDCS system may also allow predictions regarding food effects for orally dosed drugs. This is very convenient for planning clinical trials, for designing patient education strategies and for taking clinical decisions for the proper administration of oral oncolytics in countries where safe water is unavailable and medicines need to be taken with other liquids or with food.

Although the BCS and BDDCS classification systems are currently very useful tools for selecting drug formulation strategies, their application must be dynamic since it depends on the ongoing findings regarding the role of uptake and efflux transporters in oral disposition of an active substance. For example, microparticle drug delivery technologies, pelletized pulsatile delivery systems and solubility modulating hydrogel systems are strategies aimed at advancing controlled release for class I drugs. In the case of class II drugs, they benefit of the prodrug approach, micronization, solid dispersion, cyclodextrin complexation and nanosized carriers. Class III drugs enhance their deliverability by means of permeation enhancers, gastric retention and oral vaccine systems. Finally, class IV drugs take advantage of lipid based and self-microemulsifying delivery systems, polymer-based nanocarriers, self-emulsifying solid dispersions and of techniques addressing efflux transporters [33, 34]. BCS class II and IV drug products also benefit of the nanocrystal approach to increase their solubility and dissolution performance. Over the time, oral delivery has been evolving from the prodrug approach, later through the co-administration of absorption enhancers (*e.g.*, P-glycoprotein inhibitors), then by means of functional excipients (natural polymers, polyethylene glycols and derivatives, surfactants, lipids, cyclodextrins) and more recently through nanocarriers (polymeric, lipid based, nanocrystals and dendrimers) [13]. It is expected that in the era of nanotechnology, many more anticancer agents will enter the developmental pipeline of oral formulations and, of course, that new challenges and concerns will emerge.

Nanomaterials: Types and Potential Uses in Drug Delivery

As has been discussed above, one of the most important and multidisciplinary research fields being developed is drug delivery since it helps clinical scientists to reduce side effects, to enhance pharmacodynamic and pharmacokinetic parameters of drugs, and to improve patient compliance. It is of surmountable importance to develop new therapeutic strategies to overcome drug resistances and to reduce side-effects; specially in diseases such as cancer, which is why smart drug delivery systems (DDS) that could target different types of diseases (*e.g.*, infections, metabolic diseases, neurodegenerative diseases or cancers) are under development [35]. As a general principle, a drug carrier should spend maximal time in the blood to increase a drug's bioavailability and avoid high non-specific accumulation in tissues [36]. Other important preconditions for a DDS to meet are [37]: (1) that the drug carrier material is biocompatible; (2) that sufficient dosage of drug can be loaded into the system; (3) that zero premature release of drug with no leaking is achieved; (4) that the drug can be delivered to the targeted site and that it can be released in a controlled manner; and (5) that a proper release rate can be sustained to achieve an effective local drug concentration.

Nanoparticles (NPs) have many advantages that can be exploited as DDS, such as effectively protecting the encapsulated drug against enzymes and hydrolysis, having good colloidal stability, surface tailorability and multifunctionality, and that they are relatively easy to prepare. Importantly, nanoparticles can have good biocompatibility, degradation and excretion (dependent on the material used) [38]. The biocompatibility and biotranslocation of nanoparticles is directly related to the chemophysical properties of their nanomaterials including particle shape, size, surface area and structure [39]. Particle size is one of the most important parameters for the mediation of biocompatibility of nanomaterials [40, 41] as well as surface properties. It is now commonly accepted that nanoparticles with a neutral charge show favorably long circulation times and interstitial transport in tumors, while cationic charged particles are advantageous for transvascular transport in tumors but would induce more cytotoxicity and immune response [42, 43]. On the other hand, particle shape has gained attention since it was found that nonspherical particles have longer *in vivo* circulation time and reduced phagocytosis by macrophages [44, 45].

According to the definition from the NNI (*National Nanotechnology Initiative*), nanoparticles are particle structures smaller than 100 nm in at least one dimension, and can be developed from various materials, including lipids, polymers, ceramics, and carbon structures [35]. In practice, particles that are up to several hundred nanometers in size are frequently referred to with the prefix "nano" in the biomedical sciences. It is important to clarify that the term 'nanoparticle' (NP) includes polymeric nanospheres (pNSs) and nanocapsules (pNCps); and that other NPs could be polymeric micro (pMFs)- and nanofibers (pNFs), which have gained increasing attention in the past few decades. pNSs consist of a polymeric matrix in which the drug can be found built into the matrix or attached to its surface; while pNCps are small reservoirs that are surrounded by a shell in which the therapeutic substance can be connected to the surface of the particles or entrapped into the core [46]. Nano carriers (NCs) are colloidal nanostructures that can be capable of allowing for the controlled release of a drug when triggered by internal/external stimuli, loading multiple drugs with different physicochemical properties in a single carrier or providing significantly improved therapeutic efficacy, as will be explained below [47]. NCs can be classified as organic or inorganic, or into subgroups, such as: polymeric micelles, liposomes, nanoparticles, dendrimers, nanogels, and inorganic nanomaterials; among others [48, 49]. Some characteristics of these NCs are summarized in Table 3 and illustrated in Figs. (1) and (2).

Table 3. Some selected examples of organic and inorganic NCs, indicating their more important characteristics and advantages.

System	Characteristics	Refs.
Organic NCs		
Solid Lipid Nanoparticles (SLNs)	Colloidal lipidic carriers with a solid lipid interior. They can transport lipophilic drugs, have improved pharmacokinetic profile, high targeted drug delivery efficacy.	[50]
Nanosponges	Polyester based nanosized crosslinked materials. They possess a 3D architecture that can be readily functionalized.	[51]
Hydrogel nanoparticles	High stability in aqueous media, ability to contain water, good compatibility with biological systems	[52, 53]
Micelles	Easy preparation, good for transport and delivery of low permeable and poorly soluble drugs. High loading capacity.	[35]
Polymeric micelles	Self-assembled colloidal particles consisting of amphiphilic block copolymers. Can be loaded with water-insoluble drugs in the hydrophobic core, stabilized by the hydrophilic corona. Good uniformity, small size, long blood circulation time.	[54]
Polymeric nanoparticles	Improved stability, controllable drug release and drug payload. Can be prepared from natural (chitosan, albumin, hyaluronic acid) and synthetic [polyacrylamide, PAA; polylactic acid, PLA; polyglycolic acid, PGA; (poly(lactide-co-glycolide, PLGA and hyperbranched polymers]. Natural biopolymers are biodegradable, abundant, water soluble, cheap, biodegradable, biocompatible and can be chemically modified. Synthetic polymers can be engineered biodegradable, highly reproducible in their physical properties.	[55 - 63]
Liposomes	Synthetic lipid vesicles composed of concentric amphiphilic phospholipid bilayers (phospholipids and cholesterol); can be loaded with both hydrophobic and hydrophilic drugs. Can be transported across cell membranes (endocytic processes). Disadvantages: low drug encapsulating capacity, limited control of drug release, low cell uptake, unstability, short plasma half-life, expensive. Advantages: easy surface modification, tunable surface charge and size, increased circulation time and biocompatibility. Widely explored for cancer therapeutics; some products are already in the market (Doxil®, Lipusu®, DepoCyt®).	[47, 51, 64 - 68]

(Table 3) cont.....

System	Characteristics	Refs.
Dendrimers	Highly branched 3D macromolecules with controlled polymeric nanoarchitectures. They possess available functional groups for surface modification and internal cavities for molecular encapsulation where different drugs can be loaded through simple encapsulation, electrostatic interactions or covalent conjugation. Good biocompatibility, high hydrophilicity, polyvalent, precise molecular weights.	[35, 69 - 71]
Inorganic NCs		
Metal or metal oxide nanoparticles; quantum dots (QDs)	Generally, they have a core (inorganic) and shell (organic) structure. They may have unique physicochemical properties (fluorescence, high surface area, magnetism, optical absorption, catalytic activity), are easy to prepare and functionalize. Drugs can be loaded by covalent attachment to reactive surface groups or by physical adsorption, as well as by physical encasement to protect and stabilize drugs.	[72 - 75]

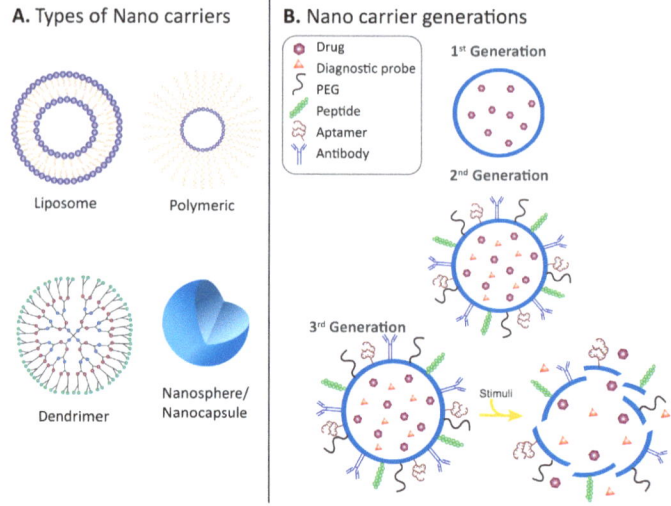

Fig. (1). Schematic representation of: (A) Types of NCs; (B) NCs generations.

In more than three decades of development of NCs for biomedical applications, major hurdles have been overcome and engineering of the properties of these systems is still of major importance to achieve the clinical translocation of the developed nanoformulations. Some challenges that NCs still face are: (1) encapsulating sufficient therapeutic agents with activated release, (2) efficient delivery of NPs to the desired location taking into account the multiple *in vivo* physiological barriers to cross, (3) toxicity of some engineered nanomaterials still requires further characterization, and (4) cost-effective and scalable fabrication of well-dispersed NPs which is a prerequisite for industrial production and clinical use [39]. Through rational design and engineering NCs have been improved artificially to adjust their specificity and level of biological interaction with target biomolecules as well as improving their pharmacokinetic and pharmacodynamic parameters, which has brought forward four distinct generations of systems [36, 76, 77].

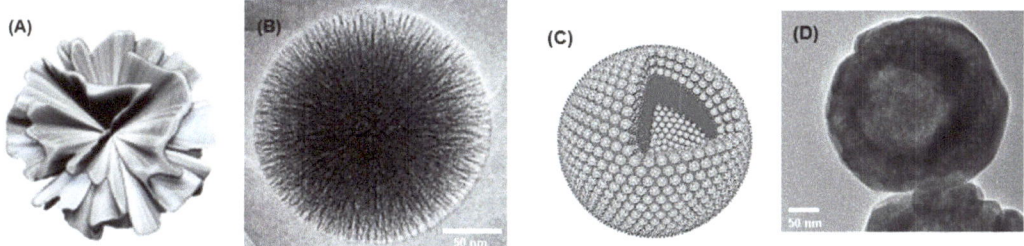

Fig. (2). Two selected inorganic mesoporous nanocarriers: (A) wrinkled mesoporous silica nanoparticles; (B) TEM of a WMS (*photo credit: Dra. Jessica Campos Delgado, UDLAP*); (C) hollow mesoporous metal oxide nanoparticle; (D) TEM of a hollow mesoporous silica nanoparticle [170].

In first generation nanostructures, nanoparticles simply encapsulate the drug and release it mainly dependent on passive diffusion that generally gives rise to a quick burst drug release; that gives rise to undesirable dose dumping and reduced long-term therapeutic efficacy, which is a long-standing formulation challenge for NCs [78]. It is important to note that NCs were themselves transported in the biological environment *via* free diffusion in a passive delivery manner; which still is the most widely utilized method in the nano-medical field [76]. Passive targeting is a result of the EPR effect, which is characteristic of leaky inflamed tissues such as tumors [79]. A representative example of passively targeted NCs that avoid unwanted filtration in the blood stream after administration are nanoparticles that are surface modified with polyethylene glycols (PEGs) [80]. The release mechanism of many biodegradable polymer-based controlled drug release systems relied on the hydrolysis-induced erosion of the carrier structure [37]. Some advantages of these first generation systems include an increase of half-life of the drug, controlled release, and the improvement of solubility of hydrophobic drugs. The main disadvantages are that these NCs are hydrophobic in nature and hardly make it into the interstitial tissue because they can be rapidly opsonized and cleared by resident macrophages [36].

Second generation nanostructures incorporate ligands that are specific to the target of interest; these are generally specifically designed peptides or aptamers that enhance cellular uptake of nano-carriers into tumor cells in a selective way, avoiding uptake by normal cells [81, 76]. These surface modifications can also enhance stability, improve biocompatibitity, half-life and biodistribution [35]. Nanoparticles can be functionalized with molecules such as Arg-Gly-Asp (RGD) peptides, folic acid (FA), or antibodies to recognize overexpressed receptors. For example, several cancer cells overexpress cell surface receptors such as epidermal growth factor receptor (EGFR) [82] and human epidermal growth factor receptor 2 (HER2) which can be targeted. Other types of specific cellular-targeting moieties have been reported, including transferrin (Tf), a glycoprotein that targets the Tf receptor (TfR) [83] and hyaluronic acid (HA), that targets the CD44 receptor [84]. Some advantages of this second generation are that these NCs can be theranostic, can be applied to tissue engineering applications, and are especially helpful for transport of therapeutic drugs across blood-brain barrier and in cancer treatments [36].

Third generation nanostructures encapsulate the drug to evade premature release at undesirable sites; these systems make use of an external stimuli (such as light or a magnetic field) or the actual disease condition, to activate the NC by local environmental changes like pH, redox state, temperature, or the presence of a particular molecule (such as gases, salts and enzymes). Redox potential is one of the major physiological differences between normal and tumor tissues, which is why redox-responsive nanostructures can be extremely advantageous as site-specific controlled delivery [36]. A second condition of extreme importance is pH because of pH changes along the gastric-intestine (GI) tract [85] as well as the fact that pH values in diseased sites such as ischemia, infection, inflammation, and cancer, tumor microenvironment is more acidic compared to normal tissues [86] which can be used to activate the NC. A major advantage of this third generation is the co-delivery of drugs which could help with multi-drug resistant (MDR) cancer [36], delivery of DNA sequences for gene treatment and personalized medicine [37, 39, 76, 81], and transport small interfering RNAs (siRNAs) and micro RNAs (miRNAs) to target genes that contribute to drug resistance by expressing, for example, drug efflux proteins [47]. For this third generation, release profiles can vary greatly; they could exhibit a long duration sustained release, pulsatile release, multiple drug release (released in sequence) or burst release [77]. The different sources of NC activation described above have been combined to develop multi-stimuli responsiveness. Generally, these systems are designed to alter their physical characteristics in a stepwise manner to control steps involved in drug-release and/or targeting [47]. Up to this moment there are dual triggered drug release systems using a combination of physiochemical stimuli (*e.g.*, electric field and pH dual-stimuli responsive chitosan-gold nanocomposite), triple triggered drug release (thermal, light and redox responsive) and a quadruple triggered drug release (pH, temperature, light, and redox responsive) [77].

What can now be called the fourth generation of nanostructures are active targeting delivery systems based on self-propelled micro/nano-carriers that can move to specific cells by themselves with appropriate guidance and self-propulsion systems [76]. This is a very recent field of research in which important and impacting advances are expected to occur in the following years.

Mesoporous Nanomaterials: Characteristics, Advantages, and Promising Role as Nanocarriers

Natural or synthetic porous materials with small pore diameters (0.3 nm to 10 μm) have found great utility in fields such as catalysis, environmental sciences, material sciences and specifically in the biomedical area as DDSs [87 - 96]. The pore structure of these materials consists of interconnected or isolated pores that may have similar or different shapes and sizes [97]. There are three basic pore models with pore shapes that roughly approximate: (a) cylindrical (b) ink-bottled and (c) slit-shaped pores [97 - 100]. IUPAC classifies these porous materials depending on the predominant pore sizes as: (1) microporous materials, having pore diameters up to 2.0 nm; (2) mesoporus materials, having pore sizes between 2.0 and 50.0 nm; and (3) macroporous materials, having pore sizes exceeding 50.0 nm (Fig. 3) [101]. These porous materials are usually defined by the ratio of the volume of pores and voids to the volume occupied by the material, which is defined as the porosity [98 - 101]; as well as in terms of their adsorption (condensation of gas on a free surface) properties [97]. Mesoporous materials range from metal sulfides, metal oxides, metal nitrides, metal organic frameworks (MOFs), carbon materials, carbonitriles, and composite materials [102]; though as for application in DDSs mesoporous silica nanocarriers (MSNs) are the most widely utilized nanomaterial. Beside silica, other materials, such as carbon, TiO_2 and ZrO_2 have been reported as the basis of a mesoporous DDSs [103 - 105]. Specifically, for the application of mesoporous materials as DDSs, it has been reported that ordered straight channels are favorable for diffusion of absorbed molecules, while disordered pores in the shell are advantageous for multi-stage and controlled drug release [39].

Prior to the late 1980's, most reported mesoporous materials were often amorphous and had broad pore size distributions. In the 1990s, the emergence of a new family of mesoporous molecular sieves based on silicate materials was reported possessing extremely high surface areas and narrow pore size distributions [106]. This family of MSNs bear a structure, composition, and pore size that can be tailored during synthesis by variation of the nature of the surfactant molecule, the reactant stoichiometry, the auxiliary chemicals, the reaction conditions, or even by post-synthesis functionalization techniques. The aforementioned is possible because MSNs are based on the concept of templating, which has been defined as a process in which an organic species functions as a central structure around which inorganic oxide units organize into a crystalline lattice that grows in a skin-tight manner [107, 108]. Upon the removal of the templating structure the geometric and electronic characteristics are replicated by the inorganic materials [108]. Besides the structural directing component of the organic template, there is a close relationship between the oxide lattice and the organic form in order that the synthesized lattice contains the organic species fixed into position; with which the lattice reflects the geometry of the organic molecule. Although structural direction requires a unique framework formed from a particular organic compound, it does not imply that the resulting oxide structure identically mimics the form of the organic molecule. Hence, the same organic molecule (surfactant template) can be used to synthesize a variety of structures where the pore size and its orientation can vary [97]. Particle morphology and size can be then controlled to from sphere-, rod-, or wormlike structures by tailoring the molar ratio of silica precursors and surfactants, as well as controlling the pH through the base catalysts [109], adding co-solvents or organic swelling agents [110], and introducing organoalkoxysilane precursors during the co-condensation reaction [111, 112]. MSNs can be classified as MCM 41 type MSN family, organically modified silica (ORMOSIL) NPs and hollow/ rattle type MSNs [113] (Fig. 3). MSNs have a solid framework, possessing a honeycomb-like structure and a very active surface distributed in various pore geometric structures (2D hexagonal, bicontinuous cubic, cage type, among others). Fig. (**4**) presents three schematic representations of the most typical MSNs structural frameworks.

MSNs are optimal for their use in drug delivery because silica has good biocompatibility and is accepted as "*Generally Recognized As Safe*" (GRAS) by the FDA [39]. Problems related to the removal of the excipient materials from the body after administration can be avoided because mesoporous silica is in an amorphous form that is degradable in aqueous solution [85]. Other advantages are that their fabrication is simple, scalable, cost-effective, and controllable and that they are heat, pH, and mechanical stress resistant. MSNs particle size can be tuned from 50 to 300 nm and they have cylindrical pores running through them that can also be tuned in diameters between of 2-50 nm; with the advantage that each cylindrical pore is an individual cargo carrier which exists completely isolated from adjacent ones [114]. Each cylindrical chamber can hold a significant amount of cargo while the release of the cargo can be regulated by modifying the openings of the pores with different materials. These features confer MSNs high loading capacity because of their high surface area (of over 700 m^2/g) and large pore volume [51], which is one of the most important advantages of MSNs over other nanocarriers because it can significantly increase the intracellular drug concentration. It has been reported that conventional MSNs can load a dose of therapeutic drug with 200-300 mg (maximally about 600 mg) drug/1 g silica

[39, 115]. For example, a MSNs known as SBA-15 loaded with cisplatin required 4 times lower doses in a B16F10 cell line to achieve the same effect as cisplatin alone [116] while against a HeLa cell line, another MSN-loaded with a cisplatin prodrug exhibited 63 times higher activity than that of cisplatin alone [117].

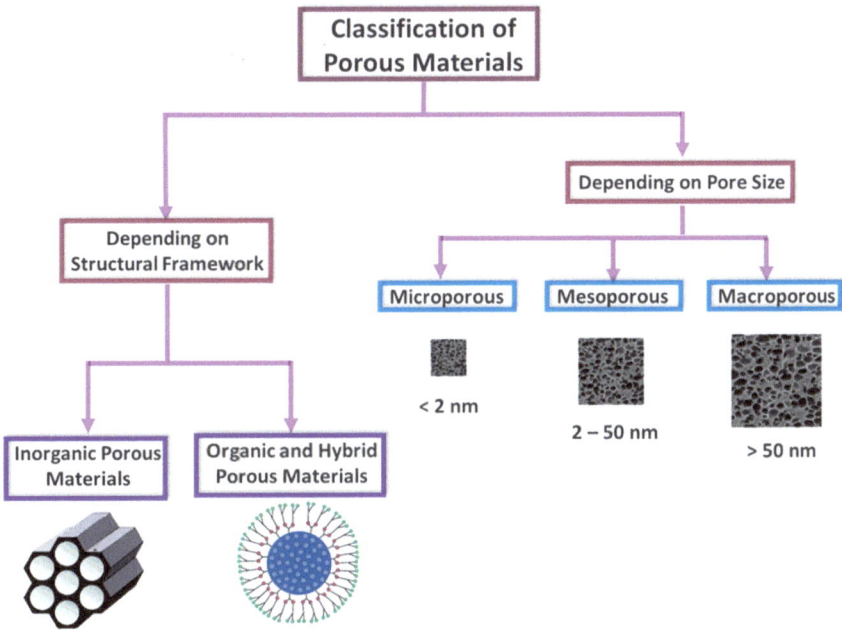

Fig. (3). Classification of most common porous materials.

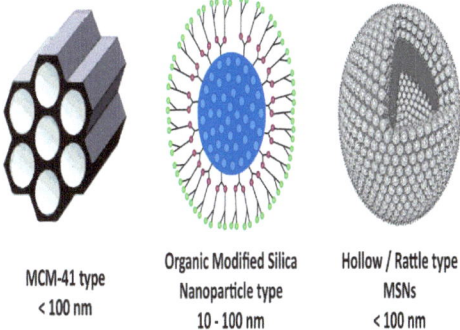

Fig. (4). Schematic representation of three types of MSNs according to their structural frameworks.

Compared to niosomes, liposomes, and dendrimers, MSNs are more stable to external response such as degradation and mechanical stress due to the strong

Si-O bond [118, 119]. Another advantage of MSNs are their silanol moieties which facilitates surface functionalization, that can be exploited to load drug molecules and functionalize with other such as antibodies, stimuli-responsive materials, luminescent or capping materials, which can lead to smart and multifunctional properties [36, 37, 39, 76, 81, 85, 115]. It has also been reported that MSNs with a diameter of 100 nm showed less inflammatory response, cytotoxicity, and contact hypersensitivity [120] as well as lower hemolytic activity [121] than colloidal solid nonporous counterparts.

Recent classes of mesoporous materials have exceptional structural and physicochemical properties, such as tunable pore and particle size, large specific surface area, high porosity, easy surface modifications, low cytotoxicity, and higher stability than classical polymer-based drug delivery vectors. An example are periodic mesoporous organosilicas (PMOs) that have organic-inorganic components homogeneously distributed inside the mesostructured framework at the molecular level [78]. Other examples are hollow/rattle-type MSNs that are ideal as new-generation drug delivery systems with extraordinarily high loading capacity because they have interstitial hollow space and a mesoporous shell that grants them low density pooled with a high specificity [39]. Hollow core-mesoporous shell structures are able to achieve a super-high drug loading capacity, typically higher than 1 g of drug/1 g of silica [115].

There are still a lot of questions on the mechanistic details to understand all the advantages related to the use of nanostructured DDS versus conventional free drug chemotherapy. Pascal and coworkers have applied first-principles cell biophysics, drug pharmacokinetics and drug pharmacodynamics to model the delivery of DOX to hepatocellular carcinoma tumor cells and predict their cytotoxicity [122]. The model developed may become useful for the optimal design of novel nanocarriers and for improving the current systems, as well as for the understanding of *in vivo* drug transport and tumor response. The design, preparation and evaluation of innovative nanocarriers as DDS is a very active field of research; although more than 2,000 papers have been published containing the keywords "nanocarrier", "drug delivery" and "release", less than 100 exploit the unique physical and chemical characteristics of mesoporous materials, specifically in applications for cancer therapy. Most of the explored nanomaterials exploited for DDSs reported in the literature (>90%) used micelles, liposomes, polymeric nanoparticles or dendrimers as the structural basis, while the remaining less than 10% considered single-walled carbon nanotubes (SWCNTs), multi-walled carbon nanotubes (MWCNTs) and inorganic nanoparticles for that application. Here, some selected examples of mesoporous NCs recently reported (2007-2018) are reviewed.

A) Mesoporous Silica Nanocarriers

MSNs are very attractive because their excellent properties can be highly useful for drug transport and delivery: tunable pore size, high drug loading, narrow porosity, surface available for chemical modification, thermal stability and biocompatibility. Size can be controlled in the range from 50 to 300 nm, obtaining very stable and rigid frameworks with pore sizes from 2 to 6 nm and high surface area and large pore volume (>900 m^2/g; >0.9 cm^3/g). Their biomedical applications, synthesis, pharmacokinetics and biocompatibility as DDS have been reviewed recently [123]. There are several methods for the preparation of mesoporous silica nanostructures (sol-gel, microwave assisted, chemical etching, templating approach, hydrothermal, emulsion) which allow control over size, shape, pore volume and structure, surface morphology and dispersibility.

Their large surface area and porosity allow loading therapeutic agents in high amounts, followed by their subsequent release, which can be controlled by chemical modification of the silanol-containing surfaces. Chemical functionalization of the external surface or the internal surface (pores), allows attaching different molecular groups that provide better drug adsorption, increased biocompatibility and/or water solubility, or changing the polarity to allow the transport of hydrophobic drugs. The fate of nanocarriers in biological media is something that may affect their potential commercial applications for the design of efficient and biocompatible DDSs. Cytotoxicity, biodegradability and biodistribution may be influenced by the nature of chemical groups derived from functionalization or type of coating used to modify the surface of the nanomaterial. Nairi and coworkers studied the interaction between bovine serum albumin and MSNs functionalized with biopolymers (hyaluronic acid, chitosan), providing evidence of the effects of the biopolymer coating [124]. It was found that different biopolymers affect in different ways the formation of a protein corona around the surface modified MSNs.

MSNs-based first, second and third generation DDSs have been prepared and explored in the last ten years. Table **4** summarizes the most important systems reported. It is clear that most of the current research is focusing on the development of third generation drug delivery systems, exploiting different strategies for drug release activation (thermal effect induced by NIR radiation absorption, hydrolysis activated by acidic pH, specific enzymatic action, redox changes, or a combination of them). However, there are still several contributions to the development of theranostic systems (second DDS generation) or simple nanocarriers (first generation).

Table 4. MSNs explored as DDSs and their main characteristics.

Drug Delivery (First Generation DDSs)		
Drug	**Characteristics**	**Ref.**
DOX / Melittin	Non-spherical MSVs consisting mainly on MSNs, chemically modified with APTES. The anti-vascular endothelial growth factor receptor 2 antibody conjugated NC produced 80% reduction in cell viability after 3 days and preferential targeting and drug delivery to human umbilical vein endothelial cells (HUVEC). The DOX loaded NC showed good efficiency against MCF6 cancer cells.	[125]
Platinum(IV) prodrug	Drug conjugated MSNs and labeled with liver-targeting lactobionic acid. NCs presented enhanced circulation time and concentrate more specifically at the liver tumor site; under the chemical environment of the tumor, Pt(IV) was reduced to Pt(II), which was released and showed improved chemotherapeutic activity.	[126]
DOX	FA or NAG conjugated MSNs. Cytotoxicity towards MCF-6 and MDA-MB-231 human breast cancer cells was evaluated. Higher cell uptake for NAG labeled MSNs was found respect FA-MSNs; cytotoxicity was higher for NAG-MSNs respect to FA-MSNs suggesting that glucosamine transporters can be used as targets for NC internalization in cancer therapy.	[127]
PTX / DOX	HMS nanospheres wrapped with a phospholipid layer. The NC was successfully internalized into A549 cancer cells and the combination of DOX (hydrophilic) and PTX (hydrophobic) showed marked synergistic effect inhibiting cancer cells proliferation.	[128]
DOX / Gefitinib	MSNs capped with cetubimax to target EGFR-mutant lung cancer cells. Treatment of a gefitinib-resistant cell line derived from PC9 cell resulted in significant cell growth inhibition, suppressing the progression of PC9 xenograft tumors.	[129]
Not specified	Vaterite particles ($CaCO_3$ nanoparticles) used as templates for the preparation of multicompartment MSNs. In comparison to HMS nanoparticles, this NC offers a cheap, accessible and green venue for the preparation of hierarchical drug nanocarriers.	[130]
Ibuprofen / 5-fluorouracil	MSNs functionalized with long organic chains, enhancing drug adhesion on the silica surface, delaying and controlling drug release.	[131]
NO / Cisplatin	WMS nanoparticles loaded with NO and cisplatin for the treatment of non-small cell lung cancer cell lines. Evaluation indicated that they were more toxic than the corresponding NCs loaded only with cisplatin.	[132]
PTX	WMS nanoparticles loaded with PTX showed improved drug loading efficiency and improved performance for sustained release, in comparison to pure MSNs.	[133]

(Table 4) cont.....

Theranostic MSNs (Second Generation DDSs)		
Use	**Characteristics**	**Ref.**
Imaging / Phototherapy	MSNs functionalized with Pd-porphyrins used as a phosphorescence probe for oxygen sensing/imaging (diagnostics) and simultaneously exploited as a nano-photosensitizer for cancer cell phototherapy against MDA-MB-231 breast cancer cells.	[134]
Imaging / DDS	FTIC labeled MSNs, coated with PEG, functionalized with anti-EpCAM antibody and loaded with lycorine, a molecule with anti-tumor activity. Evaluation on PC-3M cell line indicated good biocompatibility and cell uptake, releasing the drug and inducing cell death.	[135]
Imaging / Therapy	Eu^{3+} and Gd^{3+} doped MSNs functionalized with Cys and FA. FA-modified EuGd-MSNs increased cell uptake in HeLa cancer cells, with significant increase in red fluorescence emission and enhanced MRI response. Cys-containing EuGd-MSNs showed increased cytotoxicity against HeLa cancer cells and good biocompatibility and stability when cultivated with normal L929 cells.	[136]
PET-imaging / DDS	MCM-41 MSNs modified with CREKA (tumor homing peptide) and DTPA (Cu^{2+} ion chelating agent) and loaded with MTX. Activation of Cu^{2+} ions in a nuclear reactor to the radionuclide ^{64}Cu, allows radiotracing and doesn't affect the pharmacological action of MTX.	[137]
Radio-imaging / DDS	^{99m}Tc doped MSNs loaded with betamethasone (porous structure) or dexamethasone (surface conjugation). Cytotoxicity assays showed that dexamethasone conjugated MSNs were safer than the betamethasone loaded.	[138]
Radio-imaging/DSS	Holmium containing WMS NPs, loaded with cisplatin and coated with a phospholipid. Their chemoradiotherapeutic performance was evaluated after neutron-activation of holmium to ^{166}Ho radionuclide.	[139]
Stimuli responsive MSNs (Third Generation DDSs)		
Stimuli	**Characteristics/Advantages**	**Ref.**
DNAzyme action	Switchable DNA nanostructures (nuclei acid, hairpins, i-motif, G-quadruplex) that "open/close" the pores of drug-loaded MSN nanoplatforms for targeting cancer cells	[140]
Biotin or HAase action	Streptavidin complex with desthiobiotin grafted MSNs further functionalized with biotin-modified HA and loaded with DOX. Drug release improved in the presence of biotin or HAase. NC showed good biocompatibility (*in vitro* and *in vivo*), inducing apoptosis in cancer cells and inhibiting tumor growth with minimal systemic toxicity.	[141]
MMP-2	MSNs functionalized with MMP-2 sensitive peptides that served as nanovalves blocking the MCM-41 pores, simultaneously activating a fluorescent dye (TAMRA), improving tumor imaging and triggering drug release.	[142]
Acidic pH	Surface of MSNs was functionalized with PAsA as gatekeeper, releasing DOX in response to lysosomal/endosomal acidified environment conditions when internalized into HepG2 cells, increasing cytotoxic response in comparison to the use of free DOX or non-loaded MSNs.	[143]

(Table 4) cont.....

Stimuli	Characteristics/Advantages	Ref.
Acidic pH	Chitosan coated MSNs (<150 nm) functionalized with FA (to target folate receptors at positive tumor cells), loaded with ursolic acid. They showed good stability and inhibitory activity against HeLa cancer cells, inducing apoptosis and decreasing migration (*in vitro*) and showing suppression of lung tumor growth and metastasis (*in vivo*).	[144]
Acidic pH	β-Cyclodextrin functionalized PEGylated MSNs loaded with poorly soluble anticancer drug curcumin. The NCs showed good loading and releasing efficiencies, with maximum efficiency at pH of 5.16 after 107 h, indicating they may be good candidates for sustained drug release cancer therapy.	[145]
Acidic pH	Bilayer poly(acrylic acid-co-itaconic acid) and HAS coated MSNs (MCM-41 structure) loaded with gemcitabine. Maximum release achieved at the pH of endosomes (pH 5.5).	[146]
Acidic pH	PDA coated MSNs loaded with cationic amphiphilic drug DES. NC had high drug loading and pH sensitivity, and internalized into cells easily showing high cytotoxicity and inhibitory effects against cancer cells.	[147]
Acidic pH	HMS nanoparticles loaded with DOX containing bubble-generating agents (sodium bicarbonate, ammonium carbonate). Once internalized into tumor cells, acidic decomposition of the bicarbonate/carbonate component induces lysosomal membrane permeabilization and cancer cell apoptosis. The NC showed excellent cytotoxicity against MCF-7 cells and were efficient to overcome multidrug resistant of MCF-7/adriamycin cells.	[148]
Acidic pH	PDA and PEG coated MSNs loaded with DOX. The NC showed good stability, increased biocompatibility, good water solubility, good cellular uptake and improved anticancer effect in breast cancer models and cell cultures.	[149]
Acidic pH	A two component DDS consisting of MSNs prepared by template assisted sol-gel process and a polymerizable moiety (poly-4-vinylpyridine) attached to the mesoporous material as a gatekeeper. The MTX loaded NC exhibit "on/off" effect by controlling the environmental pH.	[150]
Acidic pH	MCM-41 type MSNs functionalized with acid-cleavable citraconic bond using "click chemistry". Exposition to acidic microenvironment (cancerous tissue or intracellular endosomes), hydrolysis o the citraconic bond releasing the drug (DOX). The NC showed good cell uptake and anti-tumor activity against human cervical cancer cells (HeLa).	[151]
Acidic pH	PAA grafted MSNs linked through an acid cleavable linker (PAA-AC--MSN) and loaded with DOX. At neutral pH the linker is stable and MSNs pores are blocked; at acidic pH, PAA is removed and DOX released in a controlled way. The NC showed good *in vitro* cytotoxicity against nasopharyngeal carcinoma cells (HNE-1), inhibiting tumor development *in vivo*.	[152]

(Table 4) cont.....

Stimuli	Characteristics/Advantages	Ref.
Acidic pH	CS-PMMA coated MSNs loaded with DOX showed good performance and biocompatibility when evaluated in two cell lines (tumor HeLa and normal somatic cells). DOX release occurs after cell uptake due to the acidic intracellular environment.	[153]
Acidic pH	HMS NCs coated with carboxylated chitosan and loaded with DOX showed good drug loading efficiency and good cell uptake in HeLa cells, inducing apoptosis, and no showing hemolytic activity in the range of 5-230 µm/ml range.	[154]
Acidic pH	Chitosan capped MSNs, chemically modified with aminosilanes on their surface, were loaded with raloxifene hydrochloride and evaluated against MCF-7 breast carcinoma cells, showing good efficiency for controlled drug release during extended periods and good biocompatibility.	[155]
NIR radiation (thermal effect) and acidic pH	DOX-loaded core-shell Au@SiO$_2$ nanorods composite with salicylic acid acid loaded PLGA based microparticles. *In vitro* evaluation in cervical cancer cells cultures showed up to 48% reduction in size of HeLa spheroids, suggesting that the dual stimuli may be useful for combined therapies on cancer treatment.	[156]
NIR radiation (thermal effect)	DOX loaded NaGdF$_4$:Yb/Er@NaGdF$_4$ nanoparticles coated with a mesoporous SiO$_2$ shell functionalized with amino groups and conjugated with Au nanoparticles. The assembled nanocomposite showed better synergistic effects against cancer cells combining chemotherapy and photothermal therapy.	[157]
NIR radiation	DOX loaded SWCNTs coated with mesoporous silica and modified with PEG. Drug loading was very efficient and after NIR stimulation the drug was released by photothermal activation resulting in a synergistic inhibitory effect on cancer cells growth.	[158]
NIR radiation (thermal effect) and HAase action	AuNBs conjugated to MSNs and the polymer formed by azobenzene and α-cyclodextrin functionalized HA. Affinity of HA in the surface of MSNs and the CD44 antigen overexpressed on tumor cells increased selectivity. Photothermal heating of hydrogen under NIR and HA degradation induced by HAase action resulted in increased drug release and delivery into tumor cells.	[159]
Redox change induced by GTH	Carboxylated MSNs caped with cross-linked DNA (Cys and 9-aminoacridine used as cross-linkers). NCs were encapsulated in a nano-network consisting of a zwitterionic amino acid (Cys), an anionic bioadhesive polymer (poly(methyl vinyl ether-alt-maleic acid) and a cationic endosomolytic polymer (polyetehieleimine). The nanocomposite was loaded with sorafenib (anticancer drug) and calcein (imaging agent), showing high-loading efficiency, low cyto- and hemo-toxicity.	[160]

There are still several surprises around the corner in the search of novel mesoporous silica nanocarriers. For example, the recent advances on the preparation of WMS nanocarriers for drug transport and delivery are very promising. WMS are spherical silica NPs with radial wrinkled structure; they have small sizes and very large surface-to-volume ratios with plenty of pore space available for drug loading or chemical functionalization. Munaweera and coworkers used WMS as nanocarriers for transport and release of nitric oxide (NO) and cisplatin, for the treatment of non-small cell lung cancer (NSCLC) [132]. The nanocarrier was characterized by different physical methods (BET, FTIR, ICP-MS, SEM and TEM) and the biological evaluation against NSCLC cell lines (H596 and A549) indicated that the NO and cisplatin loaded WMS were more toxic than the corresponding systems loaded only with cisplatin. They also explored the use of WMS NPs as vehicles for the simultaneous delivery of chemo- and radiotherapeutics [139]. The release kinetics of holmium containing WMS particles, loaded with cisplatin and coated or uncoated with the lipid 1,2-dioleyl-sn-glycero-3-phospcholine, that were prepared and fully characterized (TEM, FTIR, ^{1}H-NMR, EDS, ICP-MS and ζ-potential), was evaluated, as well as the performance as a radioactive chemoradiotherapeutic agent, after neutron-activation. Very recently, Ma and coworkers reported the preparation of highly symmetric, ultra-small inorganic silica cages ('silicages') by the self-assembly of primary silica clusters in aqueous solution on the surface of charged surfactant micelles [161]. The impressive shapes and size control of these polyhedral nanocages may find utility in the near future as nanocarriers for drugs or even genetic material, as their size is similar to some viral peptide cages, so they may become useful systems to be explored in gene therapy.

In summary, as previously stated, MSNs are currently one of the most studied and popular materials for the development of innovative DDSs. Emphasis is being placed in the development of innovative theranostic systems that allow simultaneous therapy and imaging/diagnostics. Also, several innovative third generation drug delivery systems with the ability to control the release of drugs by external stimuli (radiofrequency or electromagnetic irradiation, pH, specific enzyme activity or heat) are been designed and tested, opening the door to a more personalized medicine. Improved biocompatibility, larger surface area, easy surface functionalization and excellent drug loading efficiencies, make MSNs very attractive choices for drug delivery in cancer therapy.

B). Mesoporous Magnetic Nanocarriers

Magnetic nanomaterials are very attractive as they can be selectively targeted to cancer tissues through chemical surface functionalization or by remote manipulation applying an external magnetic field. They also can be used as contrast agents in MRI or in magnetically induced hyperthermia. Usually, MMNs are formed by two components: one mesoporous nanomaterial and an appropriate magnetic component, although in some cases both components may be the same. During the last 10 years, most of the MMNs developed can be classified as second or third generation DDSs, and most of them exploit the unique magnetic characteristics for MRI imaging, hyperthermal therapy or remotely activating drug release using an AMF (magnetic heat induction). Table **5** summarizes the most representatives works published during the present period and their main characteristics.

Table 5. MMNs explored as DDSs.

Only Drug Delivery (First Generation DDSs)		
Drug	**Characteristics**	**Ref.**
Sodium meclofenamate	Hollow magnetic iron oxide NPs prepared by a hydrothermal method. The NC showed good drug loading and release efficiencies, and were magnetically responsive.	[162]
Curcumin	Core-shell magnetic NC formed by a magnetite core coated with a mesoporous titanium dioxide/graphene oxide nanocomposite (Fe_3O_4@$mTiO_2$/GO) prepared by a simple sonochemical method. Loading and encapsulating efficiency as high as 17.8 and 72.4%, respectively and were pH responsive. MTT assay showed no cytotoxicity against human foreskin fibroblast normal cell line (HFF-2) and good inhibitory effects on Caco-2 cancerous cells.	[163]
Theranostic (Second Generation DDSs)		
Use	**Characteristics**	**Ref.**
Imaging / Target guide / DDS	The surface of a Gd^{3+} doped MSNs was modified with a lipid bilayer. It showed good stability, biocompatibility and excellent cellular uptake. The NC performed well as a T_1 contrast agent. It was loaded with the pro-apoptosis peptide KLA (HGGKLAKLAKKLAKLAK) and tested in cell cultures, inducing mitochondrial swelling and cell apoptosis.	[164]
Diagnostic / Imaging	Sandwich-structured ECL immunosensing platform consisting of CdTe QDs embedded in mesoporous silica nanospheres ($mSiO_2$/CdTe) and combined with a magnetite-silica-polystyrene nanocomposite (Fe_3O_4@SiO_2@PS). The ECL component was used as a imaging label for conjugation of secondary antibodies, while the magnetic part was used as carrier for primary antibodies due to the convenience for magnetic separation. It was able to detect carcinoembryonic antigen using cyclic voltammetry and electrochemical impedance spectroscopy with a low detection limit of 0.3 pg/mL.	[165]
Phototherapy / DDS	Core-shell PEGylated magnetic nanoparticles coated with PDA and loaded with DOX for photothermal ablation and chemotherapy of tumor cells. The NC showed strong NIR absorption and was magnetic field responsive to guide the carrier to a specific site for drug delivery. It showed great stability and biocompatibility.	[166]

(Table 5) cont.....

Use	Characteristics	Ref.
Imaging / Target guide	Core-shell magnetic MSNs (Fe_3O_4@$mSiO_2$) designed to efficiently deliver DNA-toxin anticancer drugs into targeted tumor cells. The MRI active magnetic NC was able to accumulate in tumor tissue by receptor-mediated endocytosis guided by an external magnetic field. Once internalized, the acidic pH reverses the surface charge from negative to positive, separating a charge-conversional polymer attached on the surface of the NC and exposing the nuclear-targeting TAT peptide, inducing cell apoptosis.	[167]
Imaging / Hyperthermia / DDS	Superparamagnetic Fe_3O_4 and paramagnetic MnO_x NPs composite with GO nanosheets. The magnetic composite is biocompatible, had good systemic biodistribution, and accumulate in tumor tissue *via* the EPR effect. It is MRI silent until the acidic environment in the tumor release Mn^{2+} ions, generating a strong positive contrast enhancement. DOX loaded NC inhibit metastasis and have synergistic effect for field-induced hyperthermia therapy.	[168]
Imaging / Target guide / DDS	Porous magnetic nanoclusters coated with PAA and loaded with DOX. The magnetic NC had high-drug loading and release efficiency, was MRI active as a T_2 contrast agent. It was infused *via* hepatic arteries in a rabbit model, showing good intra-tumoral delivery and MRI performance.	[169]

Stimuli responsive (Third Generation DDSs)

Stimuli	Characteristics/Advantages	Ref.
Ultrasound	Fe_3O_4 NPs embedded in a SiO_2 shell chemically modified with BNN6. BNN6 is an ultrasound-triggered NO release system. NO has been found to be able to inhibit tumor growth. The NC successfully released NO under ultrasonic activation and served as a MRI contrast agent for tumor localization.	[170]
Acidic pH / AMF	Cube shaped magnetite nanoparticles, DOX loaded, that decompose in acid medium releasing the load or can be remotely activated by an AMF inducing heating and drug release.	[171]
Acidic pH / AMF	Curcumin loaded magnetic NCs bifunctionalized (out and inside) with β-cyclodextrin hydrate, a hydrophilic non-toxic carrier for hydrophobic drugs. The NC showed pH dependent performance, and release response controlled by AMF. It was evaluated towards SK-HEP1 and HepG2 cancer cells, showing good cell uptake and increased cytotoxicity compared to the free drug.	[172]
AMF	Core-shell Fe_3O_4@$mSiO_2$ nanoparticles functionalized with thermosensitive polymer poly(N-isopropylacrylamide). The mesoporous silica shell allowed further surface modification with chitosan and rhodamine. The magnetic NC was loaded with 5-fluoroacil to evaluate target tumor cell specificity.	[173]
Acidic pH / External magnetic field	Janus nanocomposite formed by combining magnetite nanoparticles and mesoporous silica containing DOX. The magnetic nanobullets induced selective growth inhibition of cancer cells under an external AMF, releasing DOX into the acidic intracellular content. *In vivo* test in liver tumor models in mice showed remarkable tumor growth suppression and low toxicity.	[174]
Radiofrequency pulse	HMS core coated with a layer of iron oxide NPss attached to the silica surface through electrostatic charges. Application of an external AMF induced heating of the NC, achieving a heat dissipation rate of 200 W/g, activating drug release.	[175]

(Table 5) cont.....

Stimuli	Characteristics/Advantages	Ref.
External magnetic radiofrequency pulse	Mesoporous iron oxide NPs with hydrophobic pores, using a tumor-targeted lactoferrin bio-gate as cap and loaded with PTX and PFH. Under magnetic stimuli, the magnetic NC enhanced cell uptake and accumulation in deep tumors, increasing cell-killing efficiency. *In vivo* evaluation showed suppression of subcutaneous tumors after 16 days of a single magnetic frequency exposure.	[176]

C). Other Mesoporous Inorganic and Organic Nanocarriers

Aside of MSNs and MMNs, other materials based on carbon (MCNs), hydroxyapatite (MHNs), as well as ZnO, LDH nanoparticles, BN, or gold nanorods, among others, have been explored in the last decade and their performance as potential innovative DDSs has been evaluated. Mesoporous carbon materials (MCMs) are of interest for the development of DDS due to their high surface area and physicochemical properties. They can be classified on several categories, such as solid mesoporous carbon nanomaterials, hollow mesoporous carbon nanomaterials, and several types of mesoporous carbon nanocomposites. Although conventional methodologies for the preparation of MCNs usually yield randomly porous materials, with little control over the pore/size distributions, recent advances have resulted in the development of methods for the preparation of MCMs with extremely high surface areas and ordered mesostructures. Combining imaging and drug delivery is an interesting strategy for the development of innovative DDSs. On the other hand, MHNs are very attractive systems for the design of useful drug delivery system due to their inherent biocompatibility and easiness for biodegradation. A different kind of mesoporous inorganic nanocarriers are the LDH nanoparticles, which are promising due to their good biocompatibility, pH-sensitive and stimuli responsive release and high specific surface. ZnO nanostructures have been poorly investigated as potential nanocarriers for DDSs and are an interesting field of research. Other inorganic nanomaterials, nitride (BN) analogues to carbon nanomaterials, are promising platforms for biomedical applications, as they have good biocompatibility and lower cytotoxicity than their carbon counterparts do. In the other hand, organic nanocarriers based on polymeric nanostructures (nanoparticles, nanocapsules, nanospheres) or smart polymeric systems (hydrogels, dendrimers, micelles) are very attractive for their high loading efficiency and good biocompatibility. Among them, nanocapsules have been explored due to their low polymer content compared to other nanostructures. Stimuli-responsive hydrogel systems have also been explored as efficient controlled drug delivery systems. Micelles having a hydrophobic core and a cationic hydrophilic shell in water may be useful for loading hydrophobic drugs or polyanionic genes as nanocarriers. Table **6** summarizes some of the most representative examples of these miscellaneous inorganic and organic nanocarriers, classified according to their DDSs generation (first, second or third).

Table 6. Other important inorganic and organic mesoporous DDSs.

Only Drug Delivery (First Generation DDSs)		
Drug	**Characteristics**	**Ref.**
OligoDNA	MCNs with large surface area (646 m^2/g) and adjustable pore size prepared using poly(ethylene oxide)-b-polystyrene, a non-Pluronic copolymer, as template and resorcinol-formaldehyde as carbon precursor. The MCNs were able to deliver efficiently cyanine-labeled oligoDNA into human cancer cells (HCT-116), with low toxicity.	[177]
HAP	Mesoporous MgO NCs to encapsulate the anticancer candidate drug natural-based cubic HAP (loading from 0 to 60 wt%). The spherical shaped MgO NC loaded with HAP showed high activity against HepG2 liver cancer cells, inducing apoptosis even at 20 wt% HAP load.	[178]
DOX	Water soluble (2.0 mg/mL) hydroxilated, porous BN obtained by thermal substitution reaction of carbon atoms in graphitic carbon nitrides. The NC was biocompatible, and had good drug loading efficiency, up to 3 times its own weight. It showed a significant decrease in LNCap cancer cells viability.	[179]
DOX / p53 gene	Amphiphilic pullulan-stearic acid derivative with low molecular weight branched polyethyleneimine loaded with DOX and the therapeutic gene p53-encoding plasmid. The organic NC showed low cytotoxicity toward MCF-7 cells, good transfection efficiency for COS-7 cells and good co-deliver of both DOX and p53 gene into MCF-7 cells, resulting in higher tumor cell apoptosis.	[180]
DOX / hairpin RNA	A multifunctional micelle designed with an amphiphilic bifunctional pullulan-based copolymer decorated with FA, loaded with DOX and short hairpin RNA of Beclin1. The NC showed good cell uptake in HepG2 cells and significant cytotoxicity against HeLa cells, co-delivering simultaneously both DOX and the shRNA.	[181]
Theranostic (Second Generation DDSs)		
Use	**Characteristics**	**Ref.**
Diagnostics / Imaging	GO conjugated to FSHR-mAB and radiolabeled with ^{64}Cu for PET imaging. When tested on a luciferase-transfected MDA-MB-231 breast cancer lung metastasis model in female nude mice, specificity to FSHR-mAb.	[182]
Imaging / DDS	Radiolabeled (^{99m}Tc) MHNs conjugated with 2-deoxy-D-glucose and DOX. The NC was able to inhibit cell viability against MDA-MB-231, MCF-7 and MC4-L2 Balb/c mice breast cancer cells.	[183]
Imaging / DDS	Mesoporous, auto-fluorescent (440 nm emission) ZnO nanospheres (~100 nm) with 43Å pore size for drug loading.	[184]

(Table 6) cont.....

Use	Characteristics	Ref.
Imaging / DDS	Rattle-type hollow $CaWO_4:Tb^{3+}$@SiO_2 nanocapsule using a spherical Fe_3O_4 template. The NC had a large inner cavity, a biocompatible silica shell and a luminescent core. The DOX-loaded NC showed good cytotoxicity towards HeLa cells.	[185]
Imaging / DDS	PDA NPs loaded with indocyanine (green fluorescence dye), Mn^{2+} ions (for T_1-MRI) and DOX. The NC had good *in vivo* performance in a mouse tumor model, with remarkable synergistic therapeutic effect.	[186]

Stimuli responsive (Third Generation DDSs)

Stimuli	Characteristics/Advantages	Ref.
Acidic pH / Redox	HMC NCs capped with PAA *via* disulfide bonds and loaded with DOX (52% drug loading efficiency). *In vitro* evaluation showed improved drug release under acidic pH and NIR irradiation.	[187]
Acidic pH / NIR radiation	Mesoporous carbon nanospheres loaded with DOX. The carbon NCs showed good photothermal conversion and photoacoustic imaging performance, and pH and NIR drug release activation.	[188]
Acidic pH / GSH	HMC NPs grafted with photo-stable, luminescent carbon QDs immobilized on the pore's openings as gatekeepers using disulfide units to avoid premature release of DOX.	[189]
Acidic pH / Redox	MCNs capped with PAA, which acted as a gatekeeper to control DOX release. GSH induced disulfide bond dissociation and acidic pH activated drug release. The NC showed good inhibitory effect on HeLa cell cultures.	[190]
Acidic pH	HMMs constituted by nanosized HAp microcrystals synthesized from hollow $CaCO_3$ nanoparticles. Surface modification improved cell uptake. NCs were loaded with cis-diammineplatinum(II) dichloride, showing strong inhibitory growth effect on human squamous cell carcinoma *in vitro* cultures.	[191]
Acidic pH	PAA grafted MHNs and loaded with DOX. The NC had good cell uptake in HepG2 cells, low cytotoxicity and efficient intracellular pH-stimulated drug release.	[192]
Acidic pH	Hierarchal mesoporous $CaCO_3$ nanospheres loaded with anticancer drug etoposide. The NC dispersed well in a cell culture and exhibit good inhibitory effect on SGC-7901 cancer cells culture and good biocompatibility toward HEK 293 T cells.	[193]
Acidic pH	Core-shell nanocomposite with SiO_2 core and Mg/Al-LDH coating, with bevacizumab and the specific antibody to vascular endothelial growth factor immobilized on its surface and loaded with DOX. The NC showed good cell uptake, low cardiac and hepatic toxicity and significant inhibitory effect on human neuroblastoma cell line.	[194]
Acidic pH	Magnetic core coated with Al/Ni-LDH shell and loaded with a carboxy-modified DOX derivative. The surface of the LDH-shell was modified with iminodiacetic acid modified folate to target cancer cells. The NC exhibited good cytotoxicity, inhibiting HeLa growth in the acidic intracellular medium of the cancer cells.	[195]

(Table 6) cont.....

Stimuli	Characteristics/Advantages	Ref.
NIR radiation	AuNR coated with mesoporous silica, with adsorbed a phase change material (fatty alcohol or fatty acid) to increase the loading capacity to hydrophobic DOX. The NC exhibited good performance toward various cell lines.	[196]
Disulfide bond dissociation / Temperature	Polymer nanocapsules from the PMAm and NIPAAm, using the disulfide-containing cross linker BMOD. The NC surface presents several reactive alkyne groups useful for thiol-yne click chemistry and further functionalization. NCs were decorated with Cys-FA, Cys-RGD peptide and thiol-functionalized FTIC and loaded with DOX. They showed good antigrowth activity against HeLa cells.	[197]
Acidic pH / Disulfide bond dissociation	Cubic PMMA hydrogel particles prepared from sacrificial mesoporous MnO_2 particles as templates and loaded with DOX. Optima drug loading at neutral pH, and drug release at pH<6. GSH and acidic pH activates drug release.	[198]
Acidic pH / NIR radiation	Amphiphilic chitosan-g-oleic acid copolymer coated SWCNTs encapsulated in a thermos/pH sensitive hydrogel based in PEG-diacrylate den NIPPAm. The DOX loaded hydrogel showed greater cytotoxicity toward HeLa cells upon NIR radiation.	[199]
Acidic pH	Spherical and negatively charged surface hydrogel formed by self-assembly of lysozyme-pectin, loaded with MTX. After uptake in HepG2 cells, MTX loaded NC induced apoptosis.	[200]

The development of multifunctional nanocarriers is very attractive as their theranostic applications may offer several benefits. Combining imaging and drug delivery is an interesting strategy for the development of innovative DDSs. For example, Yang and coworkers conjugated a follicle stimulating hormone receptor (FSHR) monoclonal antibody (mAB) to GO in order to target angiogenic markers on tumor vasculature efficiently, and radiolabeled it with ^{64}Cu for imaging using PET [182]. When tested on a luciferase-transfected MDA-MB-231 breast cancer lung metastasis model in female nude mice, they confirmed the specificity of FSHR-mAb. They proposed that these nanocarriers may be useful for the design of GO-based platforms for early metastasis detection and targeted DDS. In another work, Wang *et al.*, prepared HMC NPs grafted with photo-stable, luminescent carbon dots synthesized from polyethylenimine by hydrothermal reaction. The carbon dots were immobilized on the pore's openings of the HMCs as gatekeepers using disulfide units to avoid premature release of the anti-cancer drug (DOX) [189]. After breaking the disulfide bond in the presence of glutathione, which triggered the release of the drug, release was accelerated by induced heating with NIR irradiation. The cleavage of the carbon dots from the HMC structure activated also their fluorescence, playing a role on monitoring the process of drug delivering. In summary, as previously discussed, several mesoporous nanocarriers have been explored during the last 10 years for the design and development of novel anti-cancer drug delivering systems. Among them, mesoporous silica nanocarriers are the most studied and explored, representing a very promising technology that may find, eventually, commercial use in pharmaceutical formulations. However, less studied mesoporous materials may also become prominent, and although not so intensively explored, they show promising properties that make them very attractive.

CONCLUDING REMARKS

There are still several challenges on the field of drug administration for cancer pharmacotherapy. During the last decades, parenteral drug administration has been the preferred choice although researchers from India recently reported that > 65% of anticancer drugs were available in oral dosage form for clinical use [13]. In Europe, as of September 2016, there were 72 licensed and commercially available oral oncolytics [29]. Availability of oral dosage forms, a reasonable use of injectable medications and the avoidance of parenteral routes when oral medication can be more appropriate have always been important components of the policies of rational use of medicines of the World Health Organization (WHO). It is well-known that oral medications maximize treatment adherence, patient compliance and safety. In addition, injections may be associated with higher costs, risk of infections, physiological and psychological pain during injection, and difficulty of titrating overdoses among other risks. Therefore, safer, cost effective and simple *oral* alternatives should be promoted. Moreover, availability of liquid and flexible solid oral dosage forms like dispersible tablets, effervescent tablets, chewable tablets, orodispersible tablets and sprinkle capsules, is important in treating pediatric cancer.

Many of those obstacles for oral administration, as well as others (limited bioavailability, low stability, and limited permeability across biological barriers, immune surveillance and target specificity), may be solved by using these novel mesoporous nanomaterials. They are excellent choices for targeted drug delivery as they could be used for the direct delivery of drugs in the organism for cancer therapy, vaccination, gene therapy or for the treatment of neurodegenerative diseases. In addition, the exploration of alternative administration routes such as intranasal drug delivery or transdermal application of drugs will expand the therapeutic choices for the treatment of different diseases. The use of multifunctional mesoporous materials with unique magnetic, optical, thermal or mechanical properties, open the chances for the design of second and third generation DDSs capable of not only carrying and delivering drugs, but also to help with imaging and diagnostics, with tunable drug release activation. The promises of nanotechnology in biomedicine are expected to be huge, not only due to the inherent health benefits, but also by the economic impacts [201]. However, the large-scale production of safe, biocompatible and economical nanomaterials suitable for pharmaceutical use is still a limitation that needs to be solved in order to have real commercial and clinical applications. A clear understanding of the interactions between nanomaterials and living organisms is necessary to the success of such applications. This comprehensive understanding is critical, particularly with respect to potential toxicological effects. The complex and diverse chemical or physical interactions among NCs and the physiological media components (proteins, sugars, ions) may change their stability, affecting their drug delivery/release kinetics. That may have a big impact on the pharmacokinetics, toxicity, biodistribution and effective internalization of the nanocarriers into the cells and tissues [202 - 204]. Surface modification of the nanocarriers may be an alternative to increase stability, solubility or biocompatibility. However, degradation of the surfactant agents may generate toxic derivatives that may negatively affect the organism. Formation of a protein corona on the nanocarrier surface that may affect its physical and chemical properties, affecting also their bioavailability, toxicity or reactivity [202, 205]. The potential toxicity of nanomaterials (nanotoxicity) is an active research field, although there is no consensus on the safety or toxicity of several nanomaterials, it is probable that their unique physical properties may produce several risks [202, 206, 207]. More research on the potential toxicity associated to nanomaterials used for pharmaceutical applications is required in order to understand their risks and potential impact [208].

There are still several questions to be answered in order to understand not only the toxicological effects of nanoformulations in living organisms but also the environmental effects of them, and the opportunities for regulatory approval and commercialization. The challenges that nanocarriers should resolve are diverse: stabilization of sensitive drugs and biomolecules, ability to cross through physiological barriers, transport to specific targets, reducing toxicity and increasing the therapeutic performance, among several others. Many of them can be addressed, partially or completely, using the different types of nanocarriers previously discussed. The potential use of mesoporous nanomaterials for pharmaceutical formulations is in the rise, and it may impact the development of a more personalized medicine, with important benefits for the patients and physicians, which currently may still be beyond our imagination.

ABBREVIATIONS

AMF	Alternating Magnetic Field
APTES	(3-Aminopropyl)triethoxysilane
AuNR	Gold nanorods
AuNBs	Gold nanobipyramids

BCS	Biopharmaceutics Classification System
BDDCS	Biopharmaceutics Drug Disposition Classification System
BMOD	Bis(2-methacryloyl)oxyethyl disulfide
BN	Boron nitride
BNN6 N	N'-di-sec-butyl-N,N'-dinitroso-1,4-phenylenediamine
CS-PMMA	Chitosan-poly(methacrylic acid)
Cys	L-cysteine
DDS	Drug delivery system
DES	Desipramine
DOX	Doxorubicin
DTPA	Diethylenetriaminepentaacetic acid
ECL	Electrochemiluminiscence
EPR	Enhanced Permeability and Retention
FA	Folic acid
FSHR-mAB	Follicle stimulating hormone receptor monoclonal antibody
FTIC	Fluorescein isothiocyanate
GO	Graphene Oxide
GTH	Glutathione
HA	Hyaluronic acic
HAP	Hydroxyapatite
HAS	Human serum albuminum
HMC	Hollow Mesoporous Carbon
HMMs	Hollow mesoporous microspheres
HMS	Hollow mesoporous silica
LDH	Layered double hydroxide
MCNs	Mesoporous carbon nanocarriers
MHNs	Mesoporous Hydroxyapatite Nanoparticles
MMNs	Mesoporous Magnetic Nanocarriers
MMP-2	Matrix metalloprotease-2
MNPs	Magnetic nanoparticles
MRI	Magnetic resonance imaging
MSNs	Mesoporous Silica Nanocarriers
MSVs	Multistage nanovectors
MTX	Methotrexate
MWCNTs	Multi-walled carbon nanotubes

NAG	N-acetyl glucosamine
NCs	Nano carriers
NIPAAm	N-isopropylacrylamide monomer
NIR	Near Infrared
NPs	Nanoparticles
PAA	Poly(acrylic acid) homopolymer
PAsA	Polyaspartic acid
PMMA	Poly(methacrylic acid)
pBN	Porous Boron Nitride
PEG	Polyethyleneglycol
PFH	Perfluorohexane
PLGA	Poly(lactic-co-glycolic acid)
PMAm	Poly(methyl acrylate) monomer
pMFs	Polymeric microfibers
pNFs	Polymeric nanofibers
pNCps	Polymeric nanocapsules
pNSs	Polymeric nanospheres
PNP	Polymer Nanoparticles
PTX	Paclitaxel
QDs	Quantum Dots
SEDDS	Self-emulsifying drug delivery systems
SWCNTs	Single-walled carbon nanotubes
TAMRA	5(6)-carboxytetramethylrhodamine hydrochloride
WMS	Wrinkled Mesoporous Silica

CONSENT FOR PUBLICATION

Not applicable.

CONFLICT OF INTEREST

The authors declare no conflict of interest, financial or otherwise.

ACKNOWLEDGEMENT

JFG is thankful to UDLAP for a Ph.D. Scholarship.

REFERENCES

[1] Siegel RL, Miller KD, Jemal A. Cancer statistics, 2018. CA Cancer J Clin 2018; 68(1): 7-30.
[http://dx.doi.org/10.3322/caac.21442] [PMID: 29313949]

[2] World Health Organization. Cancer Fact Sheets 2018 Feb 1; Available from: http://www.who.int/news-room/fact-sheets/detail/cancer

[3] Allemani C, Matsuda T, Di Carlo V, *et al.* Global surveillance of trends in cancer survival 2000-14 (CONCORD-3): analysis of individual records for 37 513 025 patients diagnosed with one of 18 cancers from 322 population-based registries in 71 countries. Lancet 2018; 391(10125): 1023-75.
[http://dx.doi.org/10.1016/S0140-6736(17)33326-3] [PMID: 29395269]

[4] Center for Drug Evaluation and Research. Advancing Health Through Innovation 2017 New Drug Therapy Approvals Silver Spring, MD: Food and Drug Administration 2018. Available from: https://www.fda.gov/downloads/AboutFDA/CentersOffices/OfficeofMedicalProductsandTobacco/CDER/ReportsBudgets/UCM591976.pdf

[5] Aitken M, Kleinrock M. Global Medicines Use in 2020 Outlook and Implications. Parsippany, NJ: IMS Institute for Healthcare Informatics 2015.

[6] Cancer.gov. A to Z list of cancer drugs National Cancer Institute June 5 2018. Available from: https://www.cancer.gov/about-cancer/treatment/drugs#V

[7] WHO Collaborating Centre for Drug Statistics Methodology, ATC classification index with DDDs, 2018. Oslo, Norway 2017. Available from: https://www.whocc.no/atc_ddd_index

[8] Ventola CL. Cancer Immunotherapy, Part 1: Current Strategies and Agents. P&T 2017; 42(6): 375-83.
[PMID: 28579724]

[9] Galluzzi L, Vacchelli E, Bravo-San Pedro JM, *et al.* Classification of current anticancer immunotherapies. Oncotarget 2014; 5(24): 12472-508.
[http://dx.doi.org/10.18632/oncotarget.2998] [PMID: 25537519]

[10] Cancer.gov. Targeted Cancer Therapies National Cancer Institute June 25 2018. Available from: https://www.cancer.gov/about-cancer/treatment/types/targeted-therapies/targeted-therapies-fact-sheet

[11] Drugs.com [Internet]. c1996-2018 [Updated: 1 June 2018, Cited: 19 July 2018] Available from: https://www.drugs.com/

[12] Cancer.org [Internet]. c4018 [Updated: 3 May 2016, Cited: 19 July 2018] 2018. Available from: https://www.cancer.org/

[13] Thanki K, Gangwal RP, Sangamwar AT, Jain S. Oral delivery of anticancer drugs: challenges and opportunities. J Control Release 2013; 170(1): 15-40.
[http://dx.doi.org/10.1016/j.jconrel.2013.04.020] [PMID: 23648832]

[14] Meng W, Garnett MC, Walker DA, Parker TL. Penetration and intracellular uptake of poly(glycerol-adipate) nanoparticles into three-dimensional brain tumour cell culture models. Exp Biol Med (Maywood) 2016; 241(5): 466-77.
[http://dx.doi.org/10.1177/1535370215610441] [PMID: 26568330]

[15] Garnett MC. Targeted drug conjugates: principles and progress. Adv Drug Deliv Rev 2001; 53(2): 171-216.
[http://dx.doi.org/10.1016/S0169-409X(01)00227-7] [PMID: 11731026]

[16] Nakamura Y, Mochida A, Choyke PL, Kobayashi H. Nanodrug delivery: Is the enhanced permeability and retention effect sufficient for curing cancer? Bioconjug Chem 2016; 27(10): 2225-38.
[http://dx.doi.org/10.1021/acs.bioconjchem.6b00437] [PMID: 27547843]

[17] Senapati S, Mahanta AK, Kumar S, Maiti P. Controlled drug delivery vehicles for cancer treatment and their performance. Signal Transduct Target Ther 2018; 3: 7.
[http://dx.doi.org/10.1038/s41392-017-0004-3] [PMID: 29560283]

[18] Mehra NK, Jain K, Jain NK. Multifunctional carbon nanotubes in cancer therapy and imaging.Nanobiomaterials in Medical Imaging. Norwich, NY: William Andrew Publishing,Elsevier 2016; pp. 421-53.
[http://dx.doi.org/10.1016/B978-0-323-41736-5.00014-5]

[19] Handbook on Injectable Drugs. Selected Revisions. 2018. © Copyright, 2018. American Society of Health-System Pharmacists, Inc., 4500 East-West Highway, Suite 900, Bethesda, Maryland 20814. MedicinesComplete © 2018 Royal Pharmaceutical Society.

[20] Thorn CF, Oshiro C, Marsh S, et al. Doxorubicin pathways: pharmacodynamics and adverse effects. Pharmacogenet Genomics 2011; 21(7): 440-6.
[http://dx.doi.org/10.1097/FPC.0b013e32833ffb56] [PMID: 21048526]

[21] Javanbakht S, Namazi H. Doxorubicin loaded carboxymethyl cellulose/graphene quantum dot nanocomposite hydrogel films as a potential anticancer drug delivery system. Mater Sci Eng C 2018; 87: 50-9.
[http://dx.doi.org/10.1016/j.msec.2018.02.010] [PMID: 29549949]

[22] Singh P, Choudhury S, Kulanthaivel S, et al. Photo-triggered destabilization of nanoscopic vehicles by dihydroindolizine for enhanced anticancer drug delivery in cervical carcinoma. Colloids Surf B Biointerfaces 2018; 162: 202-11.
[http://dx.doi.org/10.1016/j.colsurfb.2017.11.035] [PMID: 29195229]

[23] Perez-Quinones J, Jokinen J, Keinänen S, Peniche-Covas C, Brüggemann O, Ossipov D. Self-assembled hyaluronic acid-testosterone nanocarriers for delivery of anticancer drugs. Eur Polym J 2018; 99: 384-93.
[http://dx.doi.org/10.1016/j.eurpolymj.2017.12.043]

[24] Mou J, Wu Y, Bi M, Qi X, Yang J. Polyanionic holothurian glycosaminoglycans-doxorubicin nanocomplex as a delivery system for anticancer drugs. Colloids Surf B Biointerfaces 2018; 167: 364-9.
[http://dx.doi.org/10.1016/j.colsurfb.2018.04.032] [PMID: 29698785]

[25] Bajwa N, Kumar Mehra N, Jain K, Kumar Jain N. Targeted anticancer drug delivery through anthracycline antibiotic bearing functionalized quantum dots. Artif Cells Nanomed Biotechnol 2016; 44(7): 1774-82.
[http://dx.doi.org/10.3109/21691401.2015.1102740] [PMID: 26508412]

[26] Xu J, Qin B, Luan S, et al. Acid-labile poly(ethylene glycol) shell of hydrazone-containing biodegradable polymeric micelles facilitating anticancer drug delivery. J Bioact Compat Polym 2018; 33(2): 119-33.
[http://dx.doi.org/10.1177/0883911517715658]

[27] Bardajee GR, Hooshyar Z. A novel thermosensitive nanogel composing of poly(N-isopropylacrylamide) grafted onto alginate-modified graphene oxide for hydrophilic anticancer drug delivery. J Iran Chem Soc 2018; 15(1): 121-9.
[http://dx.doi.org/10.1007/s13738-017-1215-9]

[28] Hortelao AC, Patiño T, Perez-Jiménez A, Blanco A, Sánchez S. Enzyme-powered nanobots enhance anticancer drug delivery. Adv Funct Mater 2018; 28(25): 1705086.
[http://dx.doi.org/10.1002/adfm.201705086]

[29] Sawicki E, Schellens JH, Beijnen JH, Nuijen B. Inventory of oral anticancer agents: Pharmaceutical formulation aspects with focus on the solid dispersion technique. Cancer Treat Rev 2016; 50: 247-63.
[http://dx.doi.org/10.1016/j.ctrv.2016.09.012] [PMID: 27776286]

[30] WHO Drug Information. A framework for risk-based identification of essential medicine products for local manufacturing in low- and middle-income countries. WHO Drug Inf 2016; 30(1): 7-12.

[31] Wu CY, Benet LZ. Predicting drug disposition *via* application of BCS: transport/absorption/ elimination interplay and development of a biopharmaceutics drug disposition classification system.

Pharm Res 2005; 22(1): 11-23.
[http://dx.doi.org/10.1007/s11095-004-9004-4] [PMID: 15771225]

[32] Shugarts S, Benet LZ. The role of transporters in the pharmacokinetics of orally administered drugs. Pharm Res 2009; 26(9): 2039-54.
[http://dx.doi.org/10.1007/s11095-009-9924-0] [PMID: 19568696]

[33] Chavda HV, Patel CN, Anand IS. Biopharmaceutics classification system. Sys Rev Pharm 2010; 1(1): 62-9.
[http://dx.doi.org/10.4103/0975-8453.59514]

[34] Sachan NK, Bhattacharya A, Pushkar S, Mishra A. Biopharmaceutical classification system: A strategic tool for oral drug delivery technology. Asian J Pharm 2009; 3(2): 76-81.
[http://dx.doi.org/10.4103/0973-8398.55042]

[35] Mokhtarzadeh A, Tabarzad M, Ranjbari J, de la Guardia M, Hejazi M, Ramezani M. Aptamers as Smart ligands for nano-carriers targeting. TRAC-Trend Anal Chem 2016; 82: 316-27.
[http://dx.doi.org/10.1016/j.trac.2016.06.018]

[36] Sufi SA, Pajaniradje S, Mukherjee V, Rajagopalan R. Redox nano-architectures: perspectives and implications in diagnosis and treatment of human diseases. Antioxid Redox Signal in press
[PMID: 29334759]

[37] Sun R, Wang W, Wen Y, Zhang X. Recent advances on mesoporous silica nanoparticles-based controlled release system: intelligent switches open up new horizon. Nanomaterials (Basel) 2015; 5(4): 2019-53.
[http://dx.doi.org/10.3390/nano5042019] [PMID: 28347110]

[38] Chouikrat R, Seve A, Vanderesse R, *et al.* Non polymeric nanoparticles for photodynamic therapy applications: recent developments. Curr Med Chem 2012; 19(6): 781-92.
[http://dx.doi.org/10.2174/092986712799034897] [PMID: 22214454]

[39] Chen J, Gao C, Zhang Y, *et al.* Inorganic nano-targeted drugs delivery system and its application of platinum-based anticancer drugs. J Nanosci Nanotechnol 2017; 17(1): 1-17.
[http://dx.doi.org/10.1166/jnn.2017.12932] [PMID: 29616785]

[40] Seiden MV, Muggia F, Astrow A, *et al.* A phase II study of liposomal lurtotecan (OSI-211) in patients with topotecan resistant ovarian cancer. Gynecol Oncol 2004; 93(1): 229-32.
[http://dx.doi.org/10.1016/j.ygyno.2003.12.037] [PMID: 15047241]

[41] Chiang N-J, Chao T-Y, Hsieh R-K, *et al.* A phase I dose-escalation study of PEP02 (irinotecan liposome injection) in combination with 5-fluorouracil and leucovorin in advanced solid tumors. BMC Cancer 2016; 16(1): 907.
[http://dx.doi.org/10.1186/s12885-016-2933-6] [PMID: 27871319]

[42] Nel A, Xia T, Mädler L, Li N. Toxic potential of materials at the nanolevel. Science 2006; 311(5761): 622-7.
[http://dx.doi.org/10.1126/science.1114397] [PMID: 16456071]

[43] De Jong WH, Borm PJA. Drug delivery and nanoparticles:applications and hazards. Int J Nanomedicine 2008; 3(2): 133-49.
[http://dx.doi.org/10.2147/IJN.S596] [PMID: 18686775]

[44] Liu T, Wang C, Gu X, *et al.* Drug delivery with PEGylated MoS_2 nano-sheets for combined photothermal and chemotherapy of cancer. Adv Mater 2014; 26(21): 3433-40.
[http://dx.doi.org/10.1002/adma.201305256] [PMID: 24677423]

[45] Shi J, Liu Y, Wang L, *et al.* A tumoral acidic pH-responsive drug delivery system based on a novel photosensitizer (fullerene) for *in vitro* and *in vivo* chemo-photodynamic therapy. Acta Biomater 2014; 10(3): 1280-91.
[http://dx.doi.org/10.1016/j.actbio.2013.10.037] [PMID: 24211343]

[46] Szabo P, Zelko R. Formulation and stability aspects of nanosized solid drug delivery systems. Curr

Pharm Des 2015; 21(22): 3148-57.
[http://dx.doi.org/10.2174/1381612821666150531164905] [PMID: 26027571]

[47] Jeong K, Kang CS, Kim Y, Lee YD, Kwon IC, Kim S. Development of highly efficient nanocarrier-mediated delivery approaches for cancer therapy. Cancer Lett 2016; 374(1): 31-43.
[http://dx.doi.org/10.1016/j.canlet.2016.01.050] [PMID: 26854717]

[48] Peer D, Karp JM, Hong S, Farokhzad OC, Margalit R, Langer R. Nanocarriers as an emerging platform for cancer therapy. Nat Nanotechnol 2007; 2(12): 751-60.
[http://dx.doi.org/10.1038/nnano.2007.387] [PMID: 18654426]

[49] Lee D-E, Koo H, Sun I-C, Ryu JH, Kim K, Kwon IC. Multifunctional nanoparticles for multimodal imaging and theragnosis. Chem Soc Rev 2012; 41(7): 2656-72.
[http://dx.doi.org/10.1039/C2CS15261D] [PMID: 22189429]

[50] Debele TA, Peng S, Tsai HC. Drug carrier for photodynamic cancer therapy. Int J Mol Sci 2015; 16(9): 22094-136.
[http://dx.doi.org/10.3390/ijms160922094] [PMID: 26389879]

[51] Shete HK, Vyas SS, Patravale VB, Disouza JI. Pulmonary multifunctional nano-oncological modules for lung cancer treatment and prevention. J Biomed Nanotechnol 2014; 10(9): 1863-93.
[http://dx.doi.org/10.1166/jbn.2014.1900] [PMID: 25992444]

[52] Hamidi M, Azadi A, Rafiei P. Hydrogel nanoparticles in drug delivery. Adv Drug Deliv Rev 2008; 60(15): 1638-49.
[http://dx.doi.org/10.1016/j.addr.2008.08.002] [PMID: 18840488]

[53] Hoare TR, Kohane DS. Hydrogels in drug delivery: Progress and challenges. Polymer (Guildf) 2008; 49: 1993-2007.
[http://dx.doi.org/10.1016/j.polymer.2008.01.027]

[54] Torchilin VP. Micellar nanocarriers: pharmaceutical perspectives. Pharm Res 2007; 24(1): 1-16.
[http://dx.doi.org/10.1007/s11095-006-9132-0] [PMID: 17109211]

[55] Yu Y, Zhang X, Qiu L. The anti-tumor efficacy of curcumin when delivered by size/charge-changing multistage polymeric micelles based on amphiphilic poly(β-amino ester) derivates. Biomaterials 2014; 35(10): 3467-79.
[http://dx.doi.org/10.1016/j.biomaterials.2013.12.096] [PMID: 24439418]

[56] Pérez-Herrero E, Fernández-Medarde A. Advanced targeted therapies in cancer: Drug nanocarriers, the future of chemotherapy. Eur J Pharm Biopharm 2015; 93: 52-79.
[http://dx.doi.org/10.1016/j.ejpb.2015.03.018] [PMID: 25813885]

[57] Hasnain MS, Nayak AK. Chitosan as responsive polymer for drug delivery applications Stimuli Responsive Polymeric Nanocarriers for Drug Delivery Applications. Elsevier 2018; Vol. 1: pp. 581-605.
[http://dx.doi.org/10.1016/B978-0-08-101997-9.00025-4]

[58] Elzoghby AO, Samy WM, Elgindy NA. Albumin-based nanoparticles as potential controlled release drug delivery systems. J Control Release 2012; 157(2): 168-82.
[http://dx.doi.org/10.1016/j.jconrel.2011.07.031] [PMID: 21839127]

[59] Choi KY, Chung H, Min KH, et al. Self-assembled hyaluronic acid nanoparticles for active tumor targeting. Biomaterials 2010; 31(1): 106-14.
[http://dx.doi.org/10.1016/j.biomaterials.2009.09.030] [PMID: 19783037]

[60] Panyam J, Labhasetwar V. Biodegradable nanoparticles for drug and gene delivery to cells and tissue. Adv Drug Deliv Rev 2003; 55(3): 329-47.
[http://dx.doi.org/10.1016/S0169-409X(02)00228-4] [PMID: 12628320]

[61] Bugaj AM. Targeted photodynamic therapy--a promising strategy of tumor treatment. Photochem Photobiol Sci 2011; 10(7): 1097-109.
[http://dx.doi.org/10.1039/c0pp00147c] [PMID: 21547329]

[62] Liechty WB, Kryscio DR, Slaughter BV, Peppas NA. Polymers for drug delivery systems. Annu Rev Chem Biomol Eng 2010; 1: 149-73.
[http://dx.doi.org/10.1146/annurev-chembioeng-073009-100847] [PMID: 22432577]

[63] Reis AV, Moia TA, Sitta DLA, *et al.* Sustained release of potassium diclofenac from a pH-responsive hydrogel based on gum arabic conjugates into simulated intestinal fluid. J Appl Polym Sci 2016; 133: 43319.
[http://dx.doi.org/10.1002/app.43319]

[64] Mével M, Sainlos M, Chatin B, *et al.* Paromomycin and neomycin B derived cationic lipids: synthesis and transfection studies. J Control Release 2012; 158(3): 461-9.
[http://dx.doi.org/10.1016/j.jconrel.2011.12.019] [PMID: 22226775]

[65] Derycke ASL, de Witte PAM. Liposomes for photodynamic therapy. Adv Drug Deliv Rev 2004; 56(1): 17-30.
[http://dx.doi.org/10.1016/j.addr.2003.07.014] [PMID: 14706443]

[66] Caraglia M, De Rosa G, Salzano G, *et al.* Nanotech revolution for the anti-cancer drug delivery through blood-brain barrier. Curr Cancer Drug Targets 2012; 12(3): 186-96.
[http://dx.doi.org/10.2174/156800912799277421] [PMID: 22268384]

[67] Marra M, Salzano G, Leonetti C, *et al.* New self-assembly nanoparticles and stealth liposomes for the delivery of zoledronic acid: a comparative study. Biotechnol Adv 2012; 30(1): 302-9.
[http://dx.doi.org/10.1016/j.biotechadv.2011.06.018] [PMID: 21741464]

[68] Porru M, Zappavigna S, Salzano G, *et al.* Medical treatment of orthotopic glioblastoma with transferrin-conjugated nanoparticles encapsulating zoledronic acid. Oncotarget 2014; 5(21): 10446-59.
[http://dx.doi.org/10.18632/oncotarget.2182] [PMID: 25431953]

[69] Kesharwani P, Jain K, Jain NK. Dendrimer as nanocarrier for drug delivery. Prog Polym Sci 2014; 39: 268-307.
[http://dx.doi.org/10.1016/j.progpolymsci.2013.07.005]

[70] Madaan K, Kumar S, Poonia N, Lather V, Pandita D. Dendrimers in drug delivery and targeting: Drug-dendrimer interactions and toxicity issues. J Pharm Bioallied Sci 2014; 6(3): 139-50.
[http://dx.doi.org/10.4103/0975-7406.130965] [PMID: 25035633]

[71] Tomalia DA. Birth of a new macromolecular architecture: dendrimers as quantized building blocks for nanoscale synthetic polymer chemistry. Prog Polym Sci 2005; 30: 294-324.
[http://dx.doi.org/10.1016/j.progpolymsci.2005.01.007]

[72] Zhao M-X, Zhu B-J. The research and applications of quantum dots as nano-carriers for targeted drug delivery and cancer therapy. Nanoscale Res Lett 2016; 11(1): 207.
[http://dx.doi.org/10.1186/s11671-016-1394-9] [PMID: 27090658]

[73] Ahmad MZ, Akhter S, Jain GK, *et al.* Metallic nanoparticles: technology overview & drug delivery applications in oncology. Expert Opin Drug Deliv 2010; 7(8): 927-42.
[http://dx.doi.org/10.1517/17425247.2010.498473] [PMID: 20645671]

[74] Xu ZP, Zeng QH, Lu GQ, Yu AB. Inorganic nanoparticles as carriers for efficient cellular delivery. Chem Eng Sci 2006; 61: 1027-40.
[http://dx.doi.org/10.1016/j.ces.2005.06.019]

[75] Faraji AH, Wipf P. Nanoparticles in cellular drug delivery. Bioorg Med Chem 2009; 17(8): 2950-62.
[http://dx.doi.org/10.1016/j.bmc.2009.02.043] [PMID: 19299149]

[76] Ma X, Feng HH, Liang CY, Liu XJ, Zeng FY, Wang Y. Mesoporous silica as micro/nano carrier: from passive to active cargo delivery, a mini review. J Mater Sci Technol 2017; 33: 1067-74.
[http://dx.doi.org/10.1016/j.jmst.2017.06.007]

[77] Rahoui N, Jiang B, Taloub N, Huang YD. Spatio-temporal control strategy of drug delivery systems based nano structures. J Control Release 2017; 255: 176-201.

[http://dx.doi.org/10.1016/j.jconrel.2017.04.003] [PMID: 28408201]

[78] Du X, Li X, Xiong L, Zhang X, Kleitz F, Qiao SZ. Mesoporous silica nanoparticles with organo-bridged silsesquioxane framework as innovative platforms for bioimaging and therapeutic agent delivery. Biomaterials 2016; 91: 90-127.
[http://dx.doi.org/10.1016/j.biomaterials.2016.03.019] [PMID: 27017579]

[79] Prabhakar U, Maeda H, Jain RK, et al. Challenges and key considerations of the enhanced permeability and retention effect for nanomedicine drug delivery in oncology. Cancer Res 2013; 73(8): 2412-7.
[http://dx.doi.org/10.1158/0008-5472.CAN-12-4561] [PMID: 23423979]

[80] Vangara KK, Liu JL, Palakurthi S. Hyaluronic acid-decorated PLGA-PEG nanoparticles for targeted delivery of SN-38 to ovarian cancer. Anticancer Res 2013; 33(6): 2425-34.
[PMID: 23749891]

[81] Liao WC, Willner I. Synthesis and applications of stimuli-responsive DNA-based nano- and micro-sized capsules. Adv Funct Mater 2017; 41: 1702732.
[http://dx.doi.org/10.1002/adfm.201702732]

[82] Liang H, Li X, Chen B, et al. A collagen-binding EGFR single-chain Fv antibody fragment for the targeted cancer therapy. J Control Release 2015; 209: 101-9.
[http://dx.doi.org/10.1016/j.jconrel.2015.04.029] [PMID: 25916496]

[83] Choi CHJ, Alabi CA, Webster P, Davis ME. Mechanism of active targeting in solid tumors with transferrin-containing gold nanoparticles. Proc Natl Acad Sci USA 2010; 107(3): 1235-40.
[http://dx.doi.org/10.1073/pnas.0914140107] [PMID: 20080552]

[84] Yang XY, Li YX, Li M, Zhang L, Feng LX, Zhang N. Hyaluronic acid-coated nanostructured lipid carriers for targeting paclitaxel to cancer. Cancer Lett 2013; 334(2): 338-45.
[http://dx.doi.org/10.1016/j.canlet.2012.07.002] [PMID: 22776563]

[85] Shen SC, Ng WK, Chia LSO, Dong YC, Tan RBH. Applications of mesoporous materials as excipients for innovative drug delivery and formulation. Curr Pharm Des 2013; 19(35): 6270-89.
[http://dx.doi.org/10.2174/13816128113199350005] [PMID: 23470004]

[86] Yang K, Feng L, Liu Z. Stimuli responsive drug delivery systems based on nano-graphene for cancer therapy. Adv Drug Deliv Rev 2016; 105(Pt B): 228-41.
[http://dx.doi.org/10.1016/j.addr.2016.05.015] [PMID: 27233212]

[87] Knežević NZ, Kaluđerović GN. Silicon-based nanotheranostics. Nanoscale 2017; 9(35): 12821-9.
[http://dx.doi.org/10.1039/C7NR04445C] [PMID: 28853473]

[88] Chen PP, Shi BB. Supramolecular drug delivery systems based on macrocyclic hosts. Huaxue Jinzhan 2017; 29: 720-39.

[89] Porcu EP, Salis A, Gavini E, Rassu G, Maestri M, Giunchedi P. Indocyanine green delivery systems for tumour detection and treatments. Biotechnol Adv 2016; 34(5): 768-89.
[http://dx.doi.org/10.1016/j.biotechadv.2016.04.001] [PMID: 27090752]

[90] Hou XY, Jiang G, Yang CS, Tang JQ, Wei ZP, Liu YQ. Application of nanotechnology in the diagnosis and therapy of hepatocellular carcinoma. Recent Patents Anticancer Drug Discov 2016; 11(3): 322-31.
[http://dx.doi.org/10.2174/1574892811666160309121035] [PMID: 26955964]

[91] Jordan C, Shuvaev VV, Bailey M, Muzykantov VR, Dziubla TD. The role of carrier geometry in overcoming biological barriers to drug delivery. Curr Pharm Des 2016; 22(9): 1259-73.
[http://dx.doi.org/10.2174/1381612822666151216151856] [PMID: 26675218]

[92] Yang K, Feng L, Liu Z. The advancing uses of nano-graphene in drug delivery. Expert Opin Drug Deliv 2015; 12(4): 601-12.
[http://dx.doi.org/10.1517/17425247.2015.978760] [PMID: 25466364]

[93] Hao XH, Zhang CM, Liu XL, Liang XJ, Jia G, Zhang JC. Recent advances of mesoporous silica based multifunctional nano drug delivery systems. Prog Biochem Biophys 2013; 40: 1014-22.

[94] Shi JL, Chen Y, Chen HR. Progress on the multifunctional mesoporous silica-based nanotheranostics. J Inorg Mater 2013; 28: 1-11.
[http://dx.doi.org/10.3724/SP.J.1077.2012.12082]

[95] Tang F, Li L, Chen D. Mesoporous silica nanoparticles: synthesis, biocompatibility and drug delivery. Adv Mater 2012; 24(12): 1504-34.
[http://dx.doi.org/10.1002/adma.201104763] [PMID: 22378538]

[96] Zhang K, Xu ZP, Lu J, et al. Potential for layered double hydroxides-based, innovative drug delivery systems. Int J Mol Sci 2014; 15(5): 7409-28.
[http://dx.doi.org/10.3390/ijms15057409] [PMID: 24786098]

[97] Othman AL, Review ZA. Fundamental aspects of silicate mesoporous materials. Materials (Basel) 2012; 5: 2874-902.
[http://dx.doi.org/10.3390/ma5122874]

[98] Sing KSW. Reporting physisorption data for gas/solid systems with special reference to the determination of surface area and porosity (Recommendations 1984). Pure Appl Chem 1985; 57: 603-19.
[http://dx.doi.org/10.1351/pac198557040603]

[99] Broekhoff JCP. Mesopore determination from nitrogen sorption isotherms: Fundamentals, scope, limitations. Studies in surface science and catalysis 1979; 3: 663-84.

[100] Lowell S, Shields JE, Thomas MA, Thommes M. Characterization of Porous Solids and Powders: Surface Area, Pore Size and Density. Dordrecht: Springer Netherlands 2004; Vol. 16.
[http://dx.doi.org/10.1007/978-1-4020-2303-3]

[101] Zhao XS, Lu GQ. (Max), Millar GJ. Advances in mesoporous molecular sieve MCM-41. Ind Eng Chem Res 1996; 35: 2075-90.
[http://dx.doi.org/10.1021/ie950702a]

[102] Suib SL. A review of recent developments of mesoporous materials. Chem Rec 2017; 17(12): 1169-83.
[http://dx.doi.org/10.1002/tcr.201700025] [PMID: 28661074]

[103] Tang S, Huang X, Chen X, Zheng N. Hollow mesoporous zirconia nanocapsules for drug delivery. Adv Funct Mater 2010; 20: 2442-7.
[http://dx.doi.org/10.1002/adfm.201000647]

[104] Jiang H, Wang T, Wang L, Sun C, Jiang T, Cheng G, et al. Development of an amorphous mesoporous TiO_2 nanosphere as a novel carrier for poorly water-soluble drugs: Effect of different crystal forms of TiO_2 carriers on drug loading and release behaviors. Microporous Mesoporous Mater 2012; 153: 124-30.
[http://dx.doi.org/10.1016/j.micromeso.2011.12.013]

[105] Zhao P, Wang L, Sun C, et al. Uniform mesoporous carbon as a carrier for poorly water soluble drug and its cytotoxicity study. Eur J Pharm Biopharm 2012; 80(3): 535-43.
[http://dx.doi.org/10.1016/j.ejpb.2011.12.002] [PMID: 22193360]

[106] AlOthman ZA, Apblett AW. Synthesis and characterization of a hexagonal mesoporous silica with enhanced thermal and hydrothermal stabilities. Appl Surf Sci 2010; 256: 3573-80.
[http://dx.doi.org/10.1016/j.apsusc.2009.12.157]

[107] Flanigen EM, Patton RL, Wilson ST. Structural, synthetic and physicochemical concepts in aluminophosphate-based molecular sieves. Studies in surface science and catalysis 1988; 37: 13-27.

[108] Sayari A. Periodic mesoporous materials: synthesis, characterization and potential applications. Studies in Surface Science and Catalysis 1996; 102: 1-46.

[http://dx.doi.org/10.1016/S0167-2991(06)81398-4]

[109] Lin H-P, Mou C-Y. Structural and morphological control of cationic surfactant-templated mesoporous silica. Acc Chem Res 2002; 35(11): 927-35.
[http://dx.doi.org/10.1021/ar000074f] [PMID: 12437317]

[110] Anderson MT, Martin JE, Odinek JG, Newcomer PP. Surfactant-templated silica mesophases formed in water: Cosolvent mixtures. Chem Mater 1998; 10: 311-21.
[http://dx.doi.org/10.1021/cm9704600]

[111] Huh S, Wiench JW, Yoo J-C, Pruski M, Lin VS-Y. Organic functionalization and morphology control of mesoporous silicas *via* a co-condensation synthesis method. Chem Mater 2003; 15: 4247-56.
[http://dx.doi.org/10.1021/cm0210041]

[112] Huh S, Wiench JW, Trewyn BG, Song S, Pruski M, Lin VS-Y. Tuning of particle morphology and pore properties in mesoporous silicas with multiple organic functional groups. Chem Commun (Camb) 2003; (18): 2364-5.
[http://dx.doi.org/10.1039/b306255d] [PMID: 14518916]

[113] Karimi F, Shojaei AF, Tabatabaeian K, Karimi-Maleh H, Shakeri S. HAS loaded with CoFe2O4/MNPs as a high-efficienty carrier for epirubicin anticancer drug delivery. IET Nanobiotechnol 2018; 12: 336-42.
[http://dx.doi.org/10.1049/iet-nbt.2017.0057]

[114] Slowing II, Vivero-Escoto JL, Wu CW, Lin VS. Mesoporous silica nanoparticles as controlled release drug delivery and gene transfection carriers. Adv Drug Deliv Rev 2008; 60(11): 1278-88.
[http://dx.doi.org/10.1016/j.addr.2008.03.012] [PMID: 18514969]

[115] Bharti C, Nagaich U, Pal AK, Gulati N. Mesoporous silica nanoparticles in target drug delivery system: A review. Int J Pharm Investig 2015; 5(3): 124-33.
[http://dx.doi.org/10.4103/2230-973X.160844] [PMID: 26258053]

[116] Edeler D, Kaluđerović MR, Dojčinović B, Schmidt H, Kaluđerović GN. SBA-15 mesoporous silica particles loaded with cisplatin induce senescence in B16F10 cells. RSC Advances 2016; 6: 111031-40.
[http://dx.doi.org/10.1039/C6RA22596A]

[117] Ahn B, Park J, Singha K, Park H, Kim WJ. Mesoporous silica nanoparticle-based cisplatin prodrug delivery and anticancer effect under reductive cellular environment. J Mater Chem B Mater Biol Med 2013; 1: 2829.
[http://dx.doi.org/10.1039/c3tb20319k]

[118] Kwon S, Singh RK, Perez RA, Abou Neel EA, Kim H-W, Chrzanowski W. Silica-based mesoporous nanoparticles for controlled drug delivery. J Tissue Eng 2013; 4: 2041731413503357.
[http://dx.doi.org/10.1177/2041731413503357] [PMID: 24020012]

[119] Liong M, Lu J, Kovochich M, *et al.* Multifunctional inorganic nanoparticles for imaging, targeting, and drug delivery. ACS Nano 2008; 2(5): 889-96.
[http://dx.doi.org/10.1021/nn800072t] [PMID: 19206485]

[120] Lee S, Yun H-S, Kim S-H. The comparative effects of mesoporous silica nanoparticles and colloidal silica on inflammation and apoptosis. Biomaterials 2011; 32(35): 9434-43.
[http://dx.doi.org/10.1016/j.biomaterials.2011.08.042] [PMID: 21889200]

[121] Lin Y-S, Haynes CL. Impacts of mesoporous silica nanoparticle size, pore ordering, and pore integrity on hemolytic activity. J Am Chem Soc 2010; 132(13): 4834-42.
[http://dx.doi.org/10.1021/ja910846q] [PMID: 20230032]

[122] Pascal J, Ashley CE, Wang Z, *et al.* Mechanistic modeling identifies drug-uptake history as predictor of tumor drug resistance and nano-carrier-mediated response. ACS Nano 2013; 7(12): 11174-82.
[http://dx.doi.org/10.1021/nn4048974] [PMID: 24187963]

[123] He QJ, Shi JL. Mesoporous silica nanoparticles based nano drug delivery systems: synthesis, controlled drug release and delivery, pharmacokinetics and biocompatibility. J Mater Chem 2011; 21:

5845-55.
[http://dx.doi.org/10.1039/c0jm03851b]

[124] Nairi V, Medda S, Piludu M, *et al.* Interactions between bovine serum albumin and mesoporous silica nanoparticles functionalized with biopolymers. Chem Eng J 2018; 340: 42-50.
[http://dx.doi.org/10.1016/j.cej.2018.01.011]

[125] Martinez JO, Evangelopoulos M, Bhavane R, *et al.* Multistage nanovectors enhance the delivery of free and encapsulated drugs. Curr Drug Targets 2015; 16(14): 1582-90.
[http://dx.doi.org/10.2174/1389450115666141015113914] [PMID: 25316273]

[126] Wang ZG, Wu P, He ZL, *et al.* Mesoporous silica nanoparticles with lactose-mediated targeting effect to delivery platinum(IV) prodrug for liver cancer therapy. J Mater Chem B Mater Biol Med 2017; 5: 7591-7.
[http://dx.doi.org/10.1039/C7TB01704A]

[127] Kumar P, Tambe P, Paknikar KM, Gajbhiye V. Folate/N-acetyl glucosamine conjugated mesoporous silica nanoparticles for targeting breast cancer cells: A comparative study. Colloids Surf B Biointerfaces 2017; 156: 203-12.
[http://dx.doi.org/10.1016/j.colsurfb.2017.05.032] [PMID: 28531877]

[128] Qiu Y, Wu C, Jiang J, *et al.* Lipid-coated hollow mesoporous silica nanospheres for co-delivery of doxorubicin and paclitaxel: Preparation, sustained release, cellular uptake and pharmacokinetics. Mater Sci Eng C 2017; 71: 835-43.
[http://dx.doi.org/10.1016/j.msec.2016.10.081] [PMID: 27987779]

[129] Wang Y, Huang HY, Yang L, Zhang Z, Ji H. Cetuximab-modified mesoporous silica nano-medicine specifically targets EGFR-mutant lung cancer and overcomes drug resistance. Sci Rep 2016; 6: 25468.
[http://dx.doi.org/10.1038/srep25468] [PMID: 27151505]

[130] Wang A, Yang Y, Qi Y, *et al.* Fabrication of mesoporous silica nanoparticles with well-defined multicompartment structure as efficient drug carrier for cancer therapy *in vitro* and *in vivo*. ACS Appl Mater Interfaces 2016; 8(14): 8900-7.
[http://dx.doi.org/10.1021/acsami.5b12031] [PMID: 26998895]

[131] Rehman F, Ahmed K, Rahim A, *et al.* Organo-bridged silsesquioxane incorporated mesoporous silica as a carrier for the controlled delivery of ibuprofen and fluorouracil. J Mol Liq 2018; 258: 319-26.
[http://dx.doi.org/10.1016/j.molliq.2018.03.057]

[132] Munaweera I, Shi Y, Koneru B, *et al.* Nitric oxide- and cisplatin-releasing silica nanoparticles for use against non-small cell lung cancer. J Inorg Biochem 2015; 153: 23-31.
[http://dx.doi.org/10.1016/j.jinorgbio.2015.09.002] [PMID: 26402659]

[133] Munaweera I, Hong J, D'Souza A, Balkus KJ. Novel wrinkled periodic mesoporous organosilica nanoparticles for hydrophobic anticancer drug delivery. J Porous Mater 2015; 22: 1-10.
[http://dx.doi.org/10.1007/s10934-014-9897-1]

[134] Cheng SH, Lee CH, Yang CS, Tseng FG, Mou CY, Lo LW. Mesoporous silica nanoparticles functionalized with an oxygen-sensing probe for cell photodynamic therapy: potential cancer theranostics. J Mater Chem 2009; 19: 1252-7.

[135] Liu X, Kang J, Wang H, Huang T, Li C. Construction of fluorescein isothiocyanate-labeled MSNs/PEG/lycorine/antibody as drug carrier for targeting prostate cancer cells. J Nanosci Nanotechnol 2018; 18(7): 4471-7.
[http://dx.doi.org/10.1166/jnn.2018.15292] [PMID: 29442621]

[136] Hsiao SM, Peng BY, Tseng YS, Liu HT, Chen CH, Lin HM. Preparation and characterization of multifunctional mesoporous silica nanoparticles for dual magnetic resonance and fluorescence imaging in targeted cancer therapy. Microporous Mesoporous Mater 2017; 250: 210-20.
[http://dx.doi.org/10.1016/j.micromeso.2017.04.050]

[137] Freitas LBD, Corgosinho LD, Faria JAQA, *et al.* Multifunctional mesoporous silica nanoparticles for

cancer-targeted, controlled drug delivery and imaging. Microporous Mesoporous Mater 2017; 242: 271-83.
[http://dx.doi.org/10.1016/j.micromeso.2017.01.036]

[138] Pascual L, Sancenon F, Martinez-Manez R, *et al.* Mesoporous silica as multiple nanoparticles system for inflammation imaging as nano-radiopharmaceuticals. Microporous Mesoporous Mater 2017; 239: 426-31.
[http://dx.doi.org/10.1016/j.micromeso.2016.10.041]

[139] Munaweera I, Koneru B, Shi Y, DiPasqua AJ, Balkus KJ. Chemoradiotherapeutic wrinkled mesoporous silica nanoparticles for use in cancer therapy. APL Mater 2014; 2: 113315.
[http://dx.doi.org/10.1063/1.4899118]

[140] Lu CH, Willner I. Stimuli-responsive DNA-functionalized nano-/microcontainers for switchable and controlled release. Angew Chem Int Ed Engl 2015; 54(42): 12212-35.
[http://dx.doi.org/10.1002/anie.201503054] [PMID: 26296181]

[141] Zhang M, Xu C, Wen L, *et al.* A hyaluronidase-responsive nanoparticle-based drug delivery system for targeting colon cancer cells. Cancer Res 2016; 76(24): 7208-18.
[http://dx.doi.org/10.1158/0008-5472.CAN-16-1681] [PMID: 27742685]

[142] Hu JJ, Liu LH, Li ZY, Zhuo RX, Zhang XZ. MMP-responsive theranostic nanoplatform based on mesoporous silica nanoparticles for tumor imaging and targeted drug delivery. J Mater Chem B Mater Biol Med 2016; 4: 1932-40.
[http://dx.doi.org/10.1039/C5TB02490K]

[143] Hakeem A, Zahid F, Zhan G, *et al.* Polyaspartic acid-anchored mesoporous silica nanoparticles for pH-responsive doxorubicin release. Int J Nanomedicine 2018; 13: 1029-40.
[http://dx.doi.org/10.2147/IJN.S146955] [PMID: 29497295]

[144] Jiang K, Chi T, Li T, *et al.* A smart pH-responsive nano-carrier as a drug delivery system for the targeted delivery of ursolic acid: suppresses cancer growth and metastasis by modulating P53/MMP-9/PTEN/CD44 mediated multiple signaling pathways. Nanoscale 2017; 9(27): 9428-39.
[http://dx.doi.org/10.1039/C7NR01677H] [PMID: 28660943]

[145] Abdous B, Sajjadi SM, Ma'mani L. beta-Cyclodextrin modified mesoporous silica nanoparticles as a nano-carrier: response surface methodology to investigate and optimize loading and release processes for curcumin delivery. J Appl Biomed 2017; 15: 210-8.
[http://dx.doi.org/10.1016/j.jab.2017.02.004]

[146] Pourjvadi A, Tehrani ZM. Mesoporous silica nanoparticles with bilayer coating of poly(acrylic acid-co-itaconic acid) and human serum albuminum (HAS): a pH-sensitive carrier for gemcitabine delivery. Mater Sci Eng C 2016; 61: 782-90.
[http://dx.doi.org/10.1016/j.msec.2015.12.096]

[147] Chang D, Gao Y, Wang L, *et al.* Polydopamine-based surface modification of mesoporous silica nanoparticles as pH-sensitive drug delivery vehicles for cancer therapy. J Colloid Interface Sci 2016; 463: 279-87.
[http://dx.doi.org/10.1016/j.jcis.2015.11.001] [PMID: 26550786]

[148] Wen ZN, Long YJ, Yang LL, *et al.* Constructing H+-triggered bubble generating nano-drug delivery systems using bicarbonate and carbonate. RSC Advances 2016; 6: 105814-20.
[http://dx.doi.org/10.1039/C6RA19863E]

[149] Duo YH, Li Y, Chen CK, *et al.* DOX-loaded pH-sensitive mesoporous silica nanoparticles coated with PDA and PEG induce pro-death autophagy in breast cancer. RSC Advances 2017; 7: 39641-50.
[http://dx.doi.org/10.1039/C7RA05135B]

[150] Abbaszad Rafi A, Mahkam M, Davaran S, Hamishehkar H. A Smart pH-responsive Nano-Carrier as a Drug Delivery System: A hybrid system comprised of mesoporous nanosilica MCM-41 (as a nano-container) & a pH-sensitive polymer (as smart reversible gatekeepers): Preparation, characterization and *in vitro* release studies of an anti-cancer drug. Eur J Pharm Sci 2016; 93: 64-73.

[http://dx.doi.org/10.1016/j.ejps.2016.08.005] [PMID: 27497878]

[151] Yan Y, Fu J, Liu X, Wang TF, Lu XY. Acid-responsive intracelular doxorubicin reléase from click chemistry functionalized mesoporous silica nanoparticles. RSC Advances 2015; 5: 30640-6.
[http://dx.doi.org/10.1039/C5RA00059A]

[152] Chen M, He XX, Wang KM, et al. A pH-responsive polymer/mesoporous silica nano-container linked through an acid cleavable linker for intracellular controlled release and tumor therapy in vivo. J Mater Chem B Mater Biol Med 2014; 2: 428-36.
[http://dx.doi.org/10.1039/C3TB21268H]

[153] Sun Y, Ran ZP, Tang HY, et al. Continuous detection of pH-responsive drug delivery system in cells in situ by confocal laser scanning microscopy. Chin J Chem 2013; 31: 787-93.
[http://dx.doi.org/10.1002/cjoc.201300113]

[154] Liu Q, Wang J, Yang L, et al. Facile synthesis by a covalent binding reaction for pH-responsive drug release of carboxylated chitosan coated hollow mesoporous silica nanoparticles. IET Nanobiotechnol 2018; 12(4): 446-52.
[http://dx.doi.org/10.1049/iet-nbt.2017.0100] [PMID: 29768228]

[155] Shah PV, Rajput SJ. Facile synthesis of chitosan mesoporous silica nanoparticles: a pH-responsive smart delivery platform for raloxifene hydrochloride. AAPS PharmSciTech 2018; 19(3): 1344-57.
[http://dx.doi.org/10.1208/s12249-017-0949-0] [PMID: 29340980]

[156] Moreira AF, Dias DR, Costa EC, Correia IJ. Thermo- and pH-responsive nano-in-micro particles for combinatorial drug delivery to cancer cells. Eur J Pharm Sci 2017; 104: 42-51.
[http://dx.doi.org/10.1016/j.ejps.2017.03.033] [PMID: 28347775]

[157] Cai H, Shen T, Kirillov AM, et al. Self-assembled upconversion nanoparticle clusters for NIR-controlled drug release and synergistic therapy after conjugation with gold nanoparticles. Inorg Chem 2017; 56(9): 5295-304.
[http://dx.doi.org/10.1021/acs.inorgchem.7b00380] [PMID: 28402112]

[158] Liu JJ, Wang C, Wang XY, et al. Mesoporous silica coated single-walled carbon nanotubes as a multifunctional light-responsive platform for cancer combination therapy. Adv Funct Mater 2015; 25: 384-92.
[http://dx.doi.org/10.1002/adfm.201403079]

[159] Chen X, Liu Z, Parker SG, et al. Light-induced hydrogel based on tumor-targeting mesoporous silica nanoparticles as a theranostic platform for sustained cancer treatment. ACS Appl Mater Interfaces 2016; 8(25): 15857-63.
[http://dx.doi.org/10.1021/acsami.6b02562] [PMID: 27265514]

[160] Shahbazi MA, Almeida PV, Correia A, et al. Intracellular responsive dual delivery by endosomolytic polyplexes carrying DNA anchored porous silicon nanoparticles. J Control Release 2017; 249: 111-22.
[http://dx.doi.org/10.1016/j.jconrel.2017.01.046] [PMID: 28159519]

[161] Ma K, Gong Y, Aubert T, et al. Self-assembly of highly symmetrical, ultrasmall inorganic cages directed by surfactant micelles. Nature 2018; 558(7711): 577-80.
[http://dx.doi.org/10.1038/s41586-018-0221-0] [PMID: 29925942]

[162] Vargas-Gonzalez BA, Castro-Pastrana LI, Mendoza-Alvarez ME, Gonzalez-Rodriguez R, Coffer JL, Mendez-Rojas MA. Hollow magnetic iron oxide nanoparticles as sodium meclofenamate drug delivering systems. J Nanomed Res 2016; 3: 00071.

[163] Rostami M, Aghajanzadeh M, Zamani M, Manjili HK, Danafar H. Sono-chemical synthesis and characterization of Fe3O4@mTiO2-GO nanocarriers for dual-targeted colon drug delivery. Res Chem Intermed 2018; 44: 1889-904.
[http://dx.doi.org/10.1007/s11164-017-3204-0]

[164] Jin Y, Zhang N, Li C, Pu K, Ding C, Zhu Y. Nanosystem composed with MSNs, gadolinium, liposome and cytotoxic peptides for tumor theranostics. Colloids Surf B Biointerfaces 2017; 151: 240-

8.
[http://dx.doi.org/10.1016/j.colsurfb.2016.12.024] [PMID: 28024200]

[165] Dong H, Han TT, Ren LL, Ding SN. Novel sandwich-structured electrochemiluminiscence immunosensing platform *via* CdTe quantum dots-embedded mesoporous silica nanospheres as enhanced signal labels and Fe3O4@SiO2@PS nanocomposites as magnetic separable carriers. J Electroanal Chem (Lausanne Switz) 2017; 806: 32-40.
[http://dx.doi.org/10.1016/j.jelechem.2017.10.038]

[166] Xue P, Sun L, Li Q, *et al.* PEGylated polydopamine-coated magnetic nanoparticles for combined targeted chemotherapy and photothermal ablation of tumour cells. Colloids Surf B Biointerfaces 2017; 160: 11-21.
[http://dx.doi.org/10.1016/j.colsurfb.2017.09.012] [PMID: 28915497]

[167] Li ZH, Dong K, Huang S, *et al.* A smart nanoassembly for multistage targeted drug delivery and magnetic resonance imaging. Adv Funct Mater 2014; 24: 3612-20.
[http://dx.doi.org/10.1002/adfm.201303662]

[168] Chen Y, Xu PF, Shu Z, *et al.* Multifunctional graphene oxide-based triple stimuli-responsive nanotheranostics. Adv Funct Mater 2014; 24: 4386-96.
[http://dx.doi.org/10.1002/adfm.201400221]

[169] Jeon MJ, Gordon AC, Larson AC, Chung JW, Kim YI, Kim DH. Transcatheter intra-arterial infusion of doxorubicin loaded porous magnetic nano-clusters with iodinated oil for the treatment of liver cancer. Biomaterials 2016; 88: 25-33.
[http://dx.doi.org/10.1016/j.biomaterials.2016.02.021] [PMID: 26938029]

[170] Jin Z, Wen Y, Hu Y, *et al.* MRI-guided and ultrasound-triggered release of NO by advanced nanomedicine. Nanoscale 2017; 9(10): 3637-45.
[http://dx.doi.org/10.1039/C7NR00231A] [PMID: 28247895]

[171] De D, Mandal Goswami M. Shape induced acid responsive heat triggered highly facilitated drug release by cube shaped magnetite nanoparticles. Biomicrofluidics 2016; 10(6): 064112.
[http://dx.doi.org/10.1063/1.4971439] [PMID: 27990214]

[172] Huang PL, Zeng BZ, Mai ZX, *et al.* Novel drug delivery nanosystems based on out-inside bifunctionalized mesoporous silica yolk-shell magnetic nanostars used as nanocarriers for curcumin. J Mater Chem B Mater Biol Med 2016; 4: 46-56.
[http://dx.doi.org/10.1039/C5TB02184G]

[173] Shen B, Ma Y, Yu S, Ji C. Smart multifunctional magnetic nanoparticle-based drug delivery system for cancer thermos-chemotherapy and intracellular imaging. ACS Appl Mater Interfaces 2016; 8(37): 24502-8.
[http://dx.doi.org/10.1021/acsami.6b09772] [PMID: 27573061]

[174] Shao D, Li J, Zheng X, *et al.* Janus "nano-bullets" for magnetic targeting liver cancer chemotherapy. Biomaterials 2016; 100: 118-33.
[http://dx.doi.org/10.1016/j.biomaterials.2016.05.030] [PMID: 27258482]

[175] Soltys M, Kovatcik P, Lhotka M, Ulbrich P, Zadrazil A, Stepanek F. Radiofrequency controlled release from mesoporous silica nano-carriers. Microporous Mesoporous Mater 2016; 229: 14-21.
[http://dx.doi.org/10.1016/j.micromeso.2016.04.009]

[176] Su YL, Fang JH, Liao CY, Lin CT, Li YT, Hu SH. Targeted mesoporous iron oxide nanoparticles-encapsulated perfluorohexane and a hydrophobic drug for deep tumor penetration and therapy. Theranostics 2015; 5(11): 1233-48.
[http://dx.doi.org/10.7150/thno.12843] [PMID: 26379789]

[177] Liu C, Yu M, Li Y, *et al.* Synthesis of mesoporous carbon nanoparticles with large and tunable pore sizes. Nanoscale 2015; 7(27): 11580-90.
[http://dx.doi.org/10.1039/C5NR02389K] [PMID: 26087279]

[178] Awwad NS, Alshahrani AM, Saleh KA, Hamdy MS. A novel method to improve the anticancer activity of natural-based hydroxyapatite against the liver cancer cell line HepG2 using mesoporous magnesia as a micro-carrier. Molecules 2017; 22(12): 1947.
[http://dx.doi.org/10.3390/molecules22121947] [PMID: 29186752]

[179] Weng Q, Wang B, Wang X, *et al.* Highly water-soluble, porous, and biocompatible boron nitrides for anticancer drug delivery. ACS Nano 2014; 8(6): 6123-30.
[http://dx.doi.org/10.1021/nn5014808] [PMID: 24797563]

[180] Chen LL, Wang XH, Ji FL, *et al.* New bifunctional-pullulan-based micelles with good biocompatibility for efficient co-delivery of cancer suppressing p53 gene and doxorubicin to cancer cells. RSC Adv 2015; 94719-31.
[http://dx.doi.org/10.1039/C5RA17139C]

[181] Chen LL, Qian M, Zhang LW, *et al.* Co-delivery of doxorubicin and shRNA of Beclin1 by folate receptor targeted pullulan-based multifunctional nanomicelles for combinatorial cancer therapy. RSC Advances 2018; 8: 17710-22.
[http://dx.doi.org/10.1039/C8RA01679H]

[182] Yang D, Feng L, Dougherty CA, *et al. In vivo* targeting of metastatic breast cancer *via* tumor vasculature-specific nano-graphene oxide. Biomaterials 2016; 104: 361-71.
[http://dx.doi.org/10.1016/j.biomaterials.2016.07.029] [PMID: 27490486]

[183] Shamsi M, Majidi Zolbanin J, Mahmoudian B, *et al.* A study on drug delivery tracing with radiolabeled mesoporous hydroxyapatite nanoparticles conjugated with 2DG/DOX for breast tumor cells. Nucl Med Rev Cent East Eur 2018; 21(1): 32-6.
[http://dx.doi.org/10.5603/NMR.a2018.0008] [PMID: 29319137]

[184] Bakrudeen HB, Sugunalakshmi M, Reddy BSR. Auto-fluorescent mesoporous ZnO nanospheres for drug delivery carrier application. Mater Sci Eng C 2015; 56: 335-40.
[http://dx.doi.org/10.1016/j.msec.2015.06.042] [PMID: 26249598]

[185] Zhai X, Yu M, Cheng Z, *et al.* Rattle-type hollow $CaWO_4:Tb^{(3+)}@SiO_2$ nanocapsules as carriers for drug delivery. Dalton Trans 2011; 40(48): 12818-25.
[http://dx.doi.org/10.1039/c1dt10996k] [PMID: 21879092]

[186] Dong Z, Gong H, Gao M, *et al.* Polydopamine nanoparticles as a versatile molecular loading platform to enable imaging-guided cancer combination therapy. Theranostics 2016; 6(7): 1031-42.
[http://dx.doi.org/10.7150/thno.14431] [PMID: 27217836]

[187] Li X, Liu C, Wang S, *et al.* Poly(acrylic acid) conjugated hollow mesoporous carbon as a dual-stimuli triggered drug delivery system for chemo-photothermal synergistic therapy. Mater Sci Eng C 2017; 71: 594-603.
[http://dx.doi.org/10.1016/j.msec.2016.10.037] [PMID: 27987749]

[188] Zhou L, Jing Y, Liu Y, *et al.* Mesoporous carbon nanospheres as a multifunctional carrier for cancer theranostics. Theranostics 2018; 8(3): 663-75.
[http://dx.doi.org/10.7150/thno.21927] [PMID: 29344297]

[189] Wang X, Lin Y, Li X, *et al.* Fluorescent carbon dot gated hollow mesoporous carbon for chemo-photothermal synergistic therapy. J Colloid Interface Sci 2017; 507: 410-20.
[http://dx.doi.org/10.1016/j.jcis.2017.08.010] [PMID: 28806660]

[190] Zhang Y, Han L, Hu LL, *et al.* Mesoporous carbon nanoparticles capped with polyacrylic acid as drug carrier for bi-trigger continuous drug release. J Mater Chem B Mater Biol Med 2016; 4: 5178-84.
[http://dx.doi.org/10.1039/C6TB00987E]

[191] Qiao W, Lan XM, Tsoi JKH, *et al.* Biomimetic hollow mesoporous hydroxyapatite microsphere with controlled morphology, entrapment efficiency and degradability for cancer therapy. RSC Advances 2017; 7: 44788-98.
[http://dx.doi.org/10.1039/C7RA09204K]

[192] Li D, Huang X, Wu Y, *et al.* Preparation of pH-responsive mesoporous hydroxyapatite nanoparticles for intracellular controlled release of an anticancer drug. Biomater Sci 2016; 4(2): 272-80.
[http://dx.doi.org/10.1039/C5BM00228A] [PMID: 26484364]

[193] Peng H, Li K, Wang T, *et al.* Preparation of hierarchical mesoporous $CaCO_3$ by a facile binary solvent approach as anticancer drug carrier for etoposide. Nanoscale Res Lett 2013; 8(1): 321.
[http://dx.doi.org/10.1186/1556-276X-8-321] [PMID: 23849350]

[194] Zhu R, Wang Z, Liang P, *et al.* Efficient VEGF targeting delivery of DOX using Bevacizumab conjugated SiO_2@LDH for anti-neuroblastoma therapy. Acta Biomater 2017; 63: 163-80.
[http://dx.doi.org/10.1016/j.actbio.2017.09.009] [PMID: 28923539]

[195] Li D, Zhang YT, Yu M, Guo J, Chaudhary D, Wang CC. Cancer therapy and fluorescence imaging using the active release of doxorubicin from MSPs/Ni-LDH folate targeting nanoparticles. Biomaterials 2013; 34(32): 7913-22.
[http://dx.doi.org/10.1016/j.biomaterials.2013.06.046] [PMID: 23886730]

[196] Lee J, Jeong C, Kim WJ. Facile fabrication and application of near-IR light-responsive drug release system based on gold nanorods and phase change material. J Mater Chem B Mater Biol Med 2014; 2: 8338-45.
[http://dx.doi.org/10.1039/C4TB01631A]

[197] Yang WJ, Zhao TT, Zhou P, *et al.* "Click" functionalization of dual stimuli-responsive polymer nanocapsules for drug delivery systems. Polym Chem 2017; 8: 3056-65.
[http://dx.doi.org/10.1039/C7PY00161D]

[198] Xue B, Kozlovskaya V, Liu F, *et al.* Intracellular degradable hydrogel cubes and spheres for anti-cancer drug delivery. ACS Appl Mater Interfaces 2015; 7(24): 13633-44.
[http://dx.doi.org/10.1021/acsami.5b03360] [PMID: 26028158]

[199] Qin Y, Chen J, Bi Y, *et al.* Near-infrared light remote-controlled intracellular anti-cancer drug delivery using thermo/pH sensitive nanovehicle. Acta Biomater 2015; 17: 201-9.
[http://dx.doi.org/10.1016/j.actbio.2015.01.026] [PMID: 25644449]

[200] Lin L, Xu W, Liang H, *et al.* Construction of pH-sensitive lysozyme/pectin nanogel for tumor methotrexate delivery. Colloids Surf B Biointerfaces 2015; 126: 459-66.
[http://dx.doi.org/10.1016/j.colsurfb.2014.12.051] [PMID: 25601095]

[201] Mendez-Rojas MA, Angulo Molina A, Aguilera-Portillo G. Nanomedicine: small steps, big effects.CRC Concise Encyclopedia of Nanotechnology. CRC Press 2016.
[http://dx.doi.org/10.1201/b19457-64]

[202] Halappanavar S, Vogel U, Wallin H, Yauk CL. Promise and peril in nanomedicine: the challenges and needs for integrated systems biology approaches to define health risk. Wiley Interdiscip Rev Nanomed Nanobiotechnol 2018; 10(1): e1465.
[http://dx.doi.org/10.1002/wnan.1465] [PMID: 28294555]

[203] Juillerat-Jeanneret L, Dusinska M, Fjellsbø LM, Collins AR, Handy RD, Riediker M. Biological impact assessment of nanomaterial used in nanomedicine. introduction to the NanoTEST project. Nanotoxicology 2015; 9 (Suppl. 1): 5-12.
[http://dx.doi.org/10.3109/17435390.2013.826743] [PMID: 23875681]

[204] Gracssian V. Nanoscience and nanotechnology, environmental and health impact. USA: John Wiley & Sons 2008.
[http://dx.doi.org/10.1002/9780470396612]

[205] Mahmoudi M, Lynch I, Ejtehadi MR, Monopoli MP, Bombelli FB, Laurent S. Protein-nanoparticle interactions: opportunities and challenges. Chem Rev 2011; 111(9): 5610-37.
[http://dx.doi.org/10.1021/cr100440g] [PMID: 21688848]

[206] Mendez-Rojas MA, Sanchez Salas JL, Santillan-Urquiza E. Toxicity: the dawn of nanotoxicology.CRC Concise Encyclopedia of Nanotechnology. CRC Press 2016.

[http://dx.doi.org/10.1201/b19457-69]

[207] Oberdörster G, Oberdörster E, Oberdörster J. Nanotoxicology: an emerging discipline evolving from studies of ultrafine particles. Environ Health Perspect 2005; 113(7): 823-39.
[http://dx.doi.org/10.1289/ehp.7339] [PMID: 16002369]

[208] Saiyed MA, Patel RC, Patel SC. Toxicology perspective of nanopharmaceuticals: a critical review. Int J Pharm Sci Nanotech 2011; 4(1): 1287-9.

CHAPTER 7

Cutting Edge Targeting Strategies Utilizing Nanotechnology in Breast Cancer Therapy

Samipta Singh, Priyanka Maurya and **Shubhini A. Saraf**[*]

Department of Pharmaceutical Sciences, Babasaheb Bhimrao Ambedkar University, Lucknow, India

Abstract: Breast cancer is one of the major reasons for mortality and trauma amongst women. Therapy for breast cancer has various options such as, chemotherapy, hormone therapy, gene therapy, immunotherapy, and radiation therapy. Chemotherapy is the choice in most cases but is often associated with side/adverse effects. These side/adverse effects can be eliminated by delivering the drug to the target site. With the help of nanotechnology and drug delivery through a suitable carrier, targeting has become achievable. Targeting includes both, the active as well as the passive approach. Passive targeting is based on the accumulation of the drug over tumor tissues whereas active targeting is done by means of an interaction with the receptor/antigen and the targeting moiety. Nowadays, the focus is on the active targeting of drugs in which an approach to target the drug directly to the diseased cells is taken. The approaches can be broadly classified mainly into antigen-antibody, aptamers, ligand-receptors and lectin-carbohydrate based, respectively. Every targeting strategy is based on one basic concept, *i.e.* an overexpression of a biomarker on a specific diseased cell type. Hence, a suitable moiety is utilized to carry out the active targeting of drugs. Apart from chemotherapeutic agents, hormonal drugs, gene silencing molecules can also be successfully delivered through nanotechnology. Some of the nano based medicines are already in the market and there is a constant enhancement in the success of the systems. Some are in the trial phase and some approaches have been patented. However, the translational challenge yet exists and there is a need to overcome it. Thus, this chapter discusses the various delivery systems, different materials and various approaches for the active targeting of the drug, recent clinical trials, challenges and some recent patents.

Keywords: Active targeting, Aptamers, Breast cancer cells, Chemotherapy, Drug delivery, Ligand based targeting, Monoclonal antibodies, Nanomedicine, Over expression, Patents, Trials.

---

[*] **Corresponding author Shubhini A. Saraf:** Department of Pharmaceutical Sciences, Babasaheb Bhimrao Ambedkar University, Vidya Vihar, Raebareily road, Lucknow. Pin: 226025, India; Tel: 09415488410, 9628176500; Email: shubhini.saraf@gmail.com

Atta-ur-Rahman and M. Iqbal Choudhary (Eds.)
All rights reserved-© 2019 Bentham Science Publishers

INTRODUCTION

Breast cancer is a well-known cancer occurring in women worldwide. As per WHO fact sheet, this cancer impacts over 1.5 million women every year [1]. Breast cancer is a heterogeneous disease. Several processes and pathways are involved. On a molecular basis, the disease can be broadly classified into the following: luminal A, luminal B, normal breast-like, HER2 over-expressed and triple negative (basal). In the case of luminal A, there is a high level of estrogen receptor while HER2 is low. In the case of luminal B, estrogen receptor and HER2 both are low but proliferation is high. In the case of triple negative, there is an absence of estrogen, progesterone receptor and HER2 [2]. However, several subtypes can be defined by the genetic pool [3].

Conventional treatment for breast cancer includes surgery, radiotherapy and chemotherapy. The efficacy of chemotherapy in comparison to surgery has been little. Morbidity in patients of cancer is due to the subclinical metastatic disease at prognosis. Systemic therapy is the only chance for cure or prolonged survival. Major chemotherapeutic agents for breast cancer are paclitaxel, docetaxel, doxorubicin, cyclophosphamide *etc*. The limitations of conventional breast cancer chemotherapy are a low therapeutic index of a drug, side effects, therapy resistance and heterogenicity of the drug concentration within the tissue [4 - 7].

Other major treatment options are hormonal therapy, immunotherapy and targeted therapy. Hormonal therapy shows potential for the breast cancers that are hormone receptor positive. Examples of hormonal therapy are tamoxifen, aromatase inhibitors and fulvestrant [8]. However, it does not work in breast cancer other than hormonal receptor positive type of breast cancer. The treatment also fails if the cancer is resistant to hormonal therapy. In immunotherapy, medicines are used to stimulate one's own system. The therapeutics may include the tumor-antigen vaccines, activators of dendritic cells, adoptive cellar therapy, adjuvants which activate innate immunity and checkpoint blockades [9]. The targeted therapy to cancer cells involves attacking cancer cells directly or indirectly without having to affect the normal cells. Targeted therapy inhibits the mutated or overexpressed proteins which help the cancer cells to grow. Some of the examples are gefitinib for inhibiting epidermal growth factor receptor) [10]; trastuzumab, pertuzumab, lapatinib for inhibiting HER2 [11, 12]; Afinitor® (everolimus) for inhibiting mechanistic target of rapamycin [13]; palbociclib for cyclin-dependent kinases (CDK-4 and CDK-6) [14].

Gene silencing is a personalized approach to breast cancer treatment which has become a research trend and post transcriptional gene silencing most widely utilizes molecules, such as siRNA (*i.e.*, small interfering RNA) and miRNA (micro RNA) in breast cancer research. The major challenges in this therapy are the efficient delivery of these molecules to the target cells and makes these molecule reach the breast cancer cell cytoplasm, protecting it from nuclease degradation while targeting, without any adverse effects [15, 16].

With the introduction of nanotechnology, novel engineered drug delivery systems have been formulated. With the right combination nano-based science and best suitable material for the nano-based delivery system, conventional chemotherapeutic agent, hormonal drugs and gene based therapy can be efficiently delivered to the target site (*i.e.* breast cancer cells) without having to affect normal cells. Nanotechnology has a lot of potential in targeting the potent drugs to tumor cells with an increase in efficacy and with lower toxicity. Stability of the drug in the bloodstream as well as proper pharmacokinetics is important [17]. Being in nanoparticulate form may increase the circulation time of the drug in the blood, prevent the drug from early degradation and improve intracellular penetration [18, 19]. In the past few years, there have been many new approaches for targeting the drug to the breast cancer cells in a way that it does not harm normal cells. This chapter is strictly limited to different nano-based targeted delivery systems, for breast cancer therapy and their translational aspects. The major purpose of this chapter is to explain the role of nano-based delivery systems and their modifications as powerful stratagem to target the drugs to breast cancer cells, the challenges of nano-based system therapy and the limitations thereof.

DIFFERENT NANO DELIVERY SYSTEMS USED FOR THE TREATMENT OF BREAST CANCER

The preview of this chapter is strictly restricted to nano-based drug delivery systems since targeting is mostly possible only through these. There may be several materials or shapes of nanoparticles but all of these are designed with the purpose of loading the drug so that it can be delivered to cancer cell site either directly or by other means, such as conjugation or by the application of an external field. They can be categorized through multiple pathways, but the below-mentioned delivery systems have been divided on the basis of specific design or shape or uniqueness in approach:

Spherical Nanoparticles

Nanoparticles are broadly categorized into nanocapsules and nanospheres. The drug is either encapsulated or loaded within the nanoparticles. Sometimes, the drug may also be conjugated over the nanoparticles. These nanoparticles can be made of materials and can be named by the name of the materials, such as, polymers (polymeric nanoparticles), lipid (Solid lipid nanoparticles, nanostructured lipid carriers), gold (gold nanoparticles), *etc*. Nanoencapsulation of drug (doxazocin) have found to improve anti-proliferative and anti-clonogenic effects on breast cancer cells [20]. Goldman *et al.* (2016) designed two in one nanoparticles rationally and found efficient tumor killing. They also compared their work with individual nanoparticles in which they determined that cancer cells could develop adaptive resistance [21]. Nanoparticles can also be used in a combination therapy approach. Li *et al.* (2015) formulated nanoparticles which were loaded with epigenetic-targeted (decitabine) and a chemotherapeutic drug (doxorubicin) and there was high apoptotic tumor cell proportion and tumor suppressive effect [22]. Nanoparticles have also been utilized for multifunctional purposes or dual receptor targets [23]. Polymeric nanoparticles can also be employed for the sequential delivery of two drugs [24]. $Fe_3O_4@mSiO_2$ core-shell nanoparticles possess high drug loading capacity and biocompatibility. These have been researched for their effectiveness in breast cancer cells [25]. Drug-loaded core-shell nanoparticles have also been checked for the synergistic effect of cold atmospheric plasma. They can be prepared by electrospray method [26]. These can also be prepared by PLGA-casein combination approach [27].

Micelles

Pluronic micelles have been known to inhibit multi-drug resistance in cancers by interfering with P-gp. They are also known to augment apoptotic signaling and to alleviate anti-apoptotic cellular defense, thus enhancing the drug potency in MDR cells [28]. 1, 2- distearo-yl-sn-glycero-3-phosphatid-yl-ethanol-amine)-N-[methoxy(poly-ethyl-ene glycol)] micelles (DSPE-PEG-2000 micelles) are well established and sterically stable micelles. They are biodegradable, biocompatible, easy to prepare above CMC and relatively stable *in vivo*. Vinorelbine (an anti-cancer drug) can be incorporated in large quantities and the drug lies within the interface, *i.e.* between core and palisade layer of micelles [29]. Hongmei *et al.*, (2015) formulated a mixed micelle in which they used two polymers for the core-forming block, ensuring that both were responsive to similar pH conditions (PDMAEMA-b-PCDMAEMA-BMAPAA) whereas for corona block there was a variation in pH. They took 2 kDa PEG-Folic Acid and 20kDa PEG-MMP7 cleavable peptide [30]. Co-delivery of the two drugs can also be achieved using a micellar system [31, 32]. Micelles with a pH-sensitive core, PEG corona, and acid cleavable anionic shell revealed a higher intra-tumor accumulation of drug [33].

Self-emulsifying Systems

These systems are also biocompatible. Self nano/micro micellar carriers have been extensively investigated. Natural ingredients can easily be utilized with such delivery systems. Sandhu *et al.* (2017) came up with a self nano emulsifying drug delivery system (SNEDDS) where they utilized natural ingredients such as polyunsaturated fatty acids. The formulation showed complete release of drug in 30 minutes and more than 80% permeation in 45 minutes. *In vivo* studies showed remarkable improvement in the drug absorption rate. The efficacy was superior and there was an increase in the survival rate of animals [34]. Some recent works are tamoxifen citrate loaded SNEDDS [35], sofrafane-enabled SMEDDS (self-micro emulsifying drug delivery system) loaded with paclitaxel [36], *etc*. Some believe that the introduction of the term self-emulsifying is meaningless, as there is a spontaneous formation of microemulsion after shaking and physics of microemulsion is also similar [37].

Dendrimers

Dendrimers are nanoformulation with a three-dimensional structure and a central molecule; the configurational similarity can be linked with a tree and its branches. Branches are generated by polymerization of the central molecule. They can be used to load hydrophilic or hydrophobic drugs. They can also be further modified using a suitable ligand [38]. Polyamidoamine (PAMAM) dendrimers are the most common dendrimers. They can be easily cleared through the kidney. Recent studies exploded with PAMAM-siMDR1(modified with phospholipids) [39], glutaryl polyamidoamine dendrimers to overcome the resistance of cisplatin in breast cancer cells (MCF7, MCR-7/R) [40], *etc.*

Nanotubes

Nanotubes, as the name implies, are tube-like structures and are usually one-dimensional. Examples include carbon nanotubes and inorganic nanotubes like alumina nanotubes. Carbon nanotubes have been widely investigated in breast cancer research. They have reported decreasing tumor volume in breast cancer [41]. Recent works report doxorubicin loaded carbon nanotubes [42], carbon nanotube-drug (lobaplatin) complex for breast cancer, *etc*. Alumina nanotubes have been a part of the research for the examination of enhanced cancer therapy. Wang *et al.* (2015) targeted cell signaling networks (autophagic and endoplasmic reticulum stress signaling) by using thapsigargin loaded anodic alumina nanotubes. These nanotubes were co-treated with an autophagy inhibitors [43].

Vesicular Systems

Liposomes

Liposomes such as Doxil® have made significant contributions to the breast cancer research arena. Myocet has also been approved in Canada and Europe for metastatic breast cancer treatment (in combination with cyclophosphamide) [44]. In recent studies, redox-sensitive liposomes were found to escape endolysosomes and rapidly collapsed to release drugs into the cytoplasm [45]. For gene delivery, cationic lipid vesicles (*e.g.* stearyl amine) have gained great attention because of charge based interaction with negatively charged nucleic acids. They are biodegradable, biocompatible and show reduced systemic effects. Thus, it is another promising approach for breast cancer [46]. Cationic liposome nanocomplexes are also good for co-delivery of drugs and hold a promising clinical application for triple negative breast cancer [47].

Niosomes

Niosomes are the vesicular systems that have an enhanced stability in comparison to liposomes. They possess many other advantages like high dispersive nature, rigidity and biocompatibility. Recently, multilamellar gold niosomes have come to the fore, which add the advantages of a gold nanoparticle to the niosome. These gold particles loaded niosomes are an innovative approach and cationic gold favours "proton sponge effect" in the acidic environment. These nanocarriers hold a promise for potentiality against resistant breast cancer cells [48].

Exosomes

Exosomes are distinct cellular entities. These belong to the class of nanoparticle family due to their nanosize range. These are cell-derived vesicular systems. These offer advantage over other delivery system in that there is no unwanted accumulation of these delivery system in the liver and can avoid first pass metabolism. Other advantages include long-term safety and natural ability to carry molecules. Their surface can be characterized by the presence of multiple proteins like heat shock protein and lysosomal protein. Biological function of exosome remains unclear. Exosomes have delivered many agents like miRNA and have inhibited the growth of breast cancer *in vivo*. They can be loaded with drug like doxorubicin to inhibit the growth of breast carcinoma. Methods of loading the drug include electroporation, chemical-based transfection *etc*. They can be administered *via* different routes like intravenous, oral, intra-tumoral, *etc*. Before bringing them into the reality, they need to be well researched and clearly understood [49 - 51].

Polymerosomes

Polymerosomes (also referred to as "polymeric vesicles") have also gained considerable attention. They are more stable than liposomes. They can be engineered to make the delivery responsive to pH, temperature, light, enzymes or any other stimuli. They can be functionalized in order to achieve breast cancer targeting objectives [52].

Miscellaneous

Phytosomes [53, 54] and transferosomes [55] are other vesicular systems which have also been investigated for breast cancer. Phytosomes are patented technology for the conjugation of a phytochemical substance to phosphatidylcholine in order to produce a lipid compatible molecular complex. The functional group(s) present in a phytochemical is directly bound to the phosphatidyl choline's polar group whereas in case of liposomes there is no formation of chemical bond and the phytochemical is surrounded by phosphatidylcholine. This difference can result in better oral absorption and better stability profile of phytosomes in comparison to liposomes [56]. Transferosomes are deformable type of lipid vesicular system, have been investigated for breast cancer in the form of transdermal delivery of drugs [57].

Hybrid Nanosystems

These are the nanosystems consisting of combining two constituents. Several hybrid delivery systems have been attempted. Bhavasar *et al.* (2017) reported 'nano-in-nano' hybrid nanoparticles where they encapsulated poly (L-lysine--siRNA complex to silence EpCAM which is highly expressed in epithelial cancers. They developed hybrid immunoliposomes. The PEGylated liposomes were covalently linked with EpCAM antibody [58]. Several other examples are: calcium phosphate polymer hybrid nanoparticles [59], peptide/lipid hybrid systems (siRNA delivery) [60], *etc.*

Layer by Layer Nanoparticles

These are the new class of nano polymeric drug delivery systems. The structure consists of a functional core, polyelectrolyte multilayered shell and an external stealth layer for the purpose of targeting. Often, these layers are added so that a better attractive force in the case of opposite charges exists, between the delivery systems and the cells. Eric *et al.* (2015) tried to provide synergistic blockade to MAPK and PI3K pathways (most deregulated signaling pathways in human cancer) using layer by layer nanoformulations, which are toxic towards triple-negative breast cancer cells [61].

Drug Polymer/Lipid Conjugates

Drug conjugates are an emergent delivery system and may increase the selectivity towards a target (as in antibody drug conjugate) or may enhance cytotoxicity and tumor targeting (such as drug-radionuclide conjugate or drug-nanoparticle conjugate) or enhance the potency (drug-drug conjugates) [62]. As an example, polymer-drug conjugate using the polymer as poly[2-pyridin-2-yldisulfanl]-graft-polyethylene glycol and drug camptothecin with an intracellular cleavable linker has also proved its efficacy against HER2 positive breast cancer while it does not affect HER2 negative breast cancer cells [63]. Fatty acid functionalized chitosan bioconjugates have shown potential against various cell lines and are thus a promising formulation against cancer cells, including breast cancer utilizing the passive targeting approach [64].

External Field Based Delivery

Use of an external magnetic field (magnetic nanoparticles) is one of the most extensively studied approaches. On the application of physiologically acceptable magnetic fields, there has been an enhanced accumulation of magnetic nanoparticles in the breast tumor tissues [65]. Stealth magnetic siRNA nanovector also proved to be an effective approach for siRNA delivery *in vitro* as they avoid the drawbacks of siRNA delivery such as rapid degradation by nucleases and the negative charge which prevents the crossing of the cell membrane for internalization [66]. Ultrasound driven nanoparticles is another approach which has been utilized [67].

Nanostars

Nanostar is a relatively new name in terms of anti-cancer nanoparticles. Gold nanostars are anisotropic nanoparticles and offer several benefits over spherical gold nanoparticles. These have multiple branches with sharp tips. These have unique optical properties and high surface to volume ratio (due to which drug loading capacity is increased). Gold nanostars have gained some attention in cancer research [68].

Nanorods

So far, only gold nanorods have been investigated to find its application against breast cancer. Successful targeting of these nanorods to the cancer cells requires several engineering attempts in order to make them biocompatible, long-circulating, stable *in vivo,* and to be able to recognize, bind to and internalize in the cancer cells [69]. Their chemotherapeutic application is limited. Nanorods are the most extensively used for photothermal therapy because of their longitudinal structure and high efficiency. Feng *et al.* (2015) fabricated gold nanorods with the wrapping of cisplatin-polypeptide and are conjugated with folic acid for the chemotherapy as well as photothermal therapy for triple negative breast cancer. This strategy holds promise [70].

MATERIALS USED IN PREPARATION OF NANO-FORMULATIONS FOR BREAST CANCER

Selecting a suitable material for nanoformulation is one of the crucial factors, as this also governs the drug release, loading, *etc*. Some materials have additional benefits. Various materials that have been utilized to formulate nanomedicine and have been later evaluated for anti-cancer efficacy against breast cancer cells *in vitro/in vivo* have been mentioned below:

Viruses or Capsid

This material has opened up as a novel sector in the field of nanotechnology. Viruses are one of the biggest groups of biological materials of the size less than 100 nm that are also used as nanocarriers. The group originated from plant, animal or bacterial viruses. However, in order to use them, they have to be inactivated so that they are not harmful. The capsid of the filamentous viruses is generally used as the biomaterials for pharmaceutical purposes. Virus-based nanoparticles have advantages over synthetic ones, in that, they are biocompatible and biodegradable, are self-assembled, symmetric and can be synthesized inexpensively on a large scale. They also have non-toxic properties. Esfandiari *et al*. (2015) used Potato Virus X as a biomaterial and conjugated it with Herceptin. They found that this conjugation could facilitate Herceptin to be a powerful tool for HER2$^+$ Breast Cancer [71 - 73]

Cells

Exosomes are the best example in this category. These are the vesicular systems are derived from the cells. Being a nanomaterial of cellular origin, they are non-immunogenic in nature due to the similarity in composition with the body's own cells [49, 50].

Metals

Nanoparticles based on metals are mainly researched because of their rapid action. These have unique physical and chemical properties based on their quantum size. Commonly used metals are gold, silver, copper, *etc.* Silver and gold are the most prominent, flexible and reliable.

Gold

Gold is the most common form of metal that is used to formulate nanoparticles. Gold has the potential to accumulate within the tumor tissue either passively or actively *via* conjugation with some targeted molecule. Comprehensive studies of gold nanoparticle have been done by many investigators. Gold is comparatively less toxic than other metal-based nanoparticles, but it offers the disadvantage (such as, lack of clearance) which needs to be resolved before they can be brought into the clinical settings. Gold can be made into a core-shell; hollow gold nanospheres can be fabricated. Moreover, gold nanorods can also be fabricated [74]. Lee *et al.* studied the gold nanoconstructs that consisted of aptamers grafted on gold nanostars. These were then internalized by HER2 mediated endocytosis. They found that these nanoconstructs improved the targeting efficacy of aptamer [68]. Gold nanoparticles can permeate into the tumor vasculature and be retained into tumors providing EPR effect [74].

Silver

The use of silver in nanomedicine is because of its extraordinary properties, such as chemical stability and biological activities. They are extensively investigated in cancer research because of their cytotoxic potential for cancer cells [75, 76].

Other Metals

Other metals recently investigated are cadmium [77], copper [78, 79] and ruthenium [80]. In a study, copper nanoparticles alone did not show any potential cytotoxicity or antiangiogenic effect, when compared with curcumin [79].

Metal Oxide

Metal oxides have gained consideration because of their high redox cycling property and have an ability to produce cytotoxicity *via* oxidative stress on different cells.

Copper Oxide

Copper oxide nanoparticles are known to show toxic effects on a variety of cells. They can be used in case of anti-cancer therapy. Laha *et al.* (2015) reported that CuO NPs can be used after conjugation with folic acid for a therapeutic purpose [81].

Iron Oxide

Nanoparticles made up of iron oxide have been used as a magnetic contrast agent. They have also been employed in many biomedical applications. As a drug delivery system for clinical application, there were many reports of toxicity associated with them. But, iron oxide nanoparticles coated with polymer membrane have shown a promising decrease in toxicity. Swathy *et al.* (2015) developed *Centella asiatica* loaded iron oxide nanoparticles that were coated with polyvinylpyrrolidone and were found to be effective against MCF-7 cells. In the case of normal cells, there was some reduction of cytotoxicity [82]. Iron oxide can also be used to make multifunctional magnetic nanoparticles where it provides targeted delivery as well as imaging and this has shown some promising results against breast cancer [83]. Drug targeting *via* magnetic effect is based on superparamagnetic iron oxide nanoparticles and is currently widely used for theranostics. Superparamagnetic iron oxide nanoparticles (SPIO) condensed colloidal clusters in the presence of Alginate (MagAlg) can bring manipulation with an external magnetic field. Conjugation of drug to SPIO can also reduce the toxicity of the free drug [84]. SPIO nanoparticles have also been used by many researchers for the early detection of cancer [85].

Other Metal Oxide

Other metal oxides utilized are titanium dioxide [86, 87], cerium oxide [88, 89], zinc oxide [90], *etc.*

Polymers

Several examples of polymers that have been utilized for making a certain delivery system are poly (lactic-co-glycolic acid) (PLGA), polycaprolactone, chitosan *etc*. Delivery systems using polymers may simply be nanoparticles or dendrimers or micelles or polymerosome. PLGAs are the most excellent carriers. They improve the pharmacokinetic profile, efficacy, and tolerability of the drug [91]. Chitosan has been used for the stabilization of certain nanoformulations and also for passive targeting [92]. Oleanolic-bioenhancer co-loaded chitosan nanocarriers have been found to preserve female fertility along with attenuating breast cancer cells, suggesting hormone independent BC therapy [93]. Hyaluronic Acid (HA) is a water-soluble polymer and is biodegradable. Its use as a drug delivery matrix can be helpful in specific targeting [94].

Ceramics

Ceramics can be readily synthesized with the desired shape, size, and porosity at ambient temperatures [95]. They may block the drug inside the pores. Ceramics most commonly used to make nanoparticles against breast cancer are carbonic apatite (a pH-sensitive material) and mesoporous silica. Mozar and Chaudhary (2015) formulated a nanoparticle of carbonic apatite which was loaded with an anticancer drug gemcitabine. Increased cytotoxicity was observed in breast cancer cells in comparison with gemcitabine alone [96]. These can be functionalized with folic acid [97], amino-β-cyclodextrin [98], CD44-Monoclonal Antibody [99], TRC-105 [100], folic acid [101], RGD peptide [102] or dsRNA-polyinosini--polycytidylic acid [103]. Mesoporous silica nanoparticles have also proved to be effective as a theranostic agent [104].

Carbon

Carbon has been widely used in formulating many nanocarriers. Carbon nanotubes, fullerenes or graphenes are great examples of carbon-based nanomaterials. They have advantages of ease of functionalization and they themselves can also be used against breast cancer. Carbon nanomaterials have certain disadvantages like lack of solubility, lower reproduction rate, and potential toxicity. Researches to reduce the toxicity of carbon nanomaterials are trending. Increase in functionalization of carbon nanomaterials may favor solubility as well as reduce toxicity, making them viable for administration and drug delivery [105, 106]. Carbon dot nanoparticles have been found to enhance the cellular uptake of siRNA (Small interfering RNA). Carbon dot can also act as a multifunctional nanocarrier as it also enables bioimaging [107]. Carbon-based nanohybrid dots (doped and surface passivated) are good for combined chemo- and photothermal therapy and they destroy breast cancer cells [108].

Lipids

Lipids are generally well-tolerated excipient. These are biocompatible, biodegradable and less toxic than other excipients, such as polymers. These have great potential to solubilize, encapsulate, and deliver the drug molecule and to achieve good bioavailability while avoiding side effects. Some lipid-based nanoformulations can also be well utilized for delivering the two drugs simultaneously [109]. The carriers can be made up of either phospholipids, cholesterol, triglycerides or any novel lipid. Some of the examples of lipid-based nanoparticles are liposomes, solid lipid nanoparticles, nanostructured lipid carriers, *etc*. Lipid-based nanoformulations may also be microemulsion or nanoemulsion with dispersed globules instead of particles. Zhang *et al.* (2016) utilized high-density lipoproteins (HDL-lipids) to encapsulate two hydrophobic drugs (because of the previous reports which mentioned the relation of an enhanced HDL uptake in human cancer). One was an anticancer agent (paclitaxel) while the other was an agent for the reversal of P-glycoprotein mediated multidrug resistance. There was a high drug encapsulation efficiency and also, anticancer efficiency was enhanced [110]. A novel Gemini like cationic lipid (GLCL) has also been used as a delivering agent to deliver siRNA by some researchers. In this lipid, two hydrophilic heads and two hydrophobic tails were bridged with a disulfide bond. They were also compared with those bridged with carbon-carbon bonds. They found disulfide bonded GLCL to be stronger and better against MCF-7 cells [111].

Proteins

Proteins as a nanomaterial are of great advantage in being biodegradable.

metabolizable, biocompatible, easy to prepare and are easily amenable to surface modification [112, 113]. Albumin is the most commonly used protein for making a nanoformulation against breast cancer and has really made a great impact. Albumin-bound paclitaxel nanoparticle has been approved for use at the clinical level and is a well-known marketed product. Albumin is a natural protein found in the blood circulation. Most commonly used albumins include: bovine serum albumin and human serum albumin. Human serum albumin nanoparticles can accumulate in the tumor bed which facilitates the trans-cytosis of free as well as bound plasma components to the endothelial cell surfaces *via* glycoprotein 60 receptors [114]. Other protein materials as a carrier to make nanoformulation for breast cancer are gelatin [115], zein [116], gliadin [113] *etc*.

DIFFERENT SURFACE MODIFICATIONS OF THE DELIVERY SYSTEM FOR TARGETING OF DRUGS

Targeting can be achieved either passively or actively. Despite many achievements in research for cancer therapies, the delivery systems like albumin nanoparticles are able to successfully achieve EPR effect, but lack active targeting. Targeting of the drug is carried out in two ways: passive targeting and active targeting (Fig. **1**).

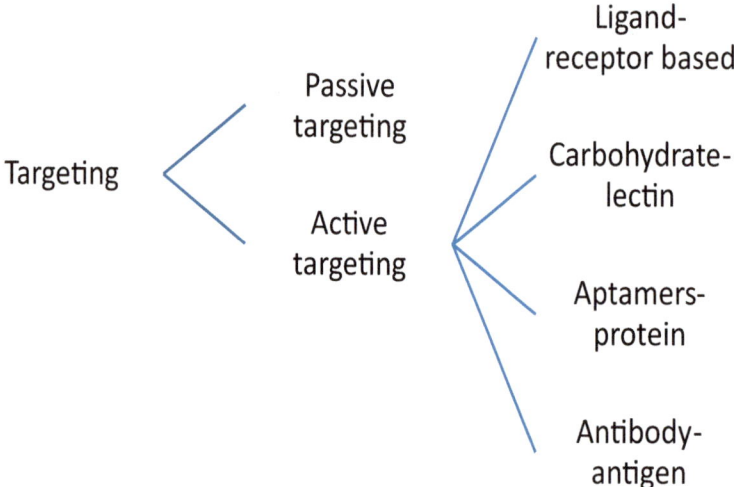

Fig. (1). Classification of targeting approaches of nanoformulations.

Passive targeting takes the advantage of tumor vasculature fenestrations and enhanced permeability and retention effect in solid tumors. PEGylation is the most widely used technique for passive targeting. It also increases the circulation time of nanoformulation in the blood [117]. The interest of this chapter is the active targeting of the drug. Some of the drugs may itself be a targeted therapy, such as monoclonal antibody or hormonal therapies. But some need to be designed in such a way that they can be targeted to the desired site. The active targeting (Fig. **2**) of the breast cancer tissue are described below.

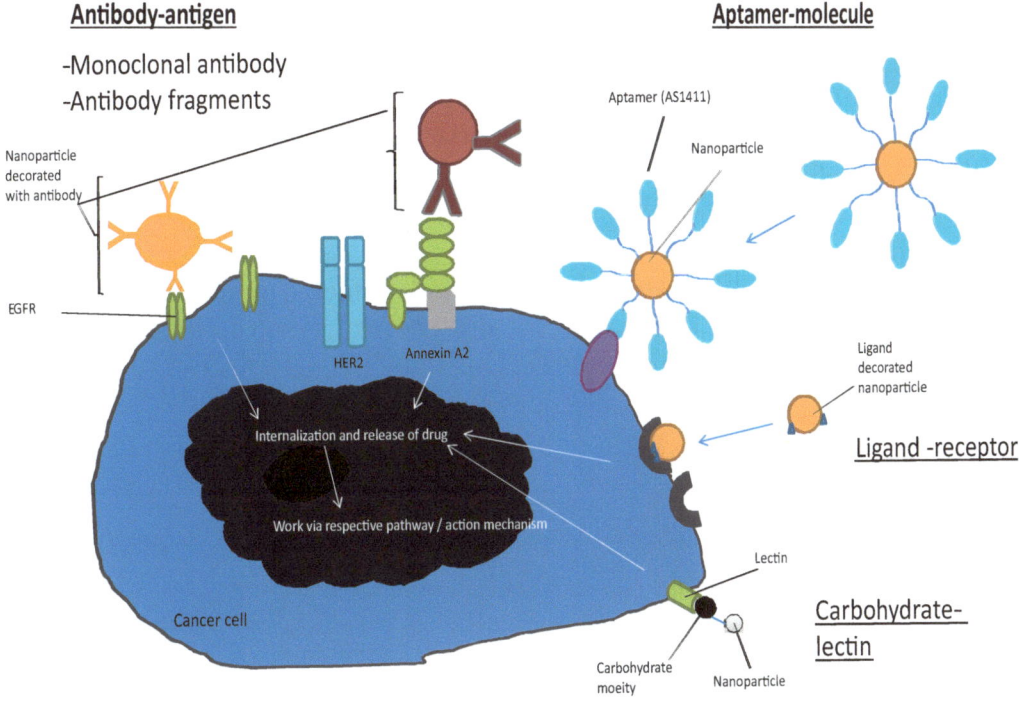

Fig. (2). Different approaches of active targeting of the drug through an activated surface modified nanoparticle.

Antibody-antigen Active Targeting

Antibodies can be conjugated to the nanosystems and targeting can be carried out without difficulty since certain antigens are over-expressed in case of breast cancer. These are the well-established and target-specific moieties in the area of breast cancer research [118]. These may be a monoclonal antibody or an antibody fragment. Monoclonal antibodies are the most effective tool for the treatment of cancer. Despite their cost, they are used in standard treatment regimes, because they have high selectivity level and positive toxicity profiles [109]. Among different potential targets, human epidermal growth factor receptor 2 (HER2), transferrin receptor, epidermal growth factor receptor (EGFR) are the most commonly investigated [119]. Few of such attempts are summarized below:

Anti HER2

HER2/neu genes are amplified in case of 25% invasive breast cancer cells but are minimally expressed in normal adult tissues [119]. Targeting HER2 has shown to be effective in HER2 positive tumors. Trastuzumab is a popular monoclonal antibody under the brand name Herceptin that has become a foundation for treating breast cancer. It is an FDA approved drug for treating breast cancer. Herceptin combined with iron oxide nanoparticles along with external magnetic field (Magnetic nanoparticles) can also have a good potential for human use [120]. Anti-HER2 antibodies can also be delivered using solid lipid nanoparticles simultaneously with paclitaxel [109] or polymerosomes [52].

SM51

SM51 is a humanized mouse monoclonal antibody which can bind to a membrane protein of about 230 kDa that is specifically overexpressed in breast and other cancer cells (hepatocellular, melanoma). This makes it a promising candidate for cancer targeted therapy [121, 122].

Other MABs/Antibody Fragments

Other antibodies are summarized in the table below (Table 1):

Table 1. Surface modification with different antibodies and their outcome.

Functionalized Nanoformulation	Strategy behind Functionalization with Specific MAB	Outcome	Reference
CD44-MAB functionalized Mesoporous Silica Nanoparticles	Overexpression of CD44 in multidrug resistant breast cancer cells	Increase in cytotoxicity More cellular uptake of Doxorubicin in resistant cells More drug retention in the tumor tissue	[99]
TRC-105 Monoclonal Antibody conjugated Hollow Mesoporous Silica Nanoparticles	TRC-105 binds to CD105 which is a marker for tumor angiogenesis and expressed on proliferating endothelial cells	3 times higher uptake than non-targeted one	[100]
VHH1-functionalized polymerosomes	VHH1 is anti-HER2 nanobody	Were able to target HER2 positive breast cancer cells	[52]

(Table 1) cont.....

Functionalized Nanoformulation	Strategy behind Functionalization with Specific MAB	Outcome	Reference
Anti-CD346 conjugated undecylenic acid thermally hydrocarbonized porous silica nanoparticles	Overexpression of CD346 in cancerous tissue	Inhibitory effect in CD346 positive MCF7 cells No difference in anti-proliferation impact of NPs on CD346 negative MDA-MB-231 cells	[123]
Anti-HB-EGF Fab' antibody conjugated lipidic nanoparticles	HB-EGF overexpressed in breast cancers	Highly taken up into MDA-MB-231 cells that overexpress HB-EGF	[124]
Tagged SWCNT conjugated with Endoglin/CD105 antibody	Ab conjugation (along with magnetic attraction) can reduce side effects associated with ineffective therapy	Enhanced therapeutic efficacy	[125]
Annexin A2 antibody conjugation over curcumin loaded PLGA nanoparticles	Annexin A2 overexpressed in breast cancer cells	Increased uptake of nanoparticles in highly metastatic breast cancer cells Inhibition of neoangiogenesis	[126]

Aptamer-Molecules

"Aptamers" is an invented term that is derived from the latin word "aptus", which means "to fit". Aptamers are the single-stranded oligonucleotide (RNA or DNA) having the ability to select specific targets, bind to their molecular target, for instance, proteins and destroy them. These are non-immunogenic. Moreover, since they are smaller in size, this property allows the specific entry into the cell [127]. Aptamers possess numerous advantages over antibody-drug conjugate. These include:

- Cost of production is low
- Equal or superior specificity and affinity for their molecular targets
- Small size of aptamers makes them more efficient for permeation to the cells
- Less immunogenic in comparison to antibodies
- Stable under a wide range of temperature and pH
- Resistant to chemical degradation
- Characterization and medication easier [128]

A lot of attempts have been tried to target breast cells using different aptamer types. Some of them are briefly described below:

AS1411

AS1411 aptamer is a guanosine-rich targeted DNA aptamer. Nucleolin is overexpressed in most of the cancers. Some attempts have been tried to check its effectiveness in breast cancer cells by functionalizing nanocarrier surface. One such example is functionalization of triblock polymer (loaded with doxorubicin) with this aptamer along with folate (for dual targeting) and checking for the potentiality. The approach enhanced the targeting efficiency and cellular uptake and a high drug payload to MCF-7 cells. Other such examples are mentioned in Table **2** [129].

EpCAM Aptamers

EpCAM (Epithelial cell adhesion molecules) are generally overexpressed in solid tumors (up to 800-fold), but are weakly expressed in normal epithelial cells (on basolateral gap junctions, making it inaccessible to drugs). Overexpression of EpCAM has been observed in approximately 98% of primary breast cancers and is also linked with poor prognosis. It is not just found in abundance in cancer cells but is also distributed across epithelial cancer cell membrane. It also marks tumor stem cells. Thus, EpCAM can be regarded as a cancer stem cell biomarker which is also been reported [130, 131].

Thioaptamer

The plasma membrane of metastatic breast cancer cells overexpresses a membrane protein, CD44. Thioaptamers are the kind of aptamers that bind specifically to the hyaluronic acid binding domain (HABD) of this membrane protein, *i.e.* CD44. CD44 targeting strategy has shown to be a powerful strategy and thioaptamer is a precious tool because of its specificity to HABD of CD44 [132].

Other Aptamers

SsDNA aptamer SRZ1 was an aptamer found by Song *et al.* (2015). In their study, they generated ten potential aptamers after multi-pool selection. Out of these, SRZ1 had the maximum and specific binding ability to 4T1 cells [133]. Few other examples are TSA1, anti-mucin1, 5TR1 *etc.*

Table 2. Different aptamers and the cells targeted with outcome.

Aptamer Taken	Approach	Drug	Cells (In Vitro) and Model for In Vivo	Result/Conclusion of the Study	Reference
AS1411	Aptamer and folate functionalized triblock polymer	Doxorubicin	MCF7	Enhanced targeting efficiency and cellular uptake. High drug payload (due to triblock)	[129]
AS1411	Aptamer conjugated gold nanospheres	-	MDA-MB-231 MCF7	Selectivity for tumour cells. Inhibition of tumour growth	[134]
AS1411	Aptamer-nanoparticle conjugate	Vinorelbine	MDA-MB-231	Enhanced cytotoxicity on nucleolin overexpressed cells	[135]
DNA Aptamer (Total DNA Aptamer)	Aptamer-modified-polymeric micelles	Paclitaxel	SK-BR-3	More cytotoxic in comparison to free paclitaxel. Micelles enhanced the binding ability of aptamer moiety at physiologic temperature	[136]
AS1411	Aptamer stabilized gold nanoparticles	Doxorubicin or AZD8055	MCF7	Increased reduction in cell viability in breast cancer cells	[137]
AS1411	Aptamer and DOX nanoparticles	Doxorubicin	MCF7S and MCF7R. For in vivo, MCF cells injected subcutaneously in mice	Effective accumulation of the drug to the tumor tissue. Nucleolin mediated endocytosis. Reversal of DOX resistance. Inhibition of tumor growth and less toxicity to the other tissues	[138]
EpCAM	PEI-Aptamer-SiRNA nanocomplex	SiRNA	MCF-7	Cytotoxicity and enhanced targeting ability on EpCAM overexpressing cells	[130]

(Table 2) cont.....

Aptamer Taken	Approach	Drug	Cells (In Vitro) and Model for In Vivo	Result/Conclusion of the Study	Reference
EpCAM	Aptamer conjugated PEG-PLGA nanopolymerosomes	Doxorubicin	MCF7	Efficient cell uptake and internalization More cytotoxic towards MCF7 in comparison to non-targeted polymerosomes	[139]
TSA 14	Aptamer modified PEGylated liposome	Doxorubicin	TUBO cells Female BALB mice injected in tumor cells	High targeting efficiency Enhanced cyto-toxicity by aptamer modification Aptamer-PL-Dox also inhibited tumor growth in the mice	[128]
SRZ1	Aptamer-functionalized (dotap: dope) liposomes	Doxorubicin	4T1 cells	Suppressed tumor growth Increased the survival rate of 4T1 bearing mice	[133]
Thioaptamer	Thioaptamer modified PEG-PAMAM (Dendrimer 5 generation)	miRNA	MDA-MB-231 MCF7 Cells injected in BALB/c mice	Thioaptamer enhanced the accumulation of nanoparticles to the breast cancer cells No impairment to the normal tissues	[132]
Anti-mucin1	Aptamer conjugated Chitosan nanoparticles	Docetaxel and siRNA	SKBR3	Decreased cell viability Reduced the genetic expression of IGF-1R, STAT3 and VEGF	[140]
5TR1	Aptamer modified with biotin CPG and Conjugated with drug	Doxorubicin	MDA-MB-231	More effective on tumor growth inhibition compared to free drug	[141]

Lectin-Carbohydrate

Carbohydrates are not only the building blocks of a living cell or a part of our diet but have wider applications. One of those applications includes utilizing it for drug delivery. Glycosylation is the process of the attachment of oligosaccharide chains covalently to lipids or proteins stepwise [142]. Glycosylation of the drug carrier can lead to a promising modified delivery system for breast cancer treatment [143]. Sugar receptors are the membrane components of many cells and are called lectins. Endogenous lectins are found on many cells and carry out various biological functions, act as specific receptors and play a role in mediating endocytosis [144]. These receptors can bind carbohydrates. All through malignant transformation, many molecular changes occur in a cell. Glycosylation of glycolipids and glycoproteins is just one such molecular transformation. This abnormal glycosylation of cancerous tissue accompanies the expression of various surface binding lectin receptors that possess high affinity for the ligands with surface carbohydrate molecules. This has become a base for finding the application of carbohydrates to target specific cancerous cells and deliver the anticancer drugs to the cancerous tissue [143]. Some of the attempts for targeting to breast cancer cells include:

Fucose

One of the important glycosylation types in cancer is fucosylation. Its alteration has been implicated in malignant transformation or metastasis of several cancer types. Approximately, 13 different fucosyltransferases have been identified. Expression of FUT8 (fucosyltransferase 8) was found to be linked with poor prognosis in breast cancer, which is highly upregulated in TGFβ-induced epithelial-mesenchymal transition (EMT) and is associated with migratory and invasive ability of aggressive breast carcinoma cell lines. It has also been demonstrated that overexpression of FUT8 stimulates EMT, whereas its knockdown suppresses the invasiveness of breast carcinoma cells that are highly aggressive [142]. *Ex vivo* evaluation of fucose decorated solid lipid nanoparticles (loaded with methotrexate) have shown augmented cellular internalization of the nanoparticles and higher cytotoxicity compared to the nanoparticle not decorated with fucose in breast cancer cells (MCF-7). *In vivo* evaluation showed efficient tumor targeting with minimal secondary drug distribution in other organs in comparison to that of a free drug [145].

Glucose

Some breast cancer cells have an overexpressed Glucose transporter membrane protein (GLUT1) and exhibit Warburg effect characteristics. Upon decorating magnetic nanoparticles with glucose, Venturelli *et al.* (2016) found a higher glucose uptake by MDA-MB-231 cells (mesenchymal-like cell line) in comparison to MCF7 (epithelial-like cell line) at lower glucose concentration [146]. Surface decoration of paclitaxel-loaded polymeric micelles with glucose enhanced its anti-cancer performance upto 14.1 fold in case of MDA-MB-231 cells and up to 1.6 fold in case of MCF-7 cells [147]. Glucose functionalized mesoporous silica nanoparticles loaded with γ-secretase inhibitors also showed promising results in breast cancer targeting, where functionalization with glucose enhanced the uptake in MDA-MB-231 cells more than MCF-10 (normal mammary epithelial) cells. Internalization of non-functionalized nanoparticles was almost up to the same degree in both cell lines (cancer and healthy) [148].

Mannose

Mannose is mainly utilized for macrophage targeting. Tumor-associated macrophages (TAMs) have been found to play a role in the invasion, proliferation, and survival of tumor cell including metastasis to local as well as distant sites. The infiltration of TAMs has been correlated with growth, metastasis and the poor prognosis in many human carcinomas, including breast cancers. Therefore, these represent an appealing target strategy for cancer (including breast) therapy. Reports suggest that TAMs possesses an elevated expression of certain membrane receptors such as mannose receptors and scavenger receptors which can be exploited to facilitate the drug by modifying the suitable delivery system using either a mannose derivative or an anti-mannose-receptor nanobody. So far, we could find a single study which utilized mannose for breast cancer targeting. Ye *et al.* (2016) synthesized amphiphilic heptamannosylated β-cyclodextrin to form nanoparticles. Multivalent mannose functionalized nanoparticles showed promising results in breast cancer targeting where mannose functionalization improved the inhibiting capability of nanoparticles against MDA-MB-231 cells with minimum side effects [149].

Ligand-Receptor

Vitamin-based Ligand Targeting

The principal advantage of using vitamins as a targeting medium is that these are inexpensive, non-immunogenic and non-toxic [150]. The most commonly used vitamins for targeting breast cancer are folic acid and biotin. However, few studies have also utilized other vitamins.

Vitamin H (Biotin)

Biotin is a form of the vitamin that is soluble in water and has one of the important roles as a micronutrient, like having a role in cell growth, signal transduction *etc*. Its internalization into the cells is *via* 'sodium-dependent multivitamin transporter' present on the cell surface. Most importantly, this transporter is highly expressed in the tumor cells. This high expression is to meet the demand of biotin for the rapid growth of tumors. Biotinylation of the delivery system is one of the logical strategies in order to fulfill the desired need of affinity. It can be a great and promising strategy to target the tumor cells that highly express these receptors. Most common breast cancers targeted using biotin is MCF-7. Biotin modification showed rapid internalization of bufalin loaded chitosan nanoparticles to MCF-7 cells in comparison to non-modified nanoparticles [151]. Guo *et al*. (2015) designed an approach based on Poly (Active Pharmaceutical Ingredient) strategy (PAPI strategy) *i.e.*, polycondensation of API or its derivative with similar bioactivity as monomer form of that API. The API was directly incorporated into the polymeric backbone instead of encapsulating it in a polymer. They formulated its nanoparticles and surface functionalized with biotin-PEG, thus making, biotin-PEG-PCDA nanoparticles and compared them against PEG-PCDA nanoparticles. They found biotin functionalized nanoparticles to be highly effective against EMT6 breast cancer cells *in vitro* and *in vivo*. Their result validated biotin in active targeting. A possible mechanism is binding to the cell surface and enhanced uptake *via* receptor-mediated endocytosis [152].

Vitamin B_9 (Folic Acid)

Folic Acid or folate, also known as Vitamin B_9 is known to play an important role in many biosynthetic mechanisms like nucleic acid metabolism (for example, synthesis of DNA and RNA), prevention of changes in DNA, and production of amino acid. Folate is notably required for the DNA replication during cell division and cell proliferation. This also includes cancer advanced stages and is also critical for the '1-carbon pathway', a key initiating step in the synthesis of nucleotide precursors as building blocks for DNA synthesis in the S-phase of the cell cycle. Cancer cells express high surface levels of folate receptors due to enormous folate requirements. Normal cells represent a significantly lower amount of this receptor [153]. Thus, using folate as a ligand is often conjugated with nanoparticles to target cancer cells. Folate receptors have high-affinity membrane folate binding proteins, which enable them to rapidly bind and be internalized by the process of endocytosis or through a hypothetical pathway involving endocytosis proposed for targeted delivery [154]. Banu *et al*. (2015) reported that MDA-MB-231 cells contain a number of folate receptors than MCF-7 cells [155]. Below are the various attempts that have been used to target breast cancer cells using this strategy and have shown promising results (Table **3**).

Table 3. Different folic acid based investigations.

Nanoformulation	Drug	Cells Targeted	Reference
Folate conjugated α-linolenic acid nanoemulsion	Doxorubicin	MCF-7	[156]
FA-conjugated- D-α-tocopheryl- PEG 1000 succinate decorated MTX conjugated Nanoparticles	Methotrexate	MCF-7	[157]
FA- conjugated Pluronic Micelles	Doxorubicin	MCF-7 and MCF-7/MDR	[28]
Curcumin polyvinyl pyrrolidone-conjugate(CurP) conjugated with Selenium nanoparticles further decorated with Folic Acid-Chitosan (forming Core shell Nanoparticles)	Doxorubicin	MCF-7	[158]
FA anchored Poly(d,l-lactide-co-glycolide) PLGA nanoparticles	Saquinavir	MCF-7	[159]
FA conjugated poly(l-γ-glutamyl glutamine) nanoparticles	Docetaxel	MCF-7, 4T1	[160]
FA conjugated core-shell micelles	Doxorubicin and SiRNA	MCF-7/ADR	[161]
FA-PEG-TiO$_2$ nanoparticles	Curcumin and Salvianolic	MCF-7, MDA-MB-231	[162]
Nanocrystals of paclitaxel and iron oxide co-encapsulated within F.A. functionalized lipid nanoparticle (low density lipoprotein mimicking nanoparticle)	Paclitaxel	MCF-7	[163]
FA conjugated gold nanorods	Cisplatin	4T1	[70]
FA conjugated polymeric gold nanoparticles	Doxorubicin	MDA-MB-231, MCF-7	[155]
FA conjugated silk fibroin nanocarriers	Doxorubicin	MDA-MB-231	[154]
PLGA-PEG-folate conjugate	Disulfiram	MCF-7	[164]
F.A. functionalized micelles with imaging dye	Orlistat	MDA-MB-231	[165]
Folate decorated human serum albumin nanoparticles	Hydroxycamptotecin	MCF-7	[166]
Folate-decorated-three star blockpolymer (nanomicelleplexes)	SiRNA and Doxorubicin	MCF-7	[167]
Folate terminated DOX polyrotaxanes along with dequalinium	Doxorubicin	MCF-7/ADR	[168]
Folate modified Lipid Polymer Hybrid Nanoparticles	Paclitaxel	EMT6	[169]
F.A. conjugated Bovine Serum Albumin nanocapsule	Radiotherapy ($^{125/131}$I)	MDA-MB-231	[170]

(Table 3) cont.....

Nanoformulation	Drug	Cells Targeted	Reference
F.A. attached liquid crystalline Nanoparticles	Docetaxel and Cisplatin	MDA-MB-231	[171]
Cholesterol-PEG$_{1000}$ - F.A.	Docetaxel	4T1	[172]
F.A. decorated dual functional nanomicelle	Doxorubicin	4T1.2, MCF-7, NCI/ADR-RES	[173]
Folate attached Nanoparticles based on BSA and Alginate-cysteine	Tamoxifen	MCF-7	[174]
Folate-decorated- albumin stabilized Silver Nanoparticles	-	MCF-7	[175]
Folate conjugated Mesoporous Silica Nanoparticles	γ-secreatase inhibitor	MDA-MB-231	[97]
Folic acid armed Mesoporous Silica Nanoparticles	Quercetin	MDA-MB-231, MCF-7	[101]
Folate modified Chitosan nanoparticles	Curcumin	MCF-7	[176]
Folic acid modified zinc oxide nanosheets	Doxorubicin	MDA-MB-231	[177]

Vitamin A

All-trans retinoic acid and its isomers are active metabolites of Vitamin A, which not only participate in a variety of functions but also useful for cancer treatment and prevention. The anti-cancer effect of all-trans retinoic acid is mainly because of its ability to activate retinoic acid receptors, which with these receptors, form heterodimers and consequently regulate the variety of gene expression, thereby inducing tumor cell differentiation, apoptosis, and cell growth arrest. Although all-trans retinoic acid alone is not sufficient to provide a therapeutic effect, combining it with another systemic chemotherapeutic agent may result in moderate responses in metastatic breast cancers. Johansson *et al.* (2013) reported the role of retinoic acid receptor alpha (high expression) in tamoxifen (a hormonal anti-breast cancer therapeutic agent) and suggested that the receptor retinoic acid alpha can be a potential target for estrogen receptor alpha-positive patients of breast cancer treated with an adjuvant tamoxifen [178]. Zhang *et al.* (2016) conjugated retinal over pH-sensitive micelles, which showed an enhanced anti-tumor efficacy by enhanced significant tumor senescence [179].

Hyaluronic Acid

Hyaluronic acid is a natural hydrophilic polysaccharide and is biocompatible, biodegradable, non-toxic and non-immunogenic in nature. It is anionic and possesses a chemical structure suitable for functionalization. The use of hyaluronic acid lies in its capability to bind specifically to cluster of differentiation 44 (CD44; which is a surface protein and principal cell surface receptor for hyaluronic acid) and RHAMM (receptor for hyaluran-mediated mobility) which are over-expressed in many cancer cell types. Coating a nano-delivery system with hyaluronic acid provides a "stealth" layer which not only targets these receptors but also may improve the uptake of drug and prevent its protein adsorption and opsonization. Aggarwal *et al.* (2017) coated lapatinib nanocrystals with hyaluronic acid to target CD44. They found higher cytotoxicity against MDA-MB-231 and 4T1 cells (cell lines for triple negative) which was assumed to be because of the active binding of the hyaluronic acid to CD44. There was also higher cellular uptake, higher apoptosis and disruption of cellular membrane potential. There was a magnificent therapeutic outcome at very low dose in 4T1 induced Xenograft model. Elzoghby *et al.* (2017) also found potential positive results against Ehrlich ascites tumor-induced model and as a targeted therapy for hormone-dependent breast cancer [180, 181].

Amino Acid

L-type amino acid transporters (LAT1, SLC7A5) are found to be abundant in many cancer types including breast cancers. The expression of LAT-1 is enhanced in response to estradiol, which activates estrogen receptor in breast cancer cells. A heterodimeric complex is formed after LAT-1 binds with a heavy chain of 4F2 cell surface antigen (CD98) *via* a disulfide bond, thus maintaining transportability by LAT-1. It preferentially transports large branched and aromatic neutral amino acids in a Na^+-independent manner, including L-leucine, L-isoleucine and L-phenylalanine. The free α-amino and α-carboxyl groups are the key components of LAT substrates. Based on the high expression of LAT1 in breast tumors, LAT1 inhibitors can be utilized to enhance the anti-tumor efficacy of a chemotherapeutic agent. An amino acid modified nanoparticle is a very good strategy. Li *et al.* (2016) utilized glutamate and conjugated them with nanoparticles to target LAT-1 [182, 183]. As per a study by Feng *et al.* (2014), modification with amino acids (lysine, aspartic acid, and valine) not only prevented the selenium nanoparticles aggregation but also enhanced the bioactivity [184].

Protein

Proteins have been utilized majorly as a potential nanocarrier. But few proteins can be utilized even as a targeting moiety. Human serum albumin has been utilized as a ligand because of its compatibility with the serum [185]. Under cellular stress conditions, as in the case of tumor tissue which is growing, albumin is taken as a source of amino acids and energy. The secreted protein, acidic and rich in cysteine protein (SPARC) binds native albumin and certain antibodies which are directed against gp60. This protein (SPARC) is found to be in a higher level in case of tumor tissue in comparison to healthy organs. Moreover, upon various tumor cell lines, albumin binding proteins are found to be expressed [186]. Overexpression of the transferrin receptor is the basis for the use of transferrin. Levels of transferring receptors are reported to be higher in the neoplastic cells that have a high metastatic potential. Transferrin is a glycoprotein (80 kDa) is available both as a human protein and as a recombinant version. It has low immunogenicity [187]. Lactoferrin is an iron-binding glycoprotein, cationic in nature and is naturally found in mammalian milk, mucosal secretion, and neutrophil granules. Lf itself has shown to possess anti-breast cancer property. Moreover, its receptor, *i.e.* LDL receptor is found to be overexpressed in breast cancer cells. Thus, its use as a ligand among proteins is another appealing moiety [116]. Ferritin is an iron storage protein and its utilization is based on the scavenger receptor class A member 5 (SCARA5) and TfR for L-ferritin and H-ferritin respectively. Ferritin can be selectively taken by the human breast cancer cells (MCF-7 cell line) *via* SCARA5 receptors [188]. Table **4** depicts the utilization of various proteins as a surface modifying agent for breast cancer.

Table 4. Various proteins used as a targeting ligand for breast cancer.

Protein	Conjugated to/Decorated Over	Drug	Outcome	Reference
Human Serum Albumin	Arginine-capped-Magnetite NPs	Paclitaxel	No side effect on the viability of cells	[185]
Human Serum Albumin	PL-PEG-Single Walled Carbon nanotubes	Paclitaxel	Greater Inhibition of MCF-7 cancer cells Increased drug efficiency (due to SWCNT mediated internalization)	[189]
Human Serum Albumin	N-hydroxy succinimide (NHS)-functionalized Microbubbles	Paclitaxel	Possibility of Early diagnosis Enhanced generation of ultrasound signal Ability of drug delivery to the preferred site (MCF-7 xenograft model) Increase in the stability in blood circulation	[114]
Bovine Serum Albumin	Copper nanoparticle	-	Suppression of viability of cancer cells (MDA-MB-231)	[78]

(Table 4) cont.....

Protein	Conjugated to/Decorated Over	Drug	Outcome	Reference
Bovine-α-lactalbumin	BLA conjugated to zinc oxide nanostructure	-	Enhanced toxicity in 2 breast cancer cell lines (MCF-7 and MDA-MB-231) Minimum toxicity to normal cells Enhanced anti-proliferative activity	[190]
Transferrin (incorporated into lipid bilayers)	PLGA nanoparticles	7-αAPTADD (Aromatase inhibitors)	Enhancement of aromatase inhibition activity (in SKBR3 cells)	[187]
Transferrin	PLGA nanoparticles	Paclitaxel	Greater anti-proliferative activity with transferring conjugation in MCF-7/Adr cells	[191]
Lactoferrin	Zein nanospheres	Exemestane and luteolin codelivery	Enhanced cytotoxicity against MCF-7 and 4T1 cells Enhanced targeting properties and internalization	[116]
Ferritin	PLGA nanoparticle	Paclitaxel	Endowed nanoparticles with targeting ability	[188]

Peptide

Use of peptide in drug targeting as a highly specific carrier or targeting moiety is structurally simple, synthetically diverse and nonantigenic [192]. Below are the most common peptides used for breast cancer targeting:

LHRH

Luteinizing hormone-releasing hormone (LHRH) is a decapeptide hormone and the LHRH receptors are highly expressed in many tumor cells such as breast, ovary cancer cells. These receptors are present in fewer amounts over the normal cells. So, this can be used as a moiety to target LHLH positive breast cancer cells. Dadras *et al.* (2016) conjugated them over polymeric nanocarriers (theranostic nanoparticles), the VEGF mRNA level expression was reduced by 83% in breast cancer cells (MCF-7) in comparison to normal cells [193]. Recently, Hu *et al.* (2018) conjugated them over PEG-coated magnetite nanoparticles and there was an enhancement in the uptake of nanoparticles by triple negative breast cancer cells [194].

RGD Peptide

$\alpha_v\beta_3$ receptor is also found to be overexpressed in some cancer cells including breast cancer cells which could be effectively and selectively recognized by arginylglycylaspartic acid (RGD) peptide. Among different breast cancer cells, this receptor is overexpressed in MDA-MB-231 and MDA-MB-435 cells while their expression is low in MCF-7 breast cancer cells. Wu *et al.* (2016) used RGD as a functionalization ligand and functionalized it over Mesoporous Silica Nanoparticles loaded with Arsenic Trioxide for triple negative breast cancer cells and it showed an improved cellular uptake [89]. Recently, this peptide has been conjugated over stealth liposomes and positive results have been reported compared to non-targeted [195].

TMT Peptide

TMT stands for tumor metastasis targeting. TMT peptides have been found to bind specifically to a series of a highly metastatic tumor while it does not bind to the non-metastatic cell lines. Hence, it holds a potential target for metastatic tumors. When conjugated to PEG-PCL nano micelles, necrosis rate was increased to 65% compared to nontargeted nano micelles (33%) and control (8%) [196].

Other Peptides

Other peptides include: GE11, L-peptide, TfR specific-7-peptide and Valreopeptide, which are listed in the table below (Table **5**).

Table 5. Different peptide functionalization over nanoparticles and their outcomes.

Formulation	Functionalized with/Targeting Moiety	Outcome	Reference
Poly(ethylene oxide)-poly(ester) micelles; PBCL cores	P18-4	Enhancement of cellular uptake due to the presence of P14-4	[197]
Hyaluronic acid-paclitaxel-Micelles	E-selectin binding peptide-PEG-1-octadecylamine	Improved drug selectivity (paclitaxel) Increased accumulation of payload Inhibition of tumor growth	[198]

(Table 5) cont.....

Formulation	Functionalized with/Targeting Moiety	Outcome	Reference
Micellar nanoparticles (loaded with aminoflavone)	GE11 peptide of 12 amino acids (targeting EGFR)	Enhanced uptake and strong inhibition of growth in triple negative breast cancer cells	[199]
Liposomal doxorubicin	L-peptide	High efficiency; minimum adverse effect	[200]
Core shell nanoparticles (siRNA)	Tfr specific-7-peptide	More efficient than non-targeted	[201]
Core shell nanoparticles (siRNA and paclitaxel co-delivery)	Valreopeptide	Higher intracellular accumulation and vascular endothelial growth factor downregulation	[202]

Miscellaneous

Targeting potential of N-acetyl glucosamine was found to be comparable to that of folate in two types of breast cancer cells (MCF-7 and MDA-MB-231). This was illustrated by Kumar *et al.* (2017) [203]. Bharti *et al.* (2017) functionalized synthetic somatostatin analogue over liposomes (because of the overexpression of somatostatin receptor in breast cancer cells). They found that the suppression of tumor growth *in vivo* in MDA-MB-231 xenograft model, suppressed angiogenesis and suppressed tumor invasion, enhanced circulation time and enhanced efficacy [204]. He *et al.* (2017) functionalized polymeric nanoparticles with bisphosphonate for treating bone metastatic breast cancer. The reason for using bisphosphonate as a functionalizing agent is that they have high affinity for bone and its uptake in bone metastatic lesion is greater in comparison to healthy bone tissue. They found 4-fold higher delivery of drug to the bone metastatic lesions than healthy bones (when administered intravenous in MDA-MB-231 induced mice) [205].

NANOFORMULATIONS AT CLINICAL LEVEL

Abraxane® (Albumin-bound paclitaxel, also called nab-paclitaxel) is a well-known nanoformulation at a clinical level. Caelyx® and Myocet® are the trade names of another nanoformulations containing liposomal doxorubicin, which has found to reduce the cardiotoxicity of doxorubicin.

RECENT CLINICAL TRIALS

Sites such as clinicaltrial.gov were utilized for finding out the current status of nanoformulations in clinical trials. Table **6** shows few of the recent clinical trials.

PEGylated liposomal doxorubicin is being analyzed in combination with cyclophosphamide followed by docetaxel prior to surgery under phase IV trial. There is also another treatment arm (which receives cyclophosphamide, epirubicin, and docetaxel. The study started in December 2016 and is estimated to be completed in 2021 (Cancer Institute, China). A monotherapy of Pegylated liposomal doxorubicin for breast neoplasms failed in the phase IV trials. The study was terminated in 2009 either due to unacceptable toxicity or unknown reason. A study (ongoing) at the fourth hospital of Hebei Medical University which is expected to be completed in December 2018, combines Doxorubicin liposome injection with pirarubicin and cyclophosphamide. Genexol-PM® is a paclitaxel-loaded polymeric micelle nanoformulation without cremophor EL. It was launched in the Korean market for breast cancer in February 2007. The phase IV trial at a Korean hospital was started in 2009. Result/ current status of the trial is unknown [206].

After countless studies, only a few targeted formulations are able to reach the stage of clinical trials, which indicates that a lot more has to be done in this direction and the complex systems have to be understood better for improved clinical outcomes.

Table 6. Recent clinical trials of targeted therapy for breast cancer treatment.

Intervention	Nanoformulation	Breast Cancer Type	Phase	Start Date	Expected Completion Date	Study Location
DS-8201a	Antibody-drug conjugate	Advanced solid tumors (including breast cancer – HER2 overexpressed)	I/II	Aug 2015 (I) Aug 2017 (II)	Sept 2019 (I) Feb 2020 (II)	Japan, United States US, Belgium, France, Italy, Japan, Korea, Spain, U.K. (95 study locations)
Trastuzumab, Atezolizumab and Pertuzumab (combination)	Targeted therapy (MABs)	HER2 positive metastatic breast cancer (CNS metastases)	II	Feb 21, 2018	Feb 2020	Dana-Farber Cancer Institute, U.S.
Nab-Paclitaxel	Nanoparticle encapsulated paclitaxel	Metastatic breast cancer	II	July 2011	Terminated because of low recruitment	GBG Forschungs GmbH, Germany
Abraxane	Nanoparticle encapsulated paclitaxel	HER2 negative high risk breast cancer	III	April 2013	Oct, 2025	Australia, Germany, Italy, Singapore and Spain (67 study locations)

(Table 6) cont.....

Intervention	Nanoformulation	Breast Cancer Type	Phase	Start Date	Expected Completion Date	Study Location
Myocet® as 2nd line (continuous v/s intermittent cycles)	Non-PEGylated liposomal doxorubicin	HER2/neu Neg metastatic breast cancer	III	Nov 2010	Oct 2019	BOOG study centre, Netherland

CHALLENGES

The major challenge in development of breast cancer lies in the proper understanding of the disease and its heterogeneity. Understanding the relation between a patient's tumor and the actual behavior of nanomedicine is another challenge. Pre-selection of patients who are likely to respond to a particular nanoformulation is another challenge. The development or exploitation of animal models that are clinically relevant and which would optimize dose, dosing schedules, properties and behavior of nanomedicine *in vivo* is also important. Moreover, clinical efficiency is not sufficient for the acceleration of its development at commercial level. Technical and cost challenges at scale-up level can either delay or necessitate further investment for the industry [207]. Thus, personalized medicine, which is now catching up, may be the answer to such therapy.

RECENT PATENTS

Table 7 is a summary of various nanoformulations that have been recently patented.

Table 7. Various recent formulations patented with (one of the) application as anti-breast cancer treatment.

Patent Number	Invention	Some Positive Outcomes of Nanoformulation	Reference
KR101875809B1	Repebody anti-cancer protein drug conjugate	Reduced the tumor volume in MDA-MB-468 gen model. Liver toxicity or nephrotoxicity did not appeared	[208]
US9974750B1	Ifflaionic acid nanopaticles	Effective in inhibiting MCF-7 breast cancer cells	[209]
US10028988B1	*Nuxia oppositifolia* nanoparticles	Effective in inhibiting MCF-7 breast cancer cells	[210]
US9789146B1	*Adansonia digitata* nanoparticles	IC_{50}=64.7 µl (against MCF-7 breast cancer cells)	[211]

(Table 7) cont.....

Patent Number	Invention	Some Positive Outcomes of Nanoformulation	Reference
CN107412196B	Orlistat nanosphere	Showed inhibition in MCF-7 cells	[212]
US9988276B2	Reduced graphene oxide synthesized from seed extract of *Nigella sativa*	IC_{50}=2.67 μl (against MCF-7 breast cancer cells)	[213]
KR101851470B1	Quercetin containing nanoformulation (MPEG-PLA-Qu nanoparticles)	Suppressed growth of cancer tissues	[214]
KR101743399B1	PEG-Triphenylphosphonium conjugate (self-assembling to form nanoparticles)	Selective targeting to mitochondria Increase in drug absorption	[215]

DISCUSSION

Targeting is a very important aspect in the field of breast cancer research. Targeting is the only strategy which can help in avoiding the side effect associated with the drug. Moreover, it also increases the efficacy and potency of the drug. A nanoparticle is usually surface decorated so that the specific targeting is achieved. For active targeting, monoclonal antibodies, aptamers or ligand are most researched (as per broad classification). Among different ligands, folate is the most extensively researched ligand. The choice of the targeting moiety is largely dependent on the type of breast cancer research in question. Hormonal therapies do not work on ER+ type of breast cancer. Similarly, for targeting moieties with which the surface modification is carried out for the purpose of targeting may not be completely cell specific to a particular organ. Folate receptors are more expressed in triple negative cells in comparison to ER+.

Based on a marker, the targeting ligand recognizes the breast cancer cell and is internalized *via* a suitable pathway. Internalization and fate are dependent on other factors, such as delivery system and material with which the nanomedicine is formulated.

Being incorporated in a nanocarrier can avoid several limitations associated with the drug. Choice of the best nanocarrier with the drug is important. There are many kinds of delivery systems, such as nanoparticles, micelles, dendrimers, liposomes, *etc.* each possessing their own special feature. This feature becomes advantageous for many anti-cancer drugs to solve the issue related to them, such as solubility, bioavailability, release, *etc.* Among different delivery system, magnetic-based delivery system is one of the most important one. This delivery system has an advantage of targeting *via* aid of external magnetic field.

Material for the delivery system is another important consideration, as it is linked with the drug stability, as it must not undergo any chemical reaction with the drug (should be compatible), are usually inert (nowadays the synergistic action is also considered), or it should diminish the drawback associated with the drug. Several materials that have been utilized to make a nanomedicine are polymers, lipids, proteins, metals, *etc.*

Many delivery systems have been invented and investigated for the breast cancer targeting. Few are patented; some of them have entered clinical trials but not most. Every research has a negative aspect which encourages further research and there is no single drug to target generic breast cancer, irrespective of its sub-classification.

Most of the target based work is supported by the overexpression of suitable protein or receptor on breast cancer cells. However, combining all the above targeting strategies, we can say that the breast cancer cells over express many such antigens/receptors which are not expressed in higher amount in case of normal tissue. There is a need to identify one specific marker and one most specific targeting agent that can work on every kind of breast cancer cells and effectively target the drug; giving an overall survival rate near to 100% and can be utilized at any stage of breast cancer cells.

CONCLUSION

Surface modification for active targeting requires overexpression of a suitable biomarker (receptor/antigen) on a particular breast cancer cell. Being overexpressed on a cancer cell, the target-specific nanoparticles move more to the target site rather than moving to the normal cells. So far, several strategies have been designed; several materials have been used and highly investigated. But there is still a gap in breast cancer research because of which the nanoformulations are neither so much in the market nor have they reached the clinical trials as much as conventional formulations have and much has yet to be done. However, there is the plethora of positive literatures for some nanoformulations, such as folate-conjugated nanoparticles, biotin conjugated nanoformulations, aptamer-conjugated nanoparticles *etc.,* which are definitely promising for future. If a drug is successfully targeted to the breast cancer cells without having to reach the normal cells, we will be able to overcome the adverse effects of the drugs which is made possible with nanoformulations. Through this, we hope that one day a multitargeted nanoformulation is developed, which is able to successfully target all types of breast cancer (irrespective of their classification and sub-classification), and is also comparatively inexpensive and available across the world. Till the time that this is achieved, we must keep exploring.

CONSENT FOR PUBLICATION

Not applicable.

CONFLICT OF INTEREST

The authors declare no conflict of interest, financial or otherwise.

ACKNOWLEDGEMENTS

We would like to acknowledge Poonam Parashar, Malti Arya and Chandra Bhushan Tripathi (Research Scholars at Department of Pharmaceutical Sciences, Babasaheb Bhimrao Ambedkar University, Lucknow) who gave more than 4 years of their time to cancer research and shared their experiences with us.

REFERENCES

[1]   World Health Organization.. Breast Cancer [cited 31st August 2018] Available at: http://www.who.int/cancer/prevention/diagnosis-screening/breast-cancer/en/

[2]   Malhotra GK, Zhao X, Band H, Band V. Histological, molecular and functional subtypes of breast cancers. Cancer Biol Ther 2010; 10(10): 955-60.
[http://dx.doi.org/10.4161/cbt.10.10.13879] [PMID: 21057215]

[3]   Curigliano G, Criscitiello C. Successes and limitations of targeted cancer therapy in breast cancer. Prog Tumor Res 2014; 41: 15-35.
[http://dx.doi.org/10.1159/000355896] [PMID: 24727984]

[4]   Drost R, Jonkers J. Opportunities and hurdles in the treatment of BRCA1-related breast cancer. Oncogene 2014; 33(29): 3753-63.
[http://dx.doi.org/10.1038/onc.2013.329] [PMID: 23955079]

[5]   Tannock IF. Conventional cancer therapy: promise broken or promise delayed? Lancet 1998; 351 (Suppl. 2): SII9-SII16.
[http://dx.doi.org/10.1016/S0140-6736(98)90327-0] [PMID: 9606361]

[6]   Verhoef MJ, Rose MS, White M, Balneaves LG. Declining conventional cancer treatment and using complementary and alternative medicine: a problem or a challenge? Curr Oncol 2008; 15 (Suppl. 2): s101-6.
[http://dx.doi.org/10.3747/co.v15i0.281] [PMID: 18769571]

[7]   Buzdar AU. Preoperative chemotherapy treatment of breast cancer: A review. Cancer 2007; 110(11): 2394-407.
[http://dx.doi.org/10.1002/cncr.23083] [PMID: 17941030]

[8]   Draganescu M, Carmocan C. Hormone therapy in breast cancer. Chirurgia (Bucharest, Romania: 1990) 2017; 112(4): 413-7.
[http://dx.doi.org/10.21614/chirurgia.112.4.413]

[9]   Ernst B, Anderson KS. Immunotherapy for the treatment of breast cancer. Curr Oncol Rep 2015; 17(2): 5.
[http://dx.doi.org/10.1007/s11912-014-0426-9] [PMID: 25677118]

[10] Geng D, Sun D, Zhang L, Zhang W. The therapy of gefitinib towards breast cancer partially through reversing breast cancer biomarker arginine. Afr Health Sci 2015; 15(2): 594-7.
[http://dx.doi.org/10.4314/ahs.v15i2.36] [PMID: 26124808]

[11] Molina MA, Codony-Servat J, Albanell J, Rojo F, Arribas J, Baselga J. Trastuzumab (herceptin), a humanized anti-Her2 receptor monoclonal antibody, inhibits basal and activated Her2 ectodomain cleavage in breast cancer cells. Cancer Res 2001; 61(12): 4744-9.
[PMID: 11406546]

[12] Rimm D, Carvajal-Hausdorf D, Harbeck N, *et al*. Abstract P2-09-07: Low levels of HER2 extracellular domain (ECD) compared to intracellular domain (ICD) in NeoALTTO may segregate benefit from lapatinib and trastuzumab in breast cancer. AACR 2018.

[13] Wang N, Wang K, Liu YT, Song FX. Everolimus plus endocrine *vs* endocrine therapy in treatment advanced ER+, HER2- breast cancer patients: A meta-analysis. Curr Probl Cancer 2018; S0147-0272(18)30247-2.
[PMID: 30220603]

[14] Messina C, Cattrini C, Buzzatti G, *et al*. CDK4/6 inhibitors in advanced hormone receptor-positive/HER2-negative breast cancer: a systematic review and meta-analysis of randomized trials. Breast Cancer Res Treat 2018; 172(1): 9-21.
[http://dx.doi.org/10.1007/s10549-018-4901-0] [PMID: 30054831]

[15] Ahmadzada T, Reid G, McKenzie DR. Fundamentals of siRNA and miRNA therapeutics and a review of targeted nanoparticle delivery systems in breast cancer. Biophys Rev 2018; 10(1): 69-86.
[http://dx.doi.org/10.1007/s12551-017-0392-1] [PMID: 29327101]

[16] Storvold GL, Andersen TI, Perou CM, Frengen E. siRNA: a potential tool for future breast cancer therapy? Critical Reviews™ in Oncogenesis 2006; 12(1-2)

[17] Marta T, Luca S, Serena M, Luisa F, Fabio C. What is the role of nanotechnology in diagnosis and treatment of metastatic breast cancer? Promising scenarios for the near future. J Nanomater 2016; 2016: 16.
[http://dx.doi.org/10.1155/2016/5436458]

[18] He C, Cai P, Li J, *et al*. Blood-brain barrier-penetrating amphiphilic polymer nanoparticles deliver docetaxel for the treatment of brain metastases of triple negative breast cancer. Journal of Controlled Release: Official Journal of the Controlled Release Society 2017; 246: 98-109.
[http://dx.doi.org/10.1016/j.jconrel.2016.12.019]

[19] Rocha M, Chaves N, Báo S. Nanobiotechnology for breast cancer treatment. Breast cancer-from biology to medicine. InTech 2017; pp. 411-23.
[http://dx.doi.org/10.5772/66989]

[20] Krai J, Beckenkamp A, Gaelzer MM, *et al*. Doxazosin nanoencapsulation improves its *in vitro* antiproliferative and anticlonogenic effects on breast cancer cells. Biomed Pharmacother 2017; 94: 10-20.
[http://dx.doi.org/10.1016/j.biopha.2017.07.048] [PMID: 28750355]

[21] Goldman A, Kulkarni A, Kohandel M, *et al*. Rationally designed 2-in-1 nanoparticles can overcome adaptive resistance in cancer. ACS Nano 2016; 10(6): 5823-34.
[http://dx.doi.org/10.1021/acsnano.6b00320] [PMID: 27257911]

[22] Peiris PM, Deb P, Doolittle E, *et al*. Vascular targeting of a gold nanoparticle to breast cancer metastasis. J Pharm Sci 2015; 104(8): 2600-10.
[http://dx.doi.org/10.1002/jps.24518] [PMID: 26036431]

[23] Liang DS, Zhang WJ, Wang AT, Su HT, Zhong HJ, Qi XR. Treating metastatic triple negative breast cancer with CD44/neuropilin dual molecular targets of multifunctional nanoparticles. Biomaterials 2017; 137: 23-36.
[http://dx.doi.org/10.1016/j.biomaterials.2017.05.022] [PMID: 28528300]

[24] Zhou Z, Kennell C, Jafari M, *et al*. Sequential delivery of erlotinib and doxorubicin for enhanced triple negative breast cancer treatment using polymeric nanoparticle. Int J Pharm 2017; 530(1-2): 300-7.
[http://dx.doi.org/10.1016/j.ijpharm.2017.07.085] [PMID: 28778627]

[25] Uribe Madrid SI, Pal U, Kang YS, Kim J, Kwon H, Kim J. Fabrication of Fe(3)O(4)@mSiO(2) core-shell composite nanoparticles for drug delivery applications. Nanoscale Res Lett 2015; 10: 217.
[http://dx.doi.org/10.1186/s11671-015-0920-5] [PMID: 26034415]

[26] Zhu W, Lee SJ, Castro NJ, Yan D, Keidar M, Zhang LG. Synergistic effect of cold atmospheric plasma and drug loaded core-shell nanoparticles on inhibiting breast cancer cell growth. Sci Rep 2016; 6: 21974.
[http://dx.doi.org/10.1038/srep21974] [PMID: 26917087]

[27] Narayanan S, Mony U, Vijaykumar DK, Koyakutty M, Paul-Prasanth B, Menon D. Sequential release of epigallocatechin gallate and paclitaxel from PLGA-casein core/shell nanoparticles sensitizes drug-resistant breast cancer cells. Nanomedicine (Lond) 2015; 11(6): 1399-406.
[http://dx.doi.org/10.1016/j.nano.2015.03.015] [PMID: 25888278]

[28] Nguyen DH, Lee JS, Bae JW, et al. Targeted doxorubicin nanotherapy strongly suppressing growth of multidrug resistant tumor in mice. Int J Pharm 2015; 495(1): 329-35.
[http://dx.doi.org/10.1016/j.ijpharm.2015.08.083] [PMID: 26325307]

[29] Bahadori F, Topçu G, Eroğlu MS, Onyüksel H. A new lipid-based nano formulation of vinorelbine. AAPS PharmSciTech 2014; 15(5): 1138-48.
[http://dx.doi.org/10.1208/s12249-014-0146-3] [PMID: 24871553]

[30] Li H, Miteva M, Kirkbride KC, et al. Dual MMP7-proximity-activated and folate receptor-targeted nanoparticles for siRNA delivery. Biomacromolecules 2015; 16(1): 192-201.
[http://dx.doi.org/10.1021/bm501394m] [PMID: 25414930]

[31] Zhang J, Kinoh H, Hespel L, et al. Effective treatment of drug resistant recurrent breast tumors harboring cancer stem-like cells by staurosporine/epirubicin co-loaded polymeric micelles. J Control Release 2017; 264: 127-35.
[http://dx.doi.org/10.1016/j.jconrel.2017.08.025] [PMID: 28842317]

[32] Wang Z, Li X, Wang D, et al. Concurrently suppressing multidrug resistance and metastasis of breast cancer by co-delivery of paclitaxel and honokiol with pH-sensitive polymeric micelles. Acta Biomater 2017; 62: 144-56.
[http://dx.doi.org/10.1016/j.actbio.2017.08.027] [PMID: 28842335]

[33] Tang S, Meng Q, Sun H, et al. Dual pH-sensitive micelles with charge-switch for controlling cellular uptake and drug release to treat metastatic breast cancer. Biomaterials 2017; 114: 44-53.
[http://dx.doi.org/10.1016/j.biomaterials.2016.06.005] [PMID: 27842234]

[34] Sandhu PS, Kumar R, Beg S, et al. Natural lipids enriched self-nano-emulsifying systems for effective co-delivery of tamoxifen and naringenin: Systematic approach for improved breast cancer therapeutics. Nanomedicine (Lond) 2017; 13(5): 1703-13.
[http://dx.doi.org/10.1016/j.nano.2017.03.003] [PMID: 28343014]

[35] Elnaggar YS, El-Massik MA, Abdallah OY. Self-nanoemulsifying drug delivery systems of tamoxifen citrate: design and optimization. Int J Pharm 2009; 380(1-2): 133-41.
[http://dx.doi.org/10.1016/j.ijpharm.2009.07.015] [PMID: 19635537]

[36] Kamal MM, Nazzal S. Novel sulforaphane-enabled self-microemulsifying delivery systems (SFN-SMEDDS) of taxanes: Formulation development and in vitro cytotoxicity against breast cancer cells. Int J Pharm 2018; 536(1): 187-98.
[http://dx.doi.org/10.1016/j.ijpharm.2017.11.063] [PMID: 29195916]

[37] Anton N, Vandamme TF. Nano-emulsions and micro-emulsions: clarifications of the critical differences. Pharm Res 2011; 28(5): 978-85.
[http://dx.doi.org/10.1007/s11095-010-0309-1] [PMID: 21057856]

[38] Olov N, Bagheri-Khoulenjani S, Mirzadeh H. Combinational drug delivery using nanocarriers for breast cancer treatments: A review. J Biomed Mater Res A 2018; 106(8): 2272-83.
[http://dx.doi.org/10.1002/jbm.a.36410] [PMID: 29577607]

[39] Liu J, Li J, Liu N, *et al. In vitro* studies of phospholipid-modified PAMAM-siMDR1 complexes for the reversal of multidrug resistance in human breast cancer cells. Int J Pharm 2017; 530(1-2): 291-9.
[http://dx.doi.org/10.1016/j.ijpharm.2017.06.026] [PMID: 28619457]

[40] Xu X, Li Y, Lu X, Sun Y, Luo J, Zhang Y. Glutaryl polyamidoamine dendrimer for overcoming cisplatin-resistance of breast cancer cells. J Nanosci Nanotechnol 2018; 18(10): 6732-9.
[http://dx.doi.org/10.1166/jnn.2018.15502] [PMID: 29954488]

[41] Kavosi A, Hosseini Ghale Noei S, Madani S, *et al.* The toxicity and therapeutic effects of single-and multi-wall carbon nanotubes on mice breast cancer. Sci Rep 2018; 8(1): 8375.
[http://dx.doi.org/10.1038/s41598-018-26790-x] [PMID: 29849103]

[42] Ünlü A, Meran M, Dinc B, Karatepe N, Bektaş M, Güner FS. Cytotoxicity of doxrubicin loaded single-walled carbon nanotubes. Mol Biol Rep 2018; 45(4): 523-31.
[http://dx.doi.org/10.1007/s11033-018-4189-5] [PMID: 29797174]

[43] Wang Y, Kaur G, Chen Y, Santos A, Losic D, Evdokiou A. Bioinert anodic alumina nanotubes for targeting of endoplasmic reticulum stress and autophagic signaling: a combinatorial nanotube-based drug delivery system for enhancing cancer therapy. ACS Appl Mater Interfaces 2015; 7(49): 27140-51.
[http://dx.doi.org/10.1021/acsami.5b07557] [PMID: 26556288]

[44] Bulbake U, Doppalapudi S, Kommineni N, Khan W. Liposomal formulations in clinical use: an updated review. Pharmaceutics 2017; 9(2): 12.
[http://dx.doi.org/10.3390/pharmaceutics9020012] [PMID: 28346375]

[45] Chen X, Zhang Y, Tang C, *et al.* Co-delivery of paclitaxel and anti-survivin siRNA *via* redox-sensitive oligopeptide liposomes for the synergistic treatment of breast cancer and metastasis. Int J Pharm 2017; 529(1-2): 102-15.
[http://dx.doi.org/10.1016/j.ijpharm.2017.06.071] [PMID: 28642204]

[46] Sharma S, Rajendran V, Kulshreshtha R, Ghosh PC. Enhanced efficacy of anti-miR-191 delivery through stearylamine liposome formulation for the treatment of breast cancer cells. Int J Pharm 2017; 530(1-2): 387-400.
[http://dx.doi.org/10.1016/j.ijpharm.2017.07.079] [PMID: 28774852]

[47] Fan Y, Wang Q, Lin G, Shi Y, Gu Z, Ding T. Combination of using prodrug-modified cationic liposome nanocomplexes and a potentiating strategy *via* targeted co-delivery of gemcitabine and docetaxel for CD44-overexpressed triple negative breast cancer therapy. Acta Biomater 2017; 62: 257-72.
[http://dx.doi.org/10.1016/j.actbio.2017.08.034] [PMID: 28859899]

[48] Rajput S, Puvvada N, Kumar BN, *et al.* Overcoming Akt induced therapeutic resistance in breast cancer through siRNA and thymoquinone encapsulated multilamellar gold niosomes. Mol Pharm 2015; 12(12): 4214-25.
[http://dx.doi.org/10.1021/acs.molpharmaceut.5b00692] [PMID: 26505213]

[49] Johnsen KB, Gudbergsson JM, Skov MN, Pilgaard L, Moos T, Duroux M. A comprehensive overview of exosomes as drug delivery vehicles - endogenous nanocarriers for targeted cancer therapy. Biochim Biophys Acta 2014; 1846(1): 75-87.
[PMID: 24747178]

[50] Ha D, Yang N, Nadithe V. Exosomes as therapeutic drug carriers and delivery vehicles across biological membranes: current perspectives and future challenges. Acta Pharm Sin B 2016; 6(4): 287-96.
[http://dx.doi.org/10.1016/j.apsb.2016.02.001] [PMID: 27471669]

[51] Théry C, Zitvogel L, Amigorena S. Exosomes: composition, biogenesis and function. Nat Rev Immunol 2002; 2(8): 569-79.
[http://dx.doi.org/10.1038/nri855] [PMID: 12154376]

[52] Zou T, Dembele F, Beugnet A, *et al.* Nanobody-functionalized PEG-b-PCL polymersomes and their targeting study. J Biotechnol 2015; 214: 147-55.
[http://dx.doi.org/10.1016/j.jbiotec.2015.09.034] [PMID: 26433047]

[53] Sabzichi M, Hamishehkar H, Ramezani F, *et al.* Luteolin-loaded phytosomes sensitize human breast carcinoma MDA-MB 231 cells to doxorubicin by suppressing Nrf2 mediated signalling. Asian Pac J Cancer Prev 2014; 15(13): 5311-6.
[http://dx.doi.org/10.7314/APJCP.2014.15.13.5311] [PMID: 25040994]

[54] Starvaggi Cucuzza L, Motta M, Miretti S, Accornero P, Baratta M. Curcuminoid-phospholipid complex induces apoptosis in mammary epithelial cells by STAT-3 signaling. Exp Mol Med 2008; 40(6): 647-57.
[http://dx.doi.org/10.3858/emm.2008.40.6.647] [PMID: 19116450]

[55] Kong M, Hou L, Wang J, *et al.* Enhanced transdermal lymphatic drug delivery of hyaluronic acid modified transfersomes for tumor metastasis therapy. Chem Commun (Camb) 2015; 51(8): 1453-6.
[http://dx.doi.org/10.1039/C4CC08746A] [PMID: 25493296]

[56] Mirzaei H, Shakeri A, Rashidi B, Jalili A, Banikazemi Z, Sahebkar A. Phytosomal curcumin: A review of pharmacokinetic, experimental and clinical studies. Biomedecine & pharmacotherapie = Biomedecine & pharmacotherapie 2017; 85: 102-12.
[http://dx.doi.org/10.1016/j.biopha.2016.11.098]

[57] Mahmood S, Taher M, Mandal UK. Experimental design and optimization of raloxifene hydrochloride loaded nanotransfersomes for transdermal application. Int J Nanomedicine 2014; 9: 4331-46.
[PMID: 25246789]

[58] Bhavsar D, Subramanian K, Sethuraman S, Krishnan UM. 'Nano-in-nano' hybrid liposomes increase target specificity and gene silencing efficiency in breast cancer induced SCID mice. Eur J Pharm Biopharm 2017; 119: 96-106.
[http://dx.doi.org/10.1016/j.ejpb.2017.06.006] [PMID: 28600223]

[59] Zhou Z, Kennell C, Lee JY, Leung YK, Tarapore P. Calcium phosphate-polymer hybrid nanoparticles for enhanced triple negative breast cancer treatment *via* co-delivery of paclitaxel and miR-221/222 inhibitors. Nanomedicine (Lond) 2017; 13(2): 403-10.
[http://dx.doi.org/10.1016/j.nano.2016.07.016] [PMID: 27520723]

[60] Wan Y, Dai W, Nevagi RJ, Toth I, Moyle PM. Multifunctional peptide-lipid nanocomplexes for efficient targeted delivery of DNA and siRNA into breast cancer cells. Acta Biomater 2017; 59: 257-68.
[http://dx.doi.org/10.1016/j.actbio.2017.06.032] [PMID: 28655658]

[61] Dreaden EC, Kong YW, Morton SW, *et al.* Tumor-targeted synergistic blockade of MAPK and PI3K from a layer-by-layer nanoparticle. Clinical cancer research: An Official Journal of the American Association for Cancer Research 2015; 21(19): 4410-9.

[62] Hasan M, Leak RK, Stratford RE, Zlotos DP, Witt-Enderby PA. Drug conjugates-an emerging approach to treat breast cancer. Pharmacol Res Perspect 2018; 6(4): e00417.
[http://dx.doi.org/10.1002/prp2.417] [PMID: 29983986]

[63] Remant BK, Chandrashekaran V, Cheng B, *et al.* Redox potential ultrasensitive nanoparticle for the targeted delivery of camptothecin to HER2-positive cancer cells. Mol Pharm 2014; 11(6): 1897-905.
[http://dx.doi.org/10.1021/mp5000482] [PMID: 24779647]

[64] Laskar K, Faisal SM, Rauf A, Ahmed A, Owais M. Undec-10-enoic acid functionalized chitosan based novel nano-conjugate: An enhanced anti-bacterial/biofilm and anti-cancer potential. Carbohydr Polym 2017; 166: 14-23.
[http://dx.doi.org/10.1016/j.carbpol.2017.02.082] [PMID: 28385217]

[65] Natesan S, Ponnusamy C, Sugumaran A, Chelladurai S, Shanmugam Palaniappan S, Palanichamy R. Artemisinin loaded chitosan magnetic nanoparticles for the efficient targeting to the breast cancer.

International Journal of Biological Macromolecules 2017; 104(Pt B): 1853-9.
[http://dx.doi.org/10.1016/j.ijbiomac.2017.03.137]

[66]   Bruniaux J, Djemaa SB, Hervé-Aubert K, Marchais H, Chourpa I, David S. Stealth magnetic nanocarriers of siRNA as platform for breast cancer theranostics. Int J Pharm 2017; 532(2): 660-8.
[http://dx.doi.org/10.1016/j.ijpharm.2017.05.022] [PMID: 28506802]

[67]   Marino A, Battaglini M, De Pasquale D, Degl'Innocenti A, Ciofani G. Ultrasound-activated piezoelectric nanoparticles inhibit proliferation of breast cancer cells. Sci Rep 2018; 8(1): 6257.
[http://dx.doi.org/10.1038/s41598-018-24697-1] [PMID: 29674690]

[68]   Lee H, Dam DH, Ha JW, Yue J, Odom TW. Enhanced human epidermal growth factor receptor 2 degradation in breast cancer cells by lysosome-targeting gold nanoconstructs. ACS Nano 2015; 9(10): 9859-67.
[http://dx.doi.org/10.1021/acsnano.5b05138] [PMID: 26335372]

[69]   Eghtedari M, Liopo AV, Copland JA, Oraevsky AA, Motamedi M. Engineering of hetero-functional gold nanorods for the *in vivo* molecular targeting of breast cancer cells. Nano Lett 2009; 9(1): 287-91.
[http://dx.doi.org/10.1021/nl802915q] [PMID: 19072129]

[70]   Feng B, Xu Z, Zhou F, *et al.* Near infrared light-actuated gold nanorods with cisplatin-polypeptide wrapping for targeted therapy of triple negative breast cancer. Nanoscale 2015; 7(36): 14854-64.
[http://dx.doi.org/10.1039/C5NR03693C] [PMID: 26222373]

[71]   Esfandiari N, Arzanani MK, Soleimani M, Kohi-Habibi M, Svendsen WE. A new application of plant virus nanoparticles as drug delivery in breast cancer. Tumour Biol 2016; 37(1): 1229-36.
[http://dx.doi.org/10.1007/s13277-015-3867-3] [PMID: 26286831]

[72]   Esfandiari N, Arzanani MK, Koohi-Habibi M. The study of toxicity and pathogenicity risk of Potato Virus X/Herceptin nanoparticles as agents for cancer therapy. Cancer Nanotechnol 2018; 9(1): 1.
[http://dx.doi.org/10.1186/s12645-018-0036-6]

[73]   Targeting breast cancer with bio-inspired virus nanoparticles 2018. [cited 3rd Sep 2018]. http://archbreastcancer.com/index.php/abc/article/view/189

[74]   Lee J, Chatterjee DK, Lee MH, Krishnan S. Gold nanoparticles in breast cancer treatment: promise and potential pitfalls. Cancer Lett 2014; 347(1): 46-53.
[http://dx.doi.org/10.1016/j.canlet.2014.02.006] [PMID: 24556077]

[75]   Rao PV, Nallappan D, Madhavi K, Rahman S, Jun Wei L, Gan SH. Phytochemicals and biogenic metallic nanoparticles as anticancer agents. Oxid Med Cell Longev 2016; 2016: 3685671.
[http://dx.doi.org/10.1155/2016/3685671] [PMID: 27057273]

[76]   Loutfy SA, Al-Ansary NA, Abdel-Ghani NT, *et al.* Anti-proliferative activities of metallic nanoparticles in an *in vitro* breast cancer model. Asian Pac J Cancer Prev 2015; 16(14): 6039-46.
[http://dx.doi.org/10.7314/APJCP.2015.16.14.6039] [PMID: 26320493]

[77]   Azizi M, Ghourchian H, Yazdian F, Alizadehzeinabad H. Albumin coated cadmium nanoparticles as chemotherapeutic agent against MDA-MB 231 human breast cancer cell line. Artif Cells Nanomed Biotechnol 2018; 1-11.
[http://dx.doi.org/10.1080/21691401.2018.1436064] [PMID: 29426245]

[78]   Azizi M, Ghourchian H, Yazdian F, Dashtestani F, AlizadehZeinabad H. Cytotoxic effect of albumin coated copper nanoparticle on human breast cancer cells of MDA-MB 231. PLoS One 2017; 12(11): e0188639.
[http://dx.doi.org/10.1371/journal.pone.0188639] [PMID: 29186208]

[79]   Kamble S, Utage B, Mogle P, *et al.* Evaluation of curcumin capped copper nanoparticles as possible inhibitors of human breast cancer cells and angiogenesis: a comparative study with native curcumin. AAPS PharmSciTech 2016; 17(5): 1030-41.
[http://dx.doi.org/10.1208/s12249-015-0435-5] [PMID: 26729534]

[80]   Irace C, Misso G, Capuozzo A, *et al.* Antiproliferative effects of ruthenium-based nucleolipidic

nanoaggregates in human models of breast cancer *in vitro*: insights into their mode of action. Sci Rep 2017; 7: 45236.
[http://dx.doi.org/10.1038/srep45236] [PMID: 28349991]

[81] Laha D, Pramanik A, Chattopadhyay S. Folic acid modified copper oxide nanoparticles for targeted delivery in *in vitro* and *in vivo* systems. RSC Advances 2015; 5(83): 68169-78.
[http://dx.doi.org/10.1039/C5RA08110F]

[82] Praseetha Pk, Swathy Js, Sakthivel G. Targeted therapy for breast cancer cells by herbal drug formulations of iron oxide nanoparticles. Asian Journal of Pharmaceutical and Clinical Research 2016; 9(1): 347-53.

[83] He Y, Zhang L, Zhu D, Song C. Design of multifunctional magnetic iron oxide nanoparticles/mitoxantrone-loaded liposomes for both magnetic resonance imaging and targeted cancer therapy. Int J Nanomedicine 2014; 9: 4055-66.
[http://dx.doi.org/10.2147/IJN.S61880] [PMID: 25187709]

[84] Tomankova K, Polakova K, Pizova K, *et al*. In vitro cytotoxicity analysis of doxorubicin-loaded/superparamagnetic iron oxide colloidal nanoassemblies on MCF7 and NIH3T3 cell lines. Int J Nanomedicine 2015; 10: 949-61.
[http://dx.doi.org/10.2147/IJN.S72590] [PMID: 25673990]

[85] Bakhtiary Z, Saei AA, Hajipour MJ, Raoufi M, Vermesh O, Mahmoudi M. Targeted superparamagnetic iron oxide nanoparticles for early detection of cancer: Possibilities and challenges. Nanomedicine (Lond) 2016; 12(2): 287-307.
[http://dx.doi.org/10.1016/j.nano.2015.10.019] [PMID: 26707817]

[86] Mund R, Panda N, Nimesh S, Biswas A. Novel titanium oxide nanoparticles for effective delivery of paclitaxel to human breast cancer cells. J Nanopart Res 2014; 16(12): 2739.
[http://dx.doi.org/10.1007/s11051-014-2739-x]

[87] Lotfian H, Nemati F. Cytotoxic effect of TiO2 nanoparticles on breast cancer cell line (MCF-7). IIOAB J 2016; 7: 219-24.

[88] Gao Y, Chen K, Ma JL, Gao F. Cerium oxide nanoparticles in cancer. OncoTargets Ther 2014; 7: 835-40.
[http://dx.doi.org/10.2147/OTT.S62057] [PMID: 24920925]

[89] Ouyang Z, Mainali MK, Sinha N, *et al*. Potential of using cerium oxide nanoparticles for protecting healthy tissue during accelerated partial breast irradiation (APBI). Physica Medica: PM: An International Journal Devoted to the Applications of Physics to Medicine and Biology: Official Journal of the Italian Association of Biomedical Physics (AIFB) 2016; 32(4): 631-5.

[90] Boroumand Moghaddam A, Moniri M, Azizi S, *et al*. Eco-friendly formulated zinc oxide nanoparticles: induction of cell cycle arrest and apoptosis in the MCF-7 cancer cell line. Genes (Basel) 2017; 8(10): 281.
[http://dx.doi.org/10.3390/genes8100281] [PMID: 29053567]

[91] Bowerman CJ, Byrne JD, Chu KS, *et al*. Docetaxel-loaded PLGA nanoparticles improve efficacy in taxane-resistant triple-negative breast cancer. Nano Lett 2017; 17(1): 242-8.
[http://dx.doi.org/10.1021/acs.nanolett.6b03971] [PMID: 27966988]

[92] Natesan S, Sugumaran A, Ponnusamy C, Thiagarajan V, Palanichamy R, Kandasamy R. Chitosan stabilized camptothecin nanoemulsions: development, evaluation and biodistribution in preclinical breast cancer animal mode. International Journal of Biological Macromolecules 2017; 104(pt B): 1846-52.
[http://dx.doi.org/10.1016/j.ijbiomac.2017.05.127]

[93] Sharma M, Sharma S, Sharma V, *et al*. Oleanolic-bioenhancer coloaded chitosan modified nanocarriers attenuate breast cancer cells by multimode mechanism and preserve female fertility. Int J Biol Macromol 2017; 104(Pt A): 1345-58.
[http://dx.doi.org/10.1016/j.ijbiomac.2017.06.005] [PMID: 28591594]

[94] Zhao Y, Zhang T, Duan S, Davies NM, Forrest ML. CD44-tropic polymeric nanocarrier for breast cancer targeted rapamycin chemotherapy. Nanomedicine (Lond) 2014; 10(6): 1221-30.
[http://dx.doi.org/10.1016/j.nano.2014.02.015] [PMID: 24637218]

[95] Biswas AK, Islam MR, Choudhury ZS, Mostafa A, Kadir MF. Nanotechnology based approaches in cancer therapeutics. Advances in Natural Sciences: Nanoscience and Nanotechnology 2014; 5(4): 043001.

[96] Mozar FS, Chowdhury EH. Gemcitabine interacts with carbonate apatite with concomitant reduction in particle diameter and enhancement of cytotoxicity in breast cancer cells. Curr Drug Deliv 2015; 12(3): 333-41.
[http://dx.doi.org/10.2174/1567201812666150120153809] [PMID: 25600981]

[97] Wittig R, Rosenholm JM, von Haartman E, *et al.* Active targeting of mesoporous silica drug carriers enhances γ-secretase inhibitor efficacy in an in vivo model for breast cancer. Nanomedicine (Lond) 2014; 9(7): 971-87.
[http://dx.doi.org/10.2217/nnm.13.62] [PMID: 23898823]

[98] Zhang Q, Wang X, Li P-Z, *et al.* Biocompatible, uniform, and redispersible mesoporous silica nanoparticles for cancer-targeted drug delivery *in vivo*. Adv Funct Mater 2014; 24(17): 2450-61.
[http://dx.doi.org/10.1002/adfm.201302988]

[99] Wang X, Liu Y, Wang S, *et al.* CD44-engineered mesoporous silica nanoparticles for overcoming multidrug resistance in breast cancer. Appl Surf Sci 2015; 332: 308-17.
[http://dx.doi.org/10.1016/j.apsusc.2015.01.204]

[100] Chen F, Hong H, Shi S, *et al.* Engineering of hollow mesoporous silica nanoparticles for remarkably enhanced tumor active targeting efficacy. Sci Rep 2014; 4: 5080.
[http://dx.doi.org/10.1038/srep05080] [PMID: 24875656]

[101] Sarkar A, Ghosh S, Chowdhury S, Pandey B, Sil PC. Targeted delivery of quercetin loaded mesoporous silica nanoparticles to the breast cancer cells. Biochim Biophys Acta 2016; 1860(10): 2065-75.
[http://dx.doi.org/10.1016/j.bbagen.2016.07.001] [PMID: 27392941]

[102] Wu X, Han Z, Schur RM, Lu ZR. Targeted mesoporous silica nanoparticles delivering arsenic trioxide with environment sensitive drug release for effective treatment of triple negative breast cancer. ACS Biomater Sci Eng 2016; 2(4): 501-7.
[http://dx.doi.org/10.1021/acsbiomaterials.5b00398]

[103] Ultimo A, Giménez C, Bartovsky P, *et al.* Targeting innate immunity with dsRNA-conjugated mesoporous silica nanoparticles promotes antitumor effects on breast cancer cells. Chemistry 2016; 22(5): 1582-6.
[http://dx.doi.org/10.1002/chem.201504629] [PMID: 26641630]

[104] Milgroom A, Intrator M, Madhavan K, *et al.* Mesoporous silica nanoparticles as a breast-cancer targeting ultrasound contrast agent. Colloids Surf B Biointerfaces 2014; 116: 652-7.
[http://dx.doi.org/10.1016/j.colsurfb.2013.10.038] [PMID: 24269054]

[105] Casais-Molina ML, Cab C, Canto G, Medina J, Tapia A. Carbon nanomaterials for breast cancer treatment. J Nanomater 2018; 2018: 9.
[http://dx.doi.org/10.1155/2018/2058613]

[106] Mahanta S, Paul S. Bovine α-lactalbumin functionalized graphene oxide nano-sheet exhibits enhanced biocompatibility: A rational strategy for graphene-based targeted cancer therapy. Colloids Surf B Biointerfaces 2015; 134: 178-87.
[http://dx.doi.org/10.1016/j.colsurfb.2015.06.061] [PMID: 26196090]

[107] Kim S, Choi Y, Park G, Won C, Park Y-J, Lee Y, *et al.* Highly efficient gene silencing and bioimaging based on fluorescent carbon dots *in vitro* and *in vivo*. Nano Res 2017; 10(2): 503-19.
[http://dx.doi.org/10.1007/s12274-016-1309-1]

[108] Ardekani SM, Dehghani A, Hassan M, Kianinia M, Aharonovich I, Gomes VG. Two-photon excitation triggers combined chemo-photothermal therapy *via* doped carbon nanohybrid dots for effective breast cancer treatment. Chem Eng J 2017; 330: 651-62.
[http://dx.doi.org/10.1016/j.cej.2017.07.165]

[109] Büyükköroğlu G, Şenel B, Gezgin S, Dinh T. The simultaneous delivery of paclitaxel and Herceptin® using solid lipid nanoparticles: *in vitro* evaluation. J Drug Deliv Sci Technol 2016; 35: 98-105.
[http://dx.doi.org/10.1016/j.jddst.2016.06.010]

[110] Zhang F, Wang X, Xu X, Li M, Zhou J, Wang W. Reconstituted high density lipoprotein mediated targeted co-delivery of HZ08 and paclitaxel enhances the efficacy of paclitaxel in multidrug-resistant MCF-7 breast cancer cells. Eur J Pharm Sci 2016; 92: 11-21.
[http://dx.doi.org/10.1016/j.ejps.2016.06.017] [PMID: 27343697]

[111] Ma X-F, Sun J, Qiu C, *et al.* The role of disulfide-bridge on the activities of H-shape gemini-like cationic lipid based siRNA delivery. J Control Release 2016; 235: 99-111.
[http://dx.doi.org/10.1016/j.jconrel.2016.05.051] [PMID: 27242198]

[112] Jahanshahi M, Babaei Z. Protein nanoparticle: a unique system as drug delivery vehicles. Afr J Biotechnol 2008; 7(25): 4926-34.

[113] Lohcharoenkal W, Wang L, Chen YC, Rojanasakul Y. Protein nanoparticles as drug delivery carriers for cancer therapy. BioMed Res Int 2014; 2014: 180549.
[http://dx.doi.org/10.1155/2014/180549] [PMID: 24772414]

[114] Moon H, Yoon C, Lee TW, *et al.* Therapeutic ultrasound contrast agents for the enhancement of tumor diagnosis and tumor therapy. J Biomed Nanotechnol 2015; 11(7): 1183-92.
[http://dx.doi.org/10.1166/jbn.2015.2056] [PMID: 26307841]

[115] Jain AP. Development of novel docetaxel-loaded gelatin nanoparticles for intravenous application: Hemolytic activity, hematological study, and biodistribution profile or *in vivo* cancer study. International Journal of Green Pharmacy 2017; 11(03) [IJGP].

[116] El-Lakany SA, Elgindy NA, Helmy MW, Abu-Serie MM, Elzoghby AO. Lactoferrin-decorated vs PEGylated zein nanospheres for combined aromatase inhibitor and herbal therapy of breast cancer. Expert Opin Drug Deliv 2018; 15(9): 835-50.
[http://dx.doi.org/10.1080/17425247.2018.1505858] [PMID: 30067113]

[117] Kydd J, Jadia R, Velpurisiva P, Gad A, Paliwal S, Rai P. Targeting strategies for the combination treatment of cancer using drug delivery systems. Pharmaceutics 2017; 9(4): 46.
[http://dx.doi.org/10.3390/pharmaceutics9040046] [PMID: 29036899]

[118] Iwamoto N, Shimomura A, Tamura K, Hamada A, Shimada T. LC-MS bioanalysis of Trastuzumab and released emtansine using nano-surface and molecular-orientation limited (nSMOL) proteolysis and liquid-liquid partition in plasma of Trastuzumab emtansine-treated breast cancer patients. J Pharm Biomed Anal 2017; 145: 33-9.
[http://dx.doi.org/10.1016/j.jpba.2017.06.032] [PMID: 28648785]

[119] Bazak R, Houri M, El Achy S, Kamel S, Refaat T. Cancer active targeting by nanoparticles: a comprehensive review of literature. J Cancer Res Clin Oncol 2015; 141(5): 769-84.
[http://dx.doi.org/10.1007/s00432-014-1767-3] [PMID: 25005786]

[120] Rasaneh S, Dadras MR. The possibility of using magnetic nanoparticles to increase the therapeutic efficiency of Herceptin antibody. Biomed Tech (Berl) 2015; 60(5): 485-90.
[http://dx.doi.org/10.1515/bmt-2014-0192] [PMID: 26146093]

[121] Li B, Wang H, Zhang D, *et al.* Construction and characterization of a high-affinity humanized SM5-1 monoclonal antibody. Biochem Biophys Res Commun 2007; 357(4): 951-6.
[http://dx.doi.org/10.1016/j.bbrc.2007.04.039] [PMID: 17451647]

[122] Ma X, Cheng Z, Jin Y, *et al.* SM5-1-conjugated PLA nanoparticles loaded with 5-fluorouracil for targeted hepatocellular carcinoma imaging and therapy. Biomaterials 2014; 35(9): 2878-89.

[http://dx.doi.org/10.1016/j.biomaterials.2013.12.045] [PMID: 24411331]

[123] Shahbazi M-A, Shrestha N, Mäkilä E, Araújo F, Correia A, Ramos T, *et al.* A prospective cancer chemo-immunotherapy approach mediated by synergistic CD326 targeted porous silicon nanovectors. Nano Res 2015; 8(5): 1505-21.
[http://dx.doi.org/10.1007/s12274-014-0635-4]

[124] Okamoto A, Asai T, Kato H, *et al.* Antibody-modified lipid nanoparticles for selective delivery of siRNA to tumors expressing membrane-anchored form of HB-EGF. Biochem Biophys Res Commun 2014; 449(4): 460-5.
[http://dx.doi.org/10.1016/j.bbrc.2014.05.043] [PMID: 24853808]

[125] Al Faraj A, Shaik AP, Shaik AS. Magnetic single-walled carbon nanotubes as efficient drug delivery nanocarriers in breast cancer murine model: noninvasive monitoring using diffusion-weighted magnetic resonance imaging as sensitive imaging biomarker. Int J Nanomedicine 2014; 10: 157-68.
[http://dx.doi.org/10.2147/IJN.S75074] [PMID: 25565811]

[126] Mukerjee A, Ranjan AP, Vishwanatha JK. Targeted nanocurcumin therapy using Annexin A2 antibody improves tumor accumulation and therapeutic efficacy against highly metastatic breast cancer. J Biomed Nanotechnol 2016; 12(7): 1374-92.
[http://dx.doi.org/10.1166/jbn.2016.2240] [PMID: 29336533]

[127] Keefe AD, Pai S, Ellington A. Aptamers as therapeutics. Nat Rev Drug Discov 2010; 9(7): 537-50.
[http://dx.doi.org/10.1038/nrd3141] [PMID: 20592747]

[128] Moosavian SA, Abnous K, Badiee A, Jaafari MR. Improvement in the drug delivery and anti-tumor efficacy of PEGylated liposomal doxorubicin by targeting RNA aptamers in mice bearing breast tumor model. Colloids Surf B Biointerfaces 2016; 139: 228-36.
[http://dx.doi.org/10.1016/j.colsurfb.2015.12.009] [PMID: 26722819]

[129] Lale SV, R G A, Aravind A, Kumar DS, Koul V. AS1411 aptamer and folic acid functionalized pH-responsive ATRP fabricated pPEGMA-PCL-pPEGMA polymeric nanoparticles for targeted drug delivery in cancer therapy. Biomacromolecules 2014; 15(5): 1737-52.
[http://dx.doi.org/10.1021/bm5001263] [PMID: 24689987]

[130] Subramanian N, Kanwar JR, Athalya PK, *et al.* EpCAM aptamer mediated cancer cell specific delivery of EpCAM siRNA using polymeric nanocomplex. J Biomed Sci 2015; 22(1): 4.
[http://dx.doi.org/10.1186/s12929-014-0108-9] [PMID: 25576037]

[131] Gilboa-Geffen A, Hamar P, Le MTN, *et al.* Gene knockdown by EpCAM aptamer–siRNA chimeras suppresses epithelial breast cancers and their tumor-initiating cells. Mol Cancer Ther 2015; 14(10): 2279-91.
[http://dx.doi.org/10.1158/1535-7163.MCT-15-0201-T] [PMID: 26264278]

[132] Fan W, Wang X, Ding B, *et al.* Thioaptamer-conjugated CD44-targeted delivery system for the treatment of breast cancer *in vitro* and *in vivo*. J Drug Target 2016; 24(4): 359-71.
[http://dx.doi.org/10.3109/1061186X.2015.1077850] [PMID: 26299192]

[133] Song X, Ren Y, Zhang J, *et al.* Targeted delivery of doxorubicin to breast cancer cells by aptamer functionalized DOTAP/DOPE liposomes. Oncol Rep 2015; 34(4): 1953-60.
[http://dx.doi.org/10.3892/or.2015.4136] [PMID: 26238192]

[134] Malik MT, O'Toole MG, Casson LK, *et al.* AS1411-conjugated gold nanospheres and their potential for breast cancer therapy. Oncotarget 2015; 6(26): 22270-81.
[http://dx.doi.org/10.18632/oncotarget.4207] [PMID: 26045302]

[135] Zhou W, Zhou Y, Wu J, *et al.* Aptamer-nanoparticle bioconjugates enhance intracellular delivery of vinorelbine to breast cancer cells. J Drug Target 2014; 22(1): 57-66.
[http://dx.doi.org/10.3109/1061186X.2013.839683] [PMID: 24156476]

[136] Nguyen KT, Le DV, Do DH, Le QH. Development of chitosan graft pluronic ® F127 copolymer nanoparticles containing DNA aptamer for paclitaxel delivery to treat breast cancer cells. Advances in

Natural Sciences: Nanoscience and Nanotechnology 2016; 7(2): 025018.

[137] Latorre A, Posch C, Garcimartín Y, *et al*. DNA and aptamer stabilized gold nanoparticles for targeted delivery of anticancer therapeutics. Nanoscale 2014; 6(13): 7436-42.
[http://dx.doi.org/10.1039/C4NR00019F] [PMID: 24882040]

[138] Liu J, Wei T, Zhao J, *et al*. Multifunctional aptamer-based nanoparticles for targeted drug delivery to circumvent cancer resistance. Biomaterials 2016; 91: 44-56.
[http://dx.doi.org/10.1016/j.biomaterials.2016.03.013] [PMID: 26994877]

[139] Alibolandi M, Ramezani M, Sadeghi F, Abnous K, Hadizadeh F. Epithelial cell adhesion molecule aptamer conjugated PEG-PLGA nanopolymersomes for targeted delivery of doxorubicin to human breast adenocarcinoma cell line *in vitro*. Int J Pharm 2015; 479(1): 241-51.
[http://dx.doi.org/10.1016/j.ijpharm.2014.12.035] [PMID: 25529433]

[140] Jafari R, Majidi Zolbanin N, Majidi J, *et al*. Anti-mucin1 aptamer-conjugated chitosan nanoparticles for targeted co-delivery of docetaxel and IGF-1R siRNA to SKBR3 metastatic breast cancer cells. Iranian Biomedical Journal 2018.

[141] Luo S, Wang S, Luo N, Chen F, Hu C, Zhang K. The application of aptamer 5TR1 in triple negative breast cancer target therapy. J Cell Biochem 2018; 119(1): 896-908.
[http://dx.doi.org/10.1002/jcb.26254] [PMID: 28671278]

[142] Tu C-F, Wu M-Y, Lin Y-C, Kannagi R, Yang R-B. FUT8 promotes breast cancer cell invasiveness by remodeling TGF-β receptor core fucosylation. Breast Cancer Res 2017; 19(1): 111.
[http://dx.doi.org/10.1186/s13058-017-0904-8] [PMID: 28982386]

[143] Jain K, Kesharwani P, Gupta U, Jain NK. A review of glycosylated carriers for drug delivery. Biomaterials 2012; 33(16): 4166-86.
[http://dx.doi.org/10.1016/j.biomaterials.2012.02.033] [PMID: 22398205]

[144] Monsigny M, Roche A-C, Midoux P, Mayer R. Glycoconjugates as carriers for specific delivery of therapeutic drugs and genes. Adv Drug Deliv Rev 1994; 14(1): 1-24.
[http://dx.doi.org/10.1016/0169-409X(94)90003-5]

[145] Garg NK, Singh B, Jain A, *et al*. Fucose decorated solid-lipid nanocarriers mediate efficient delivery of methotrexate in breast cancer therapeutics. Colloids Surf B Biointerfaces 2016; 146: 114-26.
[http://dx.doi.org/10.1016/j.colsurfb.2016.05.051] [PMID: 27268228]

[146] Venturelli L, Nappini S, Bulfoni M, *et al*. Glucose is a key driver for GLUT1-mediated nanoparticles internalization in breast cancer cells. Sci Rep 2016; 6: 21629.
[http://dx.doi.org/10.1038/srep21629] [PMID: 26899926]

[147] Moretton MA, Bernabeu E, Grotz E, Gonzalez L, Zubillaga M, Chiappetta DA. A glucose-targeted mixed micellar formulation outperforms Genexol in breast cancer cells. Eur J Pharm Biopharm 2017; 114: 305-16.
[http://dx.doi.org/10.1016/j.ejpb.2017.02.005] [PMID: 28192249]

[148] Mamaeva V, Niemi R, Beck M, *et al*. Inhibiting notch activity in breast cancer stem cells by glucose functionalized nanoparticles carrying gamma-secretase inhibitors. Molecular Therapy: The Journal of the American Society of Gene Therapy 2016; 24(5): 926-36.

[149] Ye Z, Zhang Q, Wang S, *et al*. Tumour-targeted drug delivery with mannose-functionalized nanoparticles self-assembled from amphiphilic beta-cyclodextrins. Chemistry 2016; 22(43): 15216-21.
[http://dx.doi.org/10.1002/chem.201603294] [PMID: 27714939]

[150] Thanki K, Kushwah V, Jain S. Recent advances in tumor targeting approaches.Targeted Drug Delivery:Concepts and Design: CRS. Springer 2015; p. 51.

[151] Tian X, Yin H, Zhang S, *et al*. Bufalin loaded biotinylated chitosan nanoparticles: an efficient drug delivery system for targeted chemotherapy against breast carcinoma. European Journal of Pharmaceutics and Biopharmaceutics: Official Journal of Arbeitsgemeinschaft fur Pharmazeutische Verfahrenstechnik eV 2014; 87(3): 445-53.

[http://dx.doi.org/10.1016/j.ejpb.2014.05.010]

[152] Lv L, Guo Y, Shen Y, *et al.* Intracellularly degradable, self-assembled amphiphilic block copolycurcumin nanoparticles for efficient *in vivo* cancer chemotherapy. Advanced Healthcare Materials 2015; 4(10): 1496-501.

[153] Bahrami B, Mohammadnia-Afrouzi M, Bakhshaei P, *et al.* Folate-conjugated nanoparticles as a potent therapeutic approach in targeted cancer therapy. Tumour Biol 2015; 36(8): 5727-42.
[http://dx.doi.org/10.1007/s13277-015-3706-6] [PMID: 26142733]

[154] Subia B, Chandra S, Talukdar S, Kundu SC. Folate conjugated silk fibroin nanocarriers for targeted drug delivery. Integrative Biology: Quantitative Biosciences from Nano to Macro 2014; 6(2): 203-14.
[http://dx.doi.org/10.1039/C3IB40184G]

[155] Banu H, Sethi DK, Edgar A, *et al.* Doxorubicin loaded polymeric gold nanoparticles targeted to human folate receptor upon laser photothermal therapy potentiates chemotherapy in breast cancer cell lines. J Photochem Photobiol B 2015; 149: 116-28.
[http://dx.doi.org/10.1016/j.jphotobiol.2015.05.008] [PMID: 26057021]

[156] Tripathi CB, Parashar P, Arya M, *et al.* QbD-based development of α-linolenic acid potentiated nanoemulsion for targeted delivery of doxorubicin in DMBA-induced mammary gland carcinoma: *in vitro* and *in vivo* evaluation. Drug Deliv Transl Res 2018; 8(5): 1313-34.
[http://dx.doi.org/10.1007/s13346-018-0525-5] [PMID: 29748834]

[157] Junyaprasert VB, Dhanahiranpruk S, Suksiriworapong J, Sripha K, Moongkarndi P. Enhanced toxicity and cellular uptake of methotrexate-conjugated nanoparticles in folate receptor-positive cancer cells by decorating with folic acid-conjugated d-α-tocopheryl polyethylene glycol 1000 succinate. Colloids Surf B Biointerfaces 2015; 136: 383-93.
[http://dx.doi.org/10.1016/j.colsurfb.2015.09.013] [PMID: 26433645]

[158] Yu B, Li X, Zheng W, Feng Y, Wong Y-S, Chen T. pH-responsive cancer-targeted selenium nanoparticles: a transformable drug carrier with enhanced theranostic effects. J Mater Chem B Mater Biol Med 2014; 2(33): 5409-18.
[http://dx.doi.org/10.1039/C4TB00399C]

[159] Singh R, Kesharwani P, Mehra NK, Singh S, Banerjee S, Jain NK. Development and characterization of folate anchored Saquinavir entrapped PLGA nanoparticles for anti-tumor activity. Drug Dev Ind Pharm 2015; 41(11): 1888-901.
[http://dx.doi.org/10.3109/03639045.2015.1019355] [PMID: 25738812]

[160] Tavassolian F, Kamalinia G, Rouhani H, *et al.* Targeted poly (L-γ-glutamyl glutamine) nanoparticles of docetaxel against folate over-expressed breast cancer cells. Int J Pharm 2014; 467(1-2): 123-38.
[http://dx.doi.org/10.1016/j.ijpharm.2014.03.033] [PMID: 24680951]

[161] Wu Y, Zhang Y, Zhang W, Sun C, Wu J, Tang J. Reversing of multidrug resistance breast cancer by co-delivery of P-gp siRNA and doxorubicin *via* folic acid-modified core-shell nanomicelles. Colloids Surf B Biointerfaces 2016; 138: 60-9.
[http://dx.doi.org/10.1016/j.colsurfb.2015.11.041] [PMID: 26655793]

[162] Ding L, Li J, Huang R, *et al.* Salvianolic acid B protects against myocardial damage caused by nanocarrier TiO$_2$; and synergistic anti-breast carcinoma effect with curcumin via codelivery system of folic acid-targeted and polyethylene glycol-modified TiO$_2$ nanoparticles. Int J Nanomedicine 2016; 11: 5709-27.
[http://dx.doi.org/10.2147/IJN.S107767] [PMID: 27843313]

[163] Lee JY, Kim JH, Bae KH, *et al.* Low-density lipoprotein-mimicking nanoparticles for tumor-targeted theranostic applications. Small (Weinheim an der Bergstrasse, Germany) 2015; 11(2): 222-31.
[http://dx.doi.org/10.1002/smll.201303277]

[164] Fasehee H, Dinarvand R, Ghavamzadeh A, *et al.* Delivery of disulfiram into breast cancer cells using folate-receptor-targeted PLGA-PEG nanoparticles: *in vitro* and *in vivo* investigations. J Nanobiotechnology 2016; 14(1): 32.

[http://dx.doi.org/10.1186/s12951-016-0183-z] [PMID: 27102110]

[165] Paulmurugan R, Bhethanabotla R, Mishra K, et al. Folate receptor-targeted polymeric micellar nanocarriers for delivery of orlistat as a repurposed drug against triple-negative breast cancer. Mol Cancer Ther 2016; 15(2): 221-31.
[http://dx.doi.org/10.1158/1535-7163.MCT-15-0579] [PMID: 26553061]

[166] Wang W, Liang H, Sun B, et al. Pharmacokinetics and tissue distribution of folate-decorated human serum albumin loaded with nano-hydroxycamptothecin for tumor targeting. J Pharm Sci 2016; 105(6): 1874-80.
[http://dx.doi.org/10.1016/j.xphs.2016.03.016] [PMID: 27129905]

[167] Qian J, Xu M, Suo A, et al. Folate-decorated hydrophilic three-arm star-block terpolymer as a novel nanovehicle for targeted co-delivery of doxorubicin and Bcl-2 siRNA in breast cancer therapy. Acta Biomater 2015; 15: 102-16.
[http://dx.doi.org/10.1016/j.actbio.2014.12.018] [PMID: 25545322]

[168] Wang H, Yin H, Yan F, et al. Folate-mediated mitochondrial targeting with doxorubicin-polyrotaxane nanoparticles overcomes multidrug resistance. Oncotarget 2015; 6(5): 2827-42.
[http://dx.doi.org/10.18632/oncotarget.3090] [PMID: 25605018]

[169] Zhang L, Zhu D, Dong X, et al. Folate-modified lipid-polymer hybrid nanoparticles for targeted paclitaxel delivery. Int J Nanomedicine 2015; 10: 2101-14.
[PMID: 25844039]

[170] Liang S, Jin X, Ma Y, Guo J, Wang H. Folic acid-conjugated BSA nanocapsule (n-BSA-FA) for cancer targeted radiotherapy and imaging. RSC Advances 2015; 5(108): 88560-6.
[http://dx.doi.org/10.1039/C5RA12804H]

[171] Thapa RK, Choi JY, Gupta B, et al. Liquid crystalline nanoparticles encapsulating cisplatin and docetaxel combination for targeted therapy of breast cancer. Biomater Sci 2016; 4(9): 1340-50.
[http://dx.doi.org/10.1039/C6BM00376A] [PMID: 27412822]

[172] Han MH, Li ZT, Bi DD, Guo YF, Kuang HX, Wang XT. Novel folate-targeted docetaxel-loaded nanoparticles for tumour targeting: *in vitro* and *in vivo* evaluation. RSC Advances 2016; 6(69): 64306-14.
[http://dx.doi.org/10.1039/C6RA04466B]

[173] Lu J, Zhao W, Huang Y, et al. Targeted delivery of Doxorubicin by folic acid-decorated dual functional nanocarrier. Mol Pharm 2014; 11(11): 4164-78.
[http://dx.doi.org/10.1021/mp500389v] [PMID: 25265550]

[174] Martínez A, Muñiz E, Teijón C, Iglesias I, Teijón JM, Blanco MD. Targeting tamoxifen to breast cancer xenograft tumours: preclinical efficacy of folate-attached nanoparticles based on alginate-cysteine/disulphide-bond-reduced albumin. Pharm Res 2014; 31(5): 1264-74.
[http://dx.doi.org/10.1007/s11095-013-1247-5] [PMID: 24218224]

[175] Bhushan B, Gopinath P. Tumor-targeted folate-decorated albumin-stabilised silver nanoparticles induce apoptosis at low concentration in human breast cancer cells. RSC Advances 2015; 5(105): 86242-53.
[http://dx.doi.org/10.1039/C5RA16936D]

[176] Esfandiarpour-Boroujeni S, Bagheri-Khoulenjani S, Mirzadeh H, Amanpour S. Fabrication and study of curcumin loaded nanoparticles based on folate-chitosan for breast cancer therapy application. Carbohydr Polym 2017; 168: 14-21.
[http://dx.doi.org/10.1016/j.carbpol.2017.03.031] [PMID: 28457434]

[177] Vimala K, Shanthi K, Sundarraj S, Kannan S. Synergistic effect of chemo-photothermal for breast cancer therapy using folic acid (FA) modified zinc oxide nanosheet. J Colloid Interface Sci 2017; 488: 92-108.
[http://dx.doi.org/10.1016/j.jcis.2016.10.067] [PMID: 27821343]

[178] Johansson HJ, Sanchez BC, Mundt F, *et al.* Retinoic acid receptor alpha is associated with tamoxifen resistance in breast cancer. Nat Commun 2013; 4: 2175.
[http://dx.doi.org/10.1038/ncomms3175] [PMID: 23868472]

[179] Zhang Y, Li P, Pan H, *et al.* Retinal-conjugated pH-sensitive micelles induce tumor senescence for boosting breast cancer chemotherapy. Biomaterials 2016; 83: 219-32.
[http://dx.doi.org/10.1016/j.biomaterials.2016.01.023] [PMID: 26774567]

[180] Agrawal S, Dwivedi M, Ahmad H, *et al.* CD44 targeting hyaluronic acid coated lapatinib nanocrystals foster the efficacy against triple-negative breast cancer. Nanomedicine (Lond) 2018; 14(2): 327-37.
[http://dx.doi.org/10.1016/j.nano.2017.10.010] [PMID: 29129754]

[181] Elzoghby AO, Mostafa SK, Helmy MW, ElDemellawy MA, Sheweita SA. Superiority of aromatase inhibitor and cyclooxygenase-2 inhibitor combined delivery: Hyaluronate-targeted *versus* PEGylated protamine nanocapsules for breast cancer therapy. Int J Pharm 2017; 529(1-2): 178-92.
[http://dx.doi.org/10.1016/j.ijpharm.2017.06.077] [PMID: 28663087]

[182] Li L, Di X, Wu M, *et al.* Targeting tumor highly-expressed LAT1 transporter with amino acid-modified nanoparticles: Toward a novel active targeting strategy in breast cancer therapy. Nanomedicine (Lond) 2017; 13(3): 987-98.
[http://dx.doi.org/10.1016/j.nano.2016.11.012] [PMID: 27890657]

[183] Wang Q, Holst J. L-type amino acid transport and cancer: targeting the mTORC1 pathway to inhibit neoplasia. Am J Cancer Res 2015; 5(4): 1281-94.
[PMID: 26101697]

[184] Feng Y, Su J, Zhao Z, *et al.* Differential effects of amino acid surface decoration on the anticancer efficacy of selenium nanoparticles. Dalton Trans 2014; 43(4): 1854-61.
[http://dx.doi.org/10.1039/C3DT52468J] [PMID: 24257441]

[185] Sattarahmady N, Azarpira N, Hosseinpour A, Heli H, Zare T. Albumin coated arginine-capped magnetite nanoparticles as a paclitaxel vehicle: Physicochemical characterizations and *in vitro* evaluation. J Drug Deliv Sci Technol 2016; 36: 68-74.
[http://dx.doi.org/10.1016/j.jddst.2016.07.004]

[186] Frei E. Albumin binding ligands and albumin conjugate uptake by cancer cells. Diabetol Metab Syndr 2011; 3(1): 11.
[http://dx.doi.org/10.1186/1758-5996-3-11] [PMID: 21676260]

[187] Zheng Y, Yu B, Weecharangsan W, *et al.* Transferrin-conjugated lipid-coated PLGA nanoparticles for targeted delivery of aromatase inhibitor 7α-APTADD to breast cancer cells. Int J Pharm 2010; 390(2): 234-41.
[http://dx.doi.org/10.1016/j.ijpharm.2010.02.008] [PMID: 20156537]

[188] Turino LN, Ruggiero MR, Stefanìa R, Cutrin JC, Aime S, Geninatti Crich S. Ferritin decorated PLGA/paclitaxel loaded nanoparticles endowed with an enhanced toxicity toward MCF-7 breast tumor cells. Bioconjug Chem 2017; 28(4): 1283-90.
[http://dx.doi.org/10.1021/acs.bioconjchem.7b00096] [PMID: 28301933]

[189] Shao W, Paul A, Rodes L, Prakash S. A new carbon nanotube-based breast cancer drug delivery system: preparation and *in vitro* analysis using paclitaxel. Cell Biochem Biophys 2015; 71(3): 1405-14.
[http://dx.doi.org/10.1007/s12013-014-0363-0] [PMID: 27101155]

[190] Mahanta S, Prathap S, Ban DK, Paul S. Protein functionalization of ZnO nanostructure exhibits selective and enhanced toxicity to breast cancer cells through oxidative stress-based cell death mechanism. J Photochem Photobiol B 2017; 173: 376-88.
[http://dx.doi.org/10.1016/j.jphotobiol.2017.06.015] [PMID: 28646756]

[191] Sahoo SK, Labhasetwar V. Enhanced antiproliferative activity of transferrin-conjugated paclitaxel-loaded nanoparticles is mediated *via* sustained intracellular drug retention. Mol Pharm 2005; 2(5):

373-83.
[http://dx.doi.org/10.1021/mp050032z] [PMID: 16196490]

[192] Gilad Y, Firer M, Gellerman G. Recent innovations in peptide based targeted drug delivery to cancer cells. Biomedicines 2016; 4(2): 11.
[http://dx.doi.org/10.3390/biomedicines4020011] [PMID: 28536378]

[193] Dadras P, Atyabi F, Irani S, *et al.* Formulation and evaluation of targeted nanoparticles for breast cancer theranostic system. Eur J Pharm Sci 2017; 97: 47-54.
[http://dx.doi.org/10.1016/j.ejps.2016.11.005] [PMID: 27825919]

[194] Hu J, Obayemi JD, Malatesta K, Košmrlj A, Soboyejo WO. Enhanced cellular uptake of LHRH-conjugated PEG-coated magnetite nanoparticles for specific targeting of triple negative breast cancer cells. Mater Sci Eng C 2018; 88: 32-45.
[http://dx.doi.org/10.1016/j.msec.2018.02.017] [PMID: 29636136]

[195] Wen X, Li J, Cai D, *et al.* Anticancer efficacy of targeted shikonin liposomes modified with RGD in breast cancer cells. Molecules 2018; 23(2): 268.
[http://dx.doi.org/10.3390/molecules23020268] [PMID: 29382149]

[196] Mahdaviani P, Bahadorikhalili S, Navaei-Nigjeh M, *et al.* Peptide functionalized poly ethylene glycol-poly caprolactone nanomicelles for specific cabazitaxel delivery to metastatic breast cancer cells. Mater Sci Eng C 2017; 80: 301-12.
[http://dx.doi.org/10.1016/j.msec.2017.05.126] [PMID: 28866169]

[197] Garg SM, Paiva IM, Vakili MR, *et al.* Traceable PEO-poly(ester) micelles for breast cancer targeting: The effect of core structure and targeting peptide on micellar tumor accumulation. Biomaterials 2017; 144: 17-29.
[http://dx.doi.org/10.1016/j.biomaterials.2017.08.001] [PMID: 28818703]

[198] Han X, Dong X, Li J, *et al.* Free paclitaxel-loaded E-selectin binding peptide modified micelle self-assembled from hyaluronic acid-paclitaxel conjugate inhibit breast cancer metastasis in a murine model. Int J Pharm 2017; 528(1-2): 33-46.
[http://dx.doi.org/10.1016/j.ijpharm.2017.05.063] [PMID: 28576551]

[199] Brinkman AM, Chen G, Wang Y, *et al.* Aminoflavone-loaded EGFR-targeted unimolecular micelle nanoparticles exhibit anti-cancer effects in triple negative breast cancer. Biomaterials 2016; 101: 20-31.
[http://dx.doi.org/10.1016/j.biomaterials.2016.05.041] [PMID: 27267625]

[200] Hsiao JK, Wu HC, Liu HM, Yu A, Lin CT. A multifunctional peptide for targeted imaging and chemotherapy for nasopharyngeal and breast cancers. Nanomedicine (Lond) 2015; 11(6): 1425-34.
[http://dx.doi.org/10.1016/j.nano.2015.03.011] [PMID: 25881740]

[201] Yu MZ, Pang WH, Yang T, *et al.* Systemic delivery of siRNA by T7 peptide modified core-shell nanoparticles for targeted therapy of breast cancer. European Journal of Pharmaceutical Sciences: Official Journal of the European Federation for Pharmaceutical Sciences 2016; 92: 39-48.
[http://dx.doi.org/10.1016/j.ejps.2016.06.020]

[202] Feng Q, Yu MZ, Wang JC, *et al.* Synergistic inhibition of breast cancer by co-delivery of VEGF siRNA and paclitaxel *via* vapreotide-modified core-shell nanoparticles. Biomaterials 2014; 35(18): 5028-38.
[http://dx.doi.org/10.1016/j.biomaterials.2014.03.012] [PMID: 24680191]

[203] Kumar P, Tambe P, Paknikar KM, Gajbhiye V. Folate/N-acetyl glucosamine conjugated mesoporous silica nanoparticles for targeting breast cancer cells: A comparative study. Colloids Surf B Biointerfaces 2017; 156: 203-12.
[http://dx.doi.org/10.1016/j.colsurfb.2017.05.032] [PMID: 28531877]

[204] Bharti R, Dey G, Banerjee I, *et al.* Somatostatin receptor targeted liposomes with Diacerein inhibit IL-6 for breast cancer therapy. Cancer Lett 2017; 388 (Suppl. C): 292-302.
[http://dx.doi.org/10.1016/j.canlet.2016.12.021] [PMID: 28025102]

[205] He Y, Huang Y, Huang Z, *et al.* Bisphosphonate-functionalized coordination polymer nanoparticles for the treatment of bone metastatic breast cancer. Journal of Controlled Release: Official Journal of the Controlled Release Society 2017; 264: 76-88.
[http://dx.doi.org/10.1016/j.jconrel.2017.08.024]

[206] ClinicalTrials.gov. NIH-US National Library of medicine. 2018. Available from: https://clinical trials.gov/ ct2/ home

[207] Hare JI, Lammers T, Ashford MB, Puri S, Storm G, Barry ST. Challenges and strategies in anti-cancer nanomedicine development: An industry perspective. Adv Drug Deliv Rev 2017; 108: 25-38.
[http://dx.doi.org/10.1016/j.addr.2016.04.025] [PMID: 27137110]

[208] Kim H, Jae-min J, Ryou J, Dong E, Cho D. Repebody-anticancer protein drug conjugate, preparation methods and use thereof KR101875809B1 2018.

[209] Al-Massarani SMA, El Dib RAEMK, El-Gamal AA, Awad MA. Synthesis of ifflaionic acid nanoparticles US9974750B1 2018.

[210] Awad MA, El Dib RAEMK, Al-Massarani S. Synthesis of Nuxia oppositifolia nanoparticles US10028988B1 2018.

[211] Awad MA, Awatif AH, Khalid MOO. Synthesis of adansonia digitata nanoparticles US9789146B1 2017.

[212] Zongyin Q, Yumei X, Hongwei L, Wei H, Feng YG. Orlistat nanosphere preparation method and application of anticancer drugs CN107412196B 2018.

[213] Awad MA, Ahmed AH, Ortashi KMO, Laref A. Green synthesis of reduced graphene oxide using Nigella sativa seed extract US9988276B2 2018.

[214] Sang-soo, Seog NJ. Quercetin containing breast cancer treatment composition KR101851470B1 2018.

[215] Mu H, Chang GH, Gatun J, Yeon-su C, Kim YK. Biarmed PEG-TPP conjugate as self-assembling nano-drug delivery system for targeting mitochondria KR101743399B1 2017.

SUBJECT INDEX

A

Absorption, oral 137, 186
Acetylation 92, 93, 97
Acid(s) 63, 64, 65, 66, 76, 141, 144, 149, 190, 203, 204
  all-trans retinoic 203
  ellagic 66
  gallic 66
  hyaluronic 141, 144, 149, 190, 203, 204
  organic 63
  phenolic 63, 64, 65, 76
Activity 53, 54, 117, 151, 152
  anti-tumor 117, 151, 152
  metabolic 53, 54
Adjoining sections, free 4
Aerobic glycolysis 24
Agents 76, 133
  antineoplastic 133
Albumin 141, 192, 204, 205
  human serum 192, 204, 205
Allan-Herndon-Dudley syndrome 26
Alumina nanotubes 184
Amifostine 7
Anatomical therapeutic chemical (ATC) 133, 138
Angiogenesis 24, 45, 63, 73, 77, 78, 79, 94, 97, 115, 118, 120, 122
Angiogenesis inhibitors 134
Antibodies 50, 51, 155
  primary 50, 51, 155
  secondary 50, 51, 155
Antibody fragments 193, 194
Anticancer 92, 94, 116, 118
  anti-inflammatory 92
  inflammatory 92
Anticancer efficiency 137, 191
  enhanced 137

Anticancer properties 77, 94, 96, 97
  solid 97
Antioxidant 36, 67, 76, 92, 96
Anti-proliferative assays 43, 45, 46, 47, 49, 50, 51, 55
  based 43, 46, 55
  effects 45, 46, 50
  rapid 50, 51
Apigenin 34, 69, 72, 90, 92
Apoptosis 30, 33, 34, 45, 53, 78, 79, 93, 94, 97, 100, 117, 118, 119, 120, 121, 122, 151, 152, 153, 158, 203, 204
  inducing 120, 151, 152, 153, 158
Approaches 45, 53, 55, 139
  anti-cancer drug discovery 53
  prodrug 139
Aptamers 143, 180, 189, 193, 195, 196, 197, 198, 211
Assay multiplexing 44
Astrocytomas 113
Atomic translocation 75, 96
ATP content, cellular 47
Atypical resection 5

B

Bcl-2 family protein inhibitor 117
BCS, combined 138
BDDCS system 138, 139
Beckwith-Wiedemann syndrome 1, 2
Betamethasone 151
Bevacizumab 116, 118, 134, 159
Biomarker, cancer stem cell 196
Biopharmaceutics classification system (BCS) 138, 139
Biopharmaceutics drug disposition classification system (BDDCS) 138
Biopolymers 149

Biotin 151, 200, 201
Bisphosphonate 208
Bond, disulfide 159, 160, 191, 204
Bosom cancer cells 98, 100, 101
  human 98
Brain tumor 111, 112, 113, 132, 134
BRCA1-related bosom cancer 98
BrdU assay 50, 51, 54
Breast cancer 46 98, 122, 181, 193, 199, 201, 203, 204, 206, 208, 209, 210, 212
  cell lines 122, 206
  common 201
  generic 212
  hormone-dependent 204
  human 122
  human BRCA1-related 98
  metastatic 203, 208, 209, 210
  positive metastatic 209
  stem cells 46
  tissue 193
  treatment 181, 199, 209
Breast cancer cells 94, 95, 150, 180, 182, 183, 184, 185, 186, 187, 188, 190, 191, 194 195, 196, 197, 198, 199, 204, 205, 206, 207, 208, 210, 211, 212
  attenuating 190
  destroy 191
  human 95, 150, 205
  inhibiting MCF-7 210
  invasive 194
  metastatic 195
  negative 187, 207, 208
  positive 194, 206
  resistant 185, 194
  triple-negative 186
Bumetanide 34

C

Caco-2 cancerous cells 155
Cadaveric livers 12

Cancer 26, 29, 30, 33, 43, 81, 90, 92, 93, 97, 111, 112, 114, 118, 119, 122, 132, 133, 134, 161, 186, 203
  cervical squamous cell 118
  chemoprevention 93, 97
  epithelial 186
  hormonal anti-breast 203
  medications 132, 133, 134
  metastases 81
  mortality 132
  neck 119
  pancreatic 30, 122
  skin 90, 92
  stem cells (CSCs) 111, 112, 114
  survivors 132
  thyroid 43
  tissue 26
  treating 33
  treating pediatric 161
Cancer cell(s) 24, 43, 45, 53, 94, 99, 122, 151, 152, 153, 159, 204
  apoptosis 152
  development 94
  lines 99, 122
  phototherapy 151
  proliferation 24, 43, 53, 122
  culture 159
  growth 153
  types 45, 204
Cancer prevention agent 63, 66, 70
  solid 66
  strong 63
Cancer therapy 23, 148, 150, 152, 154, 161, 184, 192
  enhanced 184
  sustained drug release 152
Cancer treatment 84, 90, 121, 153, 193, 203, 210
  anti-breast 210
Carbonic apatite 190
Carbon 131, 136, 157, 184, 191
  nanomaterials 157, 191

nanotubes 131, 136, 184, 191
Carboplatin 7, 8, 9
Carcinogenesis 67, 76, 77, 82, 88, 100
Catecholestrogens 86
Cavitron ultrasonic surgical aspirator (CUSA) 5
Cell(s) 24, 25, 26, 33, 36, 46, 47, 51, 52, 68, 80, 82, 94, 95, 97, 99, 117, 134, 137, 150, 151, 152, 155, 158, 159, 181, 194, 199, 181, 201, 206
   aerobic cancer 26, 33
   apoptosis 94, 95, 155
   attacking cancer 181
   brain cancer 97
   cancerous 24, 137, 199
   dendritic 134, 181
   endometrial cancer 47
   human cancer 158
   mind cancer 97
   mononuclear 68, 94
   nasopharyngeal carcinoma 46, 152
   oral cancer 99
   ovarian cancer 80
   pancreatic cancer 52
   resistant 117, 194
   suspension 51, 52
   survival, sustain cancer 25
   target cancer 36, 159, 201
   target EGFR-mutant lung cancer 150
Cell membranes 48, 51, 54, 196
   damaged 48, 51, 54
   epithelial cancer 196
CellTiter-Glo assays 47, 48
Cellular techniques 43
Cell viability 47, 51, 136, 150, 158, 197
   colon cancer 51
   human ovarian cancer 47
Cervical cancer cells 47, 136, 152
   human 152
Cervical cancer cells cultures 153
Chemoprevention 62, 93
Chemotherapeutics 111

Chemotherapy 1, 3, 4, 5, 6, 9, 10, 11, 12, 13, 14, 44, 97, 111, 112, 114, 115, 116, 121, 153, 155, 180, 181, 187
   adjuvant 4, 5, 6
   conventional breast cancer 181
   cycles of 4, 12
   systemic 10
Children's 1, 3, 4, 5, 6, 12, 13
   hepatic tumors international collaboration (CHIC) 4, 13
   oncology group (COG) 1, 3, 4, 5, 6, 12
Chitosan 141, 149, 152, 153, 156, 190
Chromatin 62, 89, 91
Cisplatin 6, 115, 116, 117, 147, 150, 151, 154, 184, 202
Clonogenic ability 52
Colon cancer 90, 93, 132
   cells 90, 93
   addition CaCo-2 93
Colony formation assay 52, 54
   soft agar 52
Combination, synergistic 111, 113
Combinatorial Therapy 115, 116, 117
Compounds, phenolic 67, 68
Computed tomography (CT) 11
Curcumin treatment 96, 97
Cyanidin-3-*O*-glucoside 72
Cyclin D1 79
Cyclophosphamide 6, 181, 184, 209
Cytochrome 78, 79
Cytokines 67, 68, 75
Cytoplasm, breast cancer cell 182
Cytotoxic 46, 49, 55, 115, 121
   agents 49, 55
   effects 46, 115, 121
Cytotoxicity 137, 140, 148, 149, 150, 155, 160, 186, 189, 190, 194, 197, 199, 204

D

Deacetylation 92, 93
Delivery systems 136, 182

anticancer drug 136
  nano-based 182
Demethylation 98, 99, 112, 115
Dendrimers 131, 136, 139, 141, 142, 147, 148, 157, 184, 190, 198, 211
Deoxyuridine 50
Dexamethasone 151
Diabetes mellitus 26
Dimensional shape 49
Dispersions, solid 139
Disulfide bond dissociation 160
Disulfonate 36
DNA 45, 48, 49, 54, 63, 88, 90, 94, 100, 112, 115, 119, 156, 201
  cellular 54
  damage 115, 119
  methylation 63, 88, 90, 94, 100, 112
  synthesis 45, 48, 49, 54, 201
  synthesized 49, 54
  -toxin anticancer drugs 156
DNMT 90, 91
  inhibitor 90, 91
Doxorubicin 6, 136, 181, 183, 184, 185, 194, 196, 197, 198, 202, 203, 208
DOX release 137, 153
Drug(s) 9, 23, 24, 47, 67, 111, 113, 114, 115, 121, 133, 139, 140, 141, 144, 152, 158, 159, 162, 180, 182
  anticancer candidate 158
  cationic amphiphilic 152
  efficient intracellular pH-stimulated 159
  encapsulated 140
  hormonal 180, 182
  important anti-inflammatory 67
  natural 47
  novel efficacious 9
  novel oncology 133
  psychotropic 121
  resistance 23, 24, 111, 113, 114, 115, 139, 144
  sensitive 162
  transport lipophilic 141
  water-insoluble 141
Drug transport, novel anti-cancer 131
Dye 47, 51, 54
  ethidium homodimer 54
  exclusion assays 51
  permeable 46, 47
Dysregulation 63, 115, 117

E

Edwards syndrome 1, 2
Efflux transporters 138, 139
Electric cell-substrate impedance sensing (ECIS) 49, 54
Embryonal 3
Encapsulate 143, 158, 191
Endocytosis 201
Endothelial cells 70, 73, 120, 194
Enzymes, cellular 45
EpCAM overexpressing cells 197
Epicatechin 36, 70, 71, 74, 90, 92, 100
Epicatechin-gallate 90, 92
Epidermal growth factor receptor (EGFR) 112, 119, 144, 181, 193
Epigenetic adjustments 88
Epigenetics 62, 63, 87, 88
Epigenome 112, 113
Epithelial markers 82
Epithelial-mesenchymal transition (EMT) 62, 81, 82, 83, 91, 199
Erlotinib 119, 120, 134
Esophageal cancers 90
Etoposide 8, 9, 138
Event-free survival (EFS) 3, 7, 8, 9
Exosome 185, 188
Expansion, cancer cell 94

F

Factors, annotation 4, 14
Familial adenomatous polyposis 1, 2
Fibroblast growth factor (FGF) 118

First generation DDSs 150, 151, 152, 153, 155, 156, 157, 158, 159, 160
Flavonoids 33, 34, 63, 64, 65, 68, 70, 74
Folate receptors 201, 211
Folic 144, 150, 151, 152, 158, 160, 187, 189, 190, 200, 201, 202, 203
  acid (FA) 144, 150, 151, 152, 158, 187, 189, 190, 200, 201, 202, 203
  stimulating hormone receptor (FSHR) 160
Form, phosphorylated 72
Formazan 46, 48, 53
  insoluble 46
Frameworks, structural 146, 147
Fucosyltransferases 199

G

Gastric-intestine (GI) 144
GBM 111, 112, 114, 115, 116, 117, 118, 119, 120, 122
  treatment of 111, 112, 115, 117, 119
  cell lines 117, 118, 122
  cells 112, 114, 115, 116, 117, 118, 119, 120, 122
  deficient 118
  radio sensitize 119
Gemcitabine 117, 152, 190
Gemini like cationic lipid (GLCL) 191
Genes 2, 73, 88, 91, 95, 97
  articulation 73, 88, 91, 97
  beta-catenin 2
  particular cancer-related 95
  suppression 93
Glioblastoma cells 52, 111, 121
Glioblastomas 26, 111, 112, 113, 114, 115, 120
Global cancer 132
  burden 132
  observatory 132
Glucose 23, 24, 25, 27, 33, 34, 116, 199, 200
  metabolism 24, 25, 116
  mole of 25
  transporters 33, 34

Glycolysis 24
Glycosylation 121, 199
Gold 49, 157, 182, 185, 187, 188, 189
  electrodes 49
  nanoparticles 182, 185, 188, 189
  nanorods 157, 187, 189
  nanostars 187, 189
Green tea 84, 99, 100
  extricate (GTE) 84, 100
  polyphenols (GTPs) 84, 99, 100
GSC population 114, 115
GSTP1 promoter 91, 101

H

Hallmarks of cancer 43
HB development 2
HBs 8, 9, 11, 13
  advanced 8, 9, 13
  multifocal 5, 11
HDAC 92, 93, 94, 95
  action, repressed 94
  inhibitors 92, 93, 94, 95
HeLa cancer cells 151, 152
Hepatectomy, partial 9
Hepatic arteries 12, 156
HepG2 151, 156, 158, 159, 160
  cancer cells 156
  cells 151, 158, 159, 160
  liver cancer cells 158
Herceptin 188, 194
HIFU ablation 10
High 10, 11, 45, 142, 145, 146, 149, 157
  content screening (HCS) 45
  -Intensity focused ultrasound (HIFU) 10, 11
  surface areas 142, 145, 146, 149, 157
  throughput screening (HTS) 45
Histone 90, 91, 93, 94, 95, 111, 112, 116, 119
  acetylation 90, 91, 93, 95
  alteration 94, 95
  deacetylase inhibitors (HDACi) 111, 112, 116, 119

Histone modifications 89, 91, 92
Hormonal therapies 181, 193, 211
Human umbilical vein endothelial cells (HUVEC) 75, 150
Hyaluronic acid binding domain (HABD) 196
Hybrid nanoparticles 186
Hydroxycinnamic acids 64, 65
Hydroxytyrosol 71, 75
Hyper-methylation 98, 99, 100
Hypoxia 23, 24, 26, 111, 112, 115, 118

I

Imaging agents 33, 153
Immunotherapies 44, 133, 134, 180, 181
Inflammatory processes 67, 68, 73
Information 44, 45, 53, 55, 70, 73, 86
  physiological 53
Inhibition of lactate 31
  efflux 31
  uptake 31
Inhibition of MCF-7 cancer cells 205
Inhibitors 28, 29, 33, 36, 71, 92, 98, 111, 112, 116, 118, 119, 120, 121, 134
  histone deacetylase 111, 112, 119
  signal transduction 134
Inhibitory 72, 81, 82, 83, 96, 117, 120, 121, 152, 195
  effects 81, 82, 117, 120, 121, 152, 195
  impact 72, 81, 83, 96
Inorganic NCs 141, 142
INOS articulation 69, 70, 74
Irinotecan 9, 116, 121
Iron oxide nanoparticles, superparamagnetic 190
Isoflavones 65, 87, 94
Isoforms 25, 26, 70
Isopropanol 46, 48

K

Kaempferol 34, 68, 69, 72, 75

Ketone bodies 26, 27, 29
KM12C colon cancer cells 50

L

Lactate 23, 24, 30, 31, 32, 36
  efflux 30, 31
  Shuttle 23, 24
  uptake 31, 32, 36
Lactoferrin 205, 206
LDH nanoparticles 157
Levetiracetam 117
Light microscope 52
Lignans 63, 65, 66, 77
Liposomes 135, 136, 141, 147, 148, 184, 185, 186, 191, 198, 208, 211
Live cell enzymes 53, 54
Liver 1, 3, 4, 5, 9, 10, 11, 12, 13, 150, 156
  malignancy 1
  resection 12, 13
  sectors 13
  surgery 1
  transplantation (LT) 1, 5, 9, 10, 11, 12, 13
  tumor 1, 3, 4, 150, 156
Loading 141, 146, 148, 157
  capacity, high 141, 146, 148
  hydrophobic drugs 157
Lung, colon cancer 92
Lungs cancers 90
Luteolin 34, 69, 72, 80
Lycopene 62, 75, 91, 92, 100, 101
Lysine 93, 204

M

Magnetic 154, 156, 157, 187, 190, 194, 211
  fields, external 154, 156, 187, 190, 194, 211
  nanoparticles 187, 194
  NC 156, 157
Major 53, 54, 181
  assay constituent 53, 54
Malignant transformation 43, 67, 199

Subject Index

Mannose 200
MAPK signaling 71
Materials, nanostructured 131
Medium, cell culture 50, 52
Membrane protein 194, 196
Mesenchymal markers 82
Mesoporous 145, 146, 147, 148, 149, 150, 151, 152, 153, 154, 157, 161
  carbon materials (MCMs) 146, 157
  materials 145, 148, 152
  silica nanocarriers (MSNs) 145, 146, 147, 148, 149, 150, 151, 152, 153, 154, 157, 161
Metabolism, cancer cell 30
Metal 131, 132, 145, 189, 190
  organic frameworks (MOFs) 145
  oxide 131, 132, 145, 189, 190
Metastasis 3, 4, 5, 10, 11, 13, 14, 23, 44, 62, 78, 79, 81, 82, 83, 85, 91, 97, 114, 118, 152, 156, 199, 200
  distant 3, 10, 13
Metastatic 6, 7, 8, 9, 11, 13, 85, 184, 196, 208
  breast cancer treatment 184
  cancers impervious 85
  disease 7, 8, 13
  HB 6, 8, 9, 11
  lesions 208
Methotrexate disodium 138
Methylation 62, 88, 90, 93, 98, 100
MGMT expression 116, 117
Micelles, polymeric 141
Microemulsion 184, 191
Migration, cancer cell 122
Mitogen activated protein kinase (MAPKs) 71, 72, 73, 119, 186
Molecules, organic 146
Monocarboxylic Transporters 24
Monoclonal antibodies 116, 118, 133, 160, 180, 193, 211
MTS assay 46, 53
MTT assay 45, 46, 53, 155
Multi-drug resistant (MDR) 144, 202

Multiple endocrine neoplasia type 26
Mutations, genetic 1, 2, 44
Myelosuppression 10

N

Nab-paclitaxel 208, 209
NADP-dependent oxidoreductases 48
Nanocarriers, organic 157, 158
Nano carriers (NCs) 141, 142, 143, 144, 150, 152, 153, 159, 160, 162
Nanoformulations, lipid-based 191
Natural 24, 33, 34, 35, 77, 82, 84, 85
  and Synthetic MCT Inhibitors 24
  MCT1 Inhibitors 33, 34, 35
  polyphenols 77, 82, 84, 85
Neoadjuvant chemotherapy 5, 11, 14
Neuroprotective impacts 70, 71
Non-small cell lung cancer (NSCLC) 150, 154
Novel 23, 24, 160
  anticancer agents 23
  anti-cancer drug 160
  drug combinations 23, 24
Nucleotide excision repair (NER) 115

O

Oral 137, 138, 139, 161
  disposition 138, 139
  oncolytics 137, 138, 139, 161
Ototoxicity 7, 8
Oxidative stress 71, 76, 189

P

Paclitaxel 122, 181, 184, 191, 194, 197, 202, 205, 206, 207, 209
  encapsulated 209
Pediatric 1, 3
  oncology 1, 3
  solid tumor 1

surgery 1
tumor 1
mesoporous organosilicas (PMOs) 148
Peroxisome proliferator-activated receptors (PPARs) 34
Phenotypes 83, 87
Phosphatidylcholine 186
Pirarubicin 8, 209
Pitavastatin 116, 121
Plasma membrane 25, 27, 30, 196
Poly ADP ribose polymerase (PARP) 118
Polymeric nanoparticles 136, 141, 148, 182, 183
Polymerosomes 185, 190, 194
Polyphenols 63, 67, 68, 73, 76, 77, 80, 84, 85, 86, 97, 98
  dietary 67, 73, 76, 80, 97, 98
  impacts of 68, 84, 85, 86
  regular 63, 76, 77
  in clinical trials 84
  modulate NFκB pathway 73
Population, tumor cell 114
Pore 145, 146
  diameters 145
  cylindrical 146
Porous materials 145, 157
Portal vein thrombosis 12
Potent MCT inhibitors 30, 31
Premature release 144, 159, 160
Prognosis 2, 3, 4, 6, 13, 112, 181
Pro-inflammatory cytokines 68, 72, 73, 76
Proliferation 49, 150
  epithelial cancer cells 49
  inhibiting cancer cells 150
Properties, anti-breast cancer 205
Propidium iodide (PI) 48, 51, 54
Prostate cancer 79, 84, 92, 94
  cell lines 94
  PC-3 tumor xenografts, killed 94
  xenografts 92
  unmanageable 84
Prostate cancer cells 46, 79, 95, 97 101

androgen heartless 79
inferred 101
Pulmonary metastases 9, 11
Pyruvate 24, 25, 26, 27, 29

Q

Quantum dots (QDs) 136, 137, 142
Quercetin 34, 36, 68, 69, 70, 72, 73, 75, 78, 80, 84, 86, 90, 92, 203, 211

R

Radiation therapy 117, 118, 133, 180
Radionuclide 151
Reactive oxygen species (ROS) 67, 76, 79, 120
Receptors 180, 192, 193, 199, 201, 203, 204, 205, 206, 207, 212
  death 77, 79
  estrogen 83, 181, 203, 204
  patched 120
Red blood cells (RBC) 36
Relapse 9, 14, 23, 24
Resazurin 46, 53
Response Evaluation Criteria in Solid Tumors (RECIST) 9

S

Selective serotonin reuptake inhibitors (SSRIs) 116, 121
Self nano emulsifying drug delivery system (SNEDDS) 183
SFN-treated breast cancer cells 93
Signaling 63, 70, 73, 82, 112, 114
  intrinsic molecular 114
  pathways 63, 70, 73, 82, 112, 114
Silybin 34
SiRNA delivery 186, 187
SIRTI activator 92
Sites, cancer cell 182
SK-HEP1 and HepG2 cancer cells 156

Small cell undifferentiated (SCU) 3
Solid Lipid Nanoparticles (SLNs) 141, 182, 191, 194, 199
Soluble anticancer drug curcumin 152
Stability, showed good 152, 155
Stem cell markers 114
Stilbenes 36, 63, 65, 77
Strategy 44, 55
  anti-cancer drug discovery 55
  pre-clinical anti-cancer drug development 44
Stress, mechanical 146, 147
Sulforaphane 62, 91, 92, 93
Sulforhodamine 47, 48, 49
Surgical resection 1, 3, 4, 5, 6, 10, 14
  complete 4, 6, 7, 10
Synergistic effects 67, 120, 121, 137, 153, 156, 183

T

Tamoxifen 181, 203
Target 10, 201
  breast cancer cells 201
  tumor cells 10
Targeting 30, 200
  breast cancer 200
  MCTs in cancer 30
Tea, green 62, 65, 83, 84, 85, 98, 100
Temozolomide 111, 112, 116, 118
Tetrazolium-based anti-proliferative assays 47, 48
Therapeutic agents 23, 24, 62, 142, 149, 203
Therapies 10, 111, 112, 119, 131, 134, 151, 153, 154, 161, 180, 182, 187, 191, 200, 210
  gene 154, 161, 180
  photothermal 153, 187, 191
  radio 44
Thermal effect 149, 153
Thioaptamer 196, 198
TMZ resistance 112, 114, 115

Trail 77, 78, 79
  -actuated apoptosis 77, 79
  -intervened apoptosis 78, 79
  -safe cancer cells 79
Transarterial chemoembolization (TACE) 9, 10, 11
Transcription Factors 62, 120
Transferosomes 186
Transferrin 144, 205, 206
Treatment 85, 101, 114, 200
  aggressive 114
  lycopene 101
  polyphenol-involved anti-metastatic 85
Tumors 3, 4, 5, 6, 7, 9, 10, 12, 13, 14, 44, 78, 79, 81, 83, 85, 88, 90, 91, 95, 99, 112, 113, 114, 118, 134, 135, 137, 140, 143, 144, 150, 156, 157, 180, 183, 186, 188 189, 194, 196, 197, 200, 201, 204, 207
  -associated macrophages (TAMs) 200
  metastatic 44, 81, 85, 207
  mass 112, 113
  microenvironment, complex 114
  resectability 3, 5, 6
  silencer genes 88, 90, 91, 95, 99
  stem cells 196
  tissues 135, 144, 156, 180, 188, 194, 197, 204
Tumor cells 5, 10, 77, 78, 83, 97, 114, 120, 135, 137, 138, 143, 148, 152, 153, 155, 156, 182, 197, 198, 200, 201, 206, 207, 208
  growth 67, 115, 118, 156, 197, 207, 208
  hepatocellular carcinoma 148
  human 97
  resveratrol-treated 77
  targeted 156
Tumorigenesis 2, 44, 81, 96
Tumours 23, 26, 29, 33
  solid 23, 26, 29
Tyrosol 71, 75

U

Ultra violet B (UVB) 89
Unresectable tumors 11, 12

V

Valreopeptide 207, 208
Vascular endothelial growth factor (VEGF) 72, 73, 79, 118, 150, 159, 198, 208
Vesicular systems 184, 185, 186, 188
Viable cell(s) 45, 46, 47, 52, 53, 54
  calcein 46, 54
  markers 45
Vincristine 6, 7, 9, 46
Vorinostat 93, 116, 119

W

Well-differentiated fetal (WDF) 3
WMS nanoparticles 150
Wnt signaling pathway 1, 2

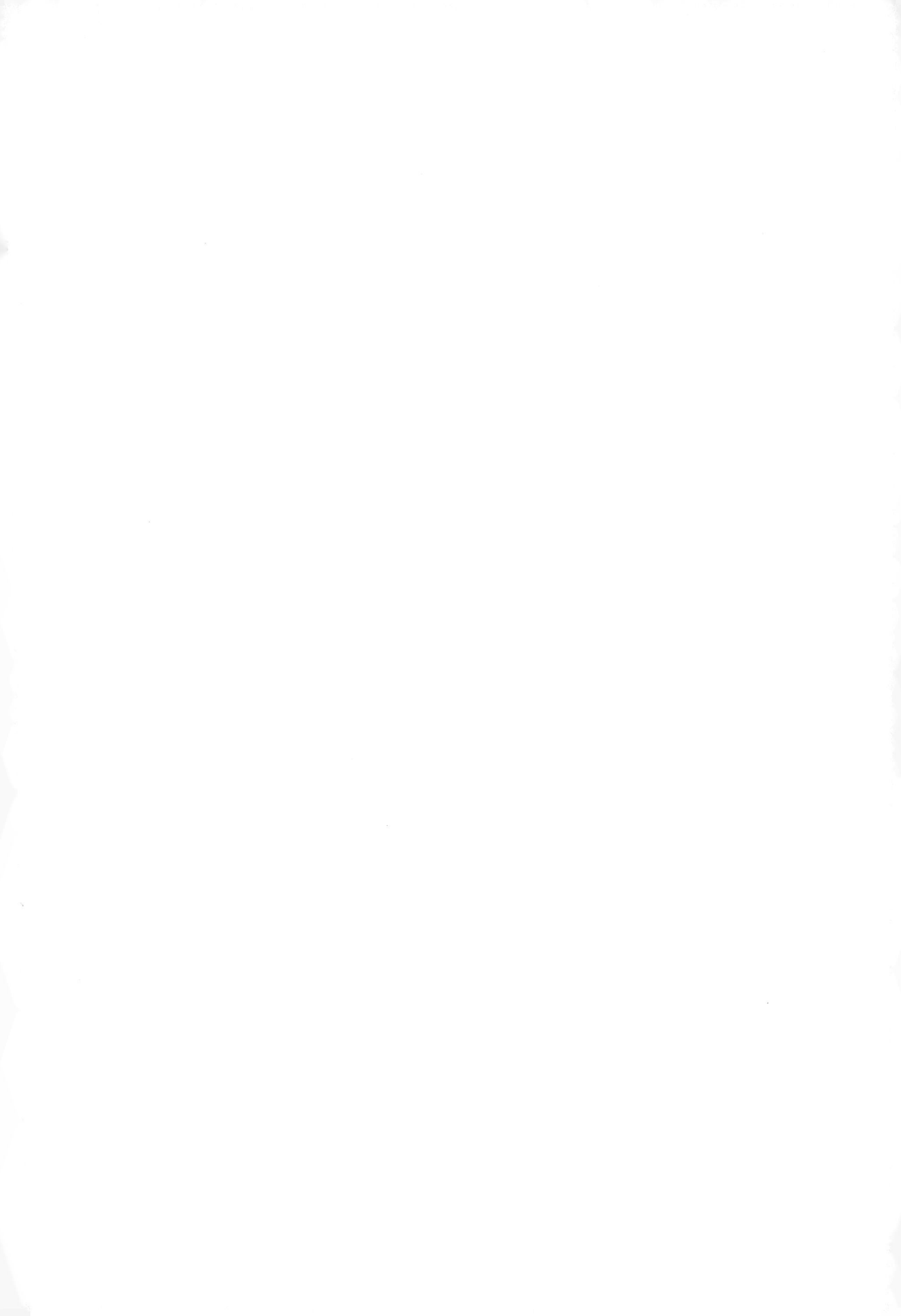

www.ingramcontent.com/pod-product-compliance
Lightning Source LLC
Chambersburg PA
CBHW051144220526
45473CB00003B/650